Proceedings of the First International Workshop on Magnetic Particle Imaging

MAGNETIC NANOPARTICLES

Particle Science, Imaging Technology, and Clinical Applications

Proceedings of the First International Workshop on Magnetic Particle Imaging

MAGNETIC NANOPARTICLES

Particle Science, Imaging Technology, and Clinical Applications

Institute of Medical Engineering, University of Lübeck, Germany

18 – 19 March 2010

Editors

T M Buzug
University of Lübeck, Germany

J Borgert
Philips Research Europe, Hamburg

T Knopp
University of Lübeck, Germany

S Biederer
University of Lübeck, Germany

T F Sattel
University of Lübeck, Germany

M Erbe
University of Lübeck, Germany

K Lüdtke-Buzug
University of Lübeck, Germany

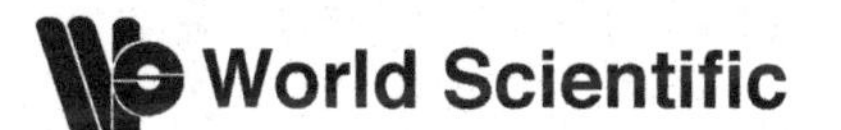

NEW JERSEY • LONDON • SINGAPORE • BEIJING • SHANGHAI • HONG KONG • TAIPEI • CHENNAI

Published by

World Scientific Publishing Co. Pte. Ltd.
5 Toh Tuck Link, Singapore 596224
USA office: 27 Warren Street, Suite 401-402, Hackensack, NJ 07601
UK office: 57 Shelton Street, Covent Garden, London WC2H 9HE

British Library Cataloguing-in-Publication Data
A catalogue record for this book is available from the British Library.

MAGNETIC NANOPARTICLES
Particle Science, Imaging Technology, and Clinical Applications
Proceedings of the First International Workshop on Magnetic Particle Imaging

ISBN-13 978-981-4324-67-0
ISBN-10 981-4324-67-1

Printed in Singapore.

FOREWORD AND ACKNOWLEDGEMENTS

This volume comprises the accepted contributions of the First International Workshop on Magnetic Particle Imaging (IWMPI). The workshop has been organized by the Institute of Medical Engineering at the University of Lübeck, Germany, in March 2010. It gives an overview on recent results of a novel imaging modality based on magnetic nanoparticles.

The magnetic particle imaging (MPI) concept falls into the category of functional imaging and, hence, the magnetic nanoparticles may serve as tracers of metabolic processes. Since the particles of choice consist of super-paramagnetic iron oxide (SPIO) cores coated with biopolymers, imaging of the metabolism may be possible without any radioactive agents. These particles are subjected to an oscillating magnetic field and, subsequently, react with a nonlinear re-magnetization. This behavior can be detected with appropriate receive coils. Due to the nonlinearity, the induced signal in the receive coils contains harmonics of the fundamental frequency of the drive field. These harmonics can be used to determine the nanoparticle concentration. For spatial encoding an additional magnetic gradient field, is superimposed onto the drive field such that a field-free point is established within the volume of interest. Only particles located at the field-free point contribute to the desired signal in the receive coils. Particles outside are saturated and do not further show any re-magnetization dynamics upon the excitation by the drive field.

Today, there are quite interesting challenges within the practical set-up of a scanning device and also in the design of new MPI nanoparticles. Scientists from chemical engineering, biology, electrical engineering, physics, computer sciences and medicine (see Fig. 1) discussed the promises and challenges of magnetic particle imaging during the workshop in spring 2010.

As chair of the workshop I would like the thank my co-chair, J. Borgert, Philips Research Hamburg, and the members of the program committee for the selection of works included in this book: C. Alexiou, University Erlangen; J. Barkhausen, University Clinics Schleswig-Holstein, Campus Lübeck; J. Borgert, Philips Research Hamburg; J. Bulte, Johns Hopkins University, School of Medicine, Baltimore; T. M. Buzug, University of Lübeck; S. Conolly, UC Berkeley; O. Dössel, University of Karlsruhe; S. Dutz, IPHT Jena; Z. A. Fayad, Mount Sinai School of Medicine, NY; D. Finas, University Clinics Schleswig-Holstein, Campus

Lübeck; V. Fuster, Mount Sinai School of Medicine, NY; B. Gleich, Philips Research Hamburg; J. Haueisen, Technical University Ilmenau; K. Krishnan, University of Washington; M. Kuhn, Philips Healthcare Hamburg; M. Magnani, Università degli Studi di Urbino; M. Port, Guerbet Roissy CDG; M. Schilling, TU Braunschweig; G. Schütz, Bayer Schering Pharma Berlin; M. Taupitz, Charité Berlin; L. Trahms, PTB Berlin; J. B. Weaver, Dartmouth Medical School; J. Weizenecker, University of Applied Sciences Karlsruhe.

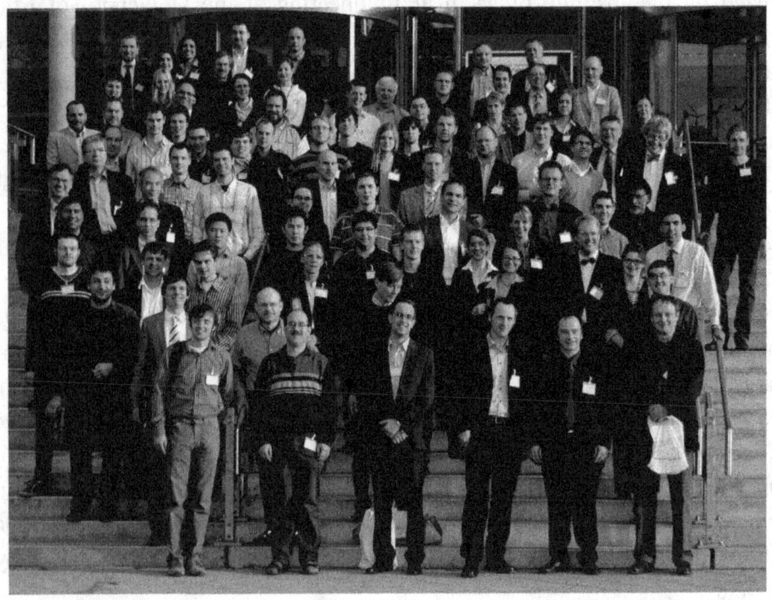

Fig. 1. Participants of the First International Workshop on Magnetic Particle Imaging, University of Lübeck, March 2010.

For supporting the workshop I have to thank the German Society of Biomedical Engineering (DGBMT) and the Arbeitsgemeinschaft Medizintechnik Schleswig-Holstein (AGMT). For financial support I would like to thank Philips Health Care, Bruker BioSpin, Bayer-Schering, Lanxess and Olympus.

Last but not least warm thanks go to the members of the local organization team at the Institute of Medical Engineering, University of Lübeck.

Thorsten M. Buzug
Workshop Chair
Lübeck, March 2010

Institute of Medical Engineering
University of Lübeck
buzug@imt.uni-luebeck.de

CONTENTS

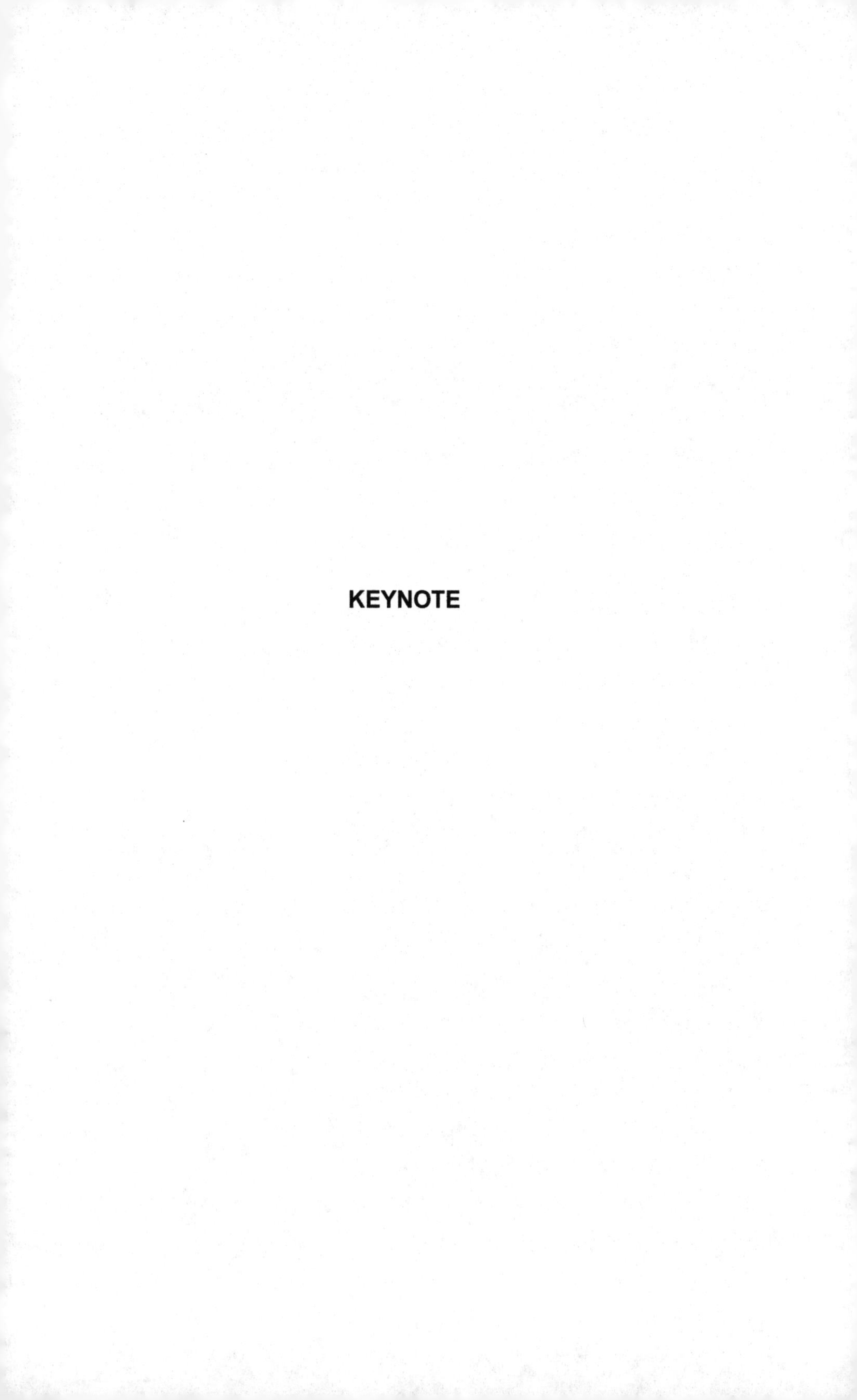

KEYNOTE

PARTICLE DYNAMICS OF MONO-DOMAIN PARTICLES IN MAGNETIC PARTICLE IMAGING

JÜRGEN WEIZENECKER
Department of Electrical Engineering, University of Applied Science,
Moltkestrasse 30, 76133 Karlsruhe, Germany
Email: juergen.weizenecker@hs-karlsruhe.de

BERNHARD GLEICH, JÜRGEN RAHMER, JÖRN BORGERT
Philips Research Europe – Hamburg,
Röntgenstraße 24-26, 22335 Hamburg, Germany
Email: bernhard.gleich@philips.com

In this report we present a detailed model of Brownian, Néel and combined rotation of magnetic mono domain particles in Magnetic Particle Imaging (MPI)[5]. The magnetization and rotational movement is predicted using a set of Langevin equations. The stochastic differential equations were solved numerically and applied to MPI for a simple sequence. At 25 kHz and with moderate anisotropies, the Néel rotation dominates the signal. Nevertheless, the Brownian motion modulates the signal in a model of combined motion.

1. INTRODUCTION

Magnetic Particle Imaging (MPI) does not provide any natural contrast and thus needs a tracer to perform imaging, the performance of which is of crucial importance. In order to understand the behaviour of the tracer in the various applied magnetic fields a suitable model has to be provided. It has been shown, that the simple Langevin Theory of magnetism is capable of describing the important features of the imaging process[7,13]. In a real experiment, of course, the tracer will always contain different types of particles (in terms of size and anisotropy). Nevertheless, the above-mentioned theory can still be used as an approximation in which distributions of parameters are modelled by effective values, like mean diameter and magnetization[8].

However, in order to evaluate ways to increase the performance of the particles and to understand experimental data, a more detailed model has to be provided. The model should contain relevant input parameters like particle diameter, arbitrary time varying magnetic fields, magnetic particle anisotropy, magnetization relaxation, and thermodynamic equilibrium.

There are two relevant mechanisms to change the magnetization of magnetic particles in an external field (figure 1). The first one is based on the reorientation of the magnetic particles and is named Brownian rotation. The second one is based on the change of magnetization in the fixed particle and is named Néel rotation. This report will present a detailed theory, which describes both effects separately, as well as in combination.

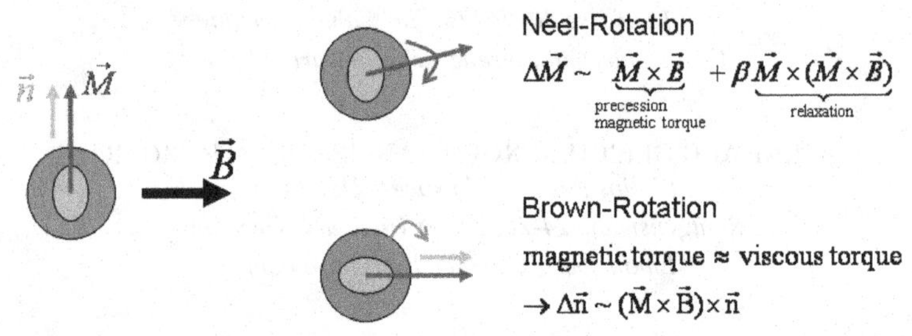

Fig. 1. Magnetization change of a single particle. In case of Néel rotation, the magnetization changes inside the particle. The magnetization can also change due to particle reorientation, referred to as Brownian rotation.

2. THEORY

2.1. Brownian Rotation

The behaviour of a spherical magnetic particle for the case of Brownian rotation in an external field $\vec{B}$ can be described[5] by

$$\frac{d\vec{n}}{dt} = \frac{V_{core}M_s}{6\eta V_{Hydro}}\left(\vec{n}\times\vec{B}\right)\times\vec{n} + \vec{N}(t)\times\vec{n}$$

Here the unit vector $\vec{n}$ represents a fixed direction of the particle; its direction is the same as the direction of the magnetization of the particle, as within the particle, the magnetization is assumed to be fixed. The parameter η is the viscosity, $V_{core}(V_{Hydro})$ is the core (hydrodynamic) volume of the particle, and M_s is the saturation magnetization of the particle. The term $\mathcal{N}(t)$ is proportional to a random torque describing the thermal impact on the microscopic particles. The above equation is quite similar to the differential description of Brownian motion of particles. For the components of the random vector field the following conditions are valid.

$$\langle N_i(t)\rangle = 0 \qquad \langle N_i(t)N_j(t')\rangle = \frac{2k_BT}{6\eta V_{Hydro}}\delta(t-t')\delta_{ij} \quad i,j=1,2,3$$

Such an equation is named Langevin equation and describes the particle direction by a stochastic differential equation. It can be interpreted in the Ito or Stratonovitch calculus[3,6]. The numerical solution will in general differ depending on the interpretation. For physical reasons[3] we chose the Stratonovitch interpretation and transform the above equation according to the transformation rules between Stratonovitch and Ito calculus[6]. This adds an additional diffusion term and the final equation becomes

$$d\vec{n} = \left[\frac{V_{core}M_s}{6\eta V_{Hydro}}\left(\vec{n}\times\vec{B}\right)\times\vec{n} - \frac{2k_BT}{6\eta V_{Hydro}}\vec{n}\right]dt + \sqrt{\frac{2k_BT}{6\eta V_{Hydro}}}d\vec{W}\times\vec{n} \quad . \tag{1}$$

For a numerical solution, $d\vec{n}$, dt, $d\vec{W}$ are replaced by $\vec{n}(t_k+\Delta t)-\vec{n}(t_k)$, Δt and $\vec{W}\sqrt{\Delta t}$, respectively. The random numbers W_j, $j = 1,2,3$ have zero mean value and unit standard deviation. The three coupled stochastic differential equations are solved using a Heun[11] scheme. To derive a mean value, the differential equations have to be solved multiple times and the results averaged.
As in this case the single particle magnetization is assumed to always face in particle direction $\vec{n}$, the mean (single particle) magnetization for P solutions of equation (1) is

$$\frac{1}{P}\sum_{i=1}^{P} M_s\vec{n}_i \ .$$

The mean (single particle) magnetic moment is obtained by multiplication with the particle core volume V_{core}. The first part of equation (1) describes the change of magnetization due to the external magnetic field. Within a certain time constant, it drives the direction of the magnetic moment into the field direction. The term containing the random torques describes the relaxation into equilibrium. Figure 2 shows a numerical solution of equation (1) with respect to the mean magnetic moment for the two limiting cases. For the parameters chosen, the field-induced rotation dominates the thermal relaxation.

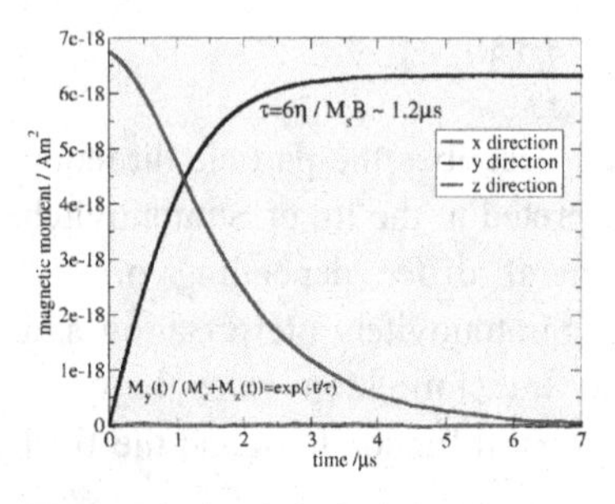

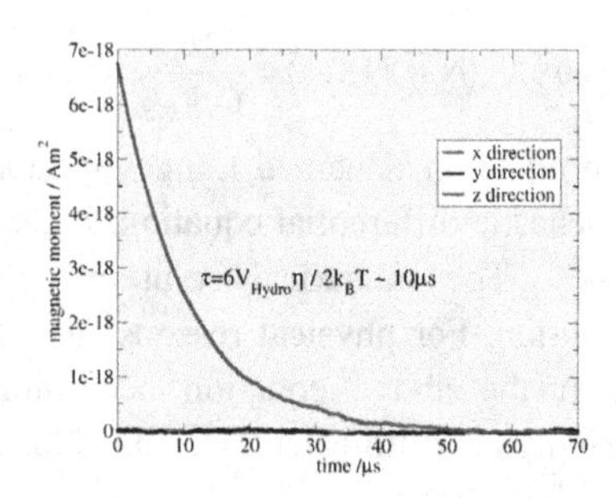

Fig. 2. Calculated single particle mean magnetic moment for 10^4 particles of 30nm diameter, with η=1 mPa s, M_s=0.6T/μ_0 at T=300K. At t=0s all particles are aligned in z direction. On the left side a constant field of B=10mT is applied in y direction at t=0 s. On the right side, no magnetic field is present. The theoretical time constants τ are taken from[12].

If an oscillating magnetic field is applied, both time constants will be noticeable. Relaxation will take place for small field values and rotation towards the field direction will dominate for large fields. If the change of the external magnetic field is faster than the internal time constants, a delay of magnetization alignment with respect to the field will occur. This fact is illustrated in figure 3, where 1000 solutions of equation (1) are visualized. Each dot represents the tip of a single particle magnetization vector $M_s\vec{n}$, projected to the xy-plane for T=300 K. At the very beginning, all particles are aligned in vertical direction (y-direction). The orange line is the mean value of the magnetization. Some dephasing due to thermal relaxation can already be seen after a few microseconds in the upper left image. An oscillating magnetic field in horizontal direction (x-direction) with frequency f=1/T=25 kHz[5,13] is switched on, as indicated by the green line. With increasing field, the particles are forced to rotate in the direction of the field (see first row, second image). After t=T/4, the magnetic field amplitude decreases, but due to the time constants τ, the magnetization remains aligned, even if the magnetic field passes zero (see second row, second image). Finally, the magnetic field increases in the negative direction forcing the particles to rotate back in field direction. At some point in time, the total magnetization will therefore be zero, indicating that a hysteresis loop is passed by the magnetization (second row, last image and third row). This process of relaxation and delayed magnetization alignment will occur periodically and after some cycles an equilibrium state will be reached. The width of the hysteresis loop will depend on the time constant τ, the frequency $\omega=2\pi f$ and the temperature T.

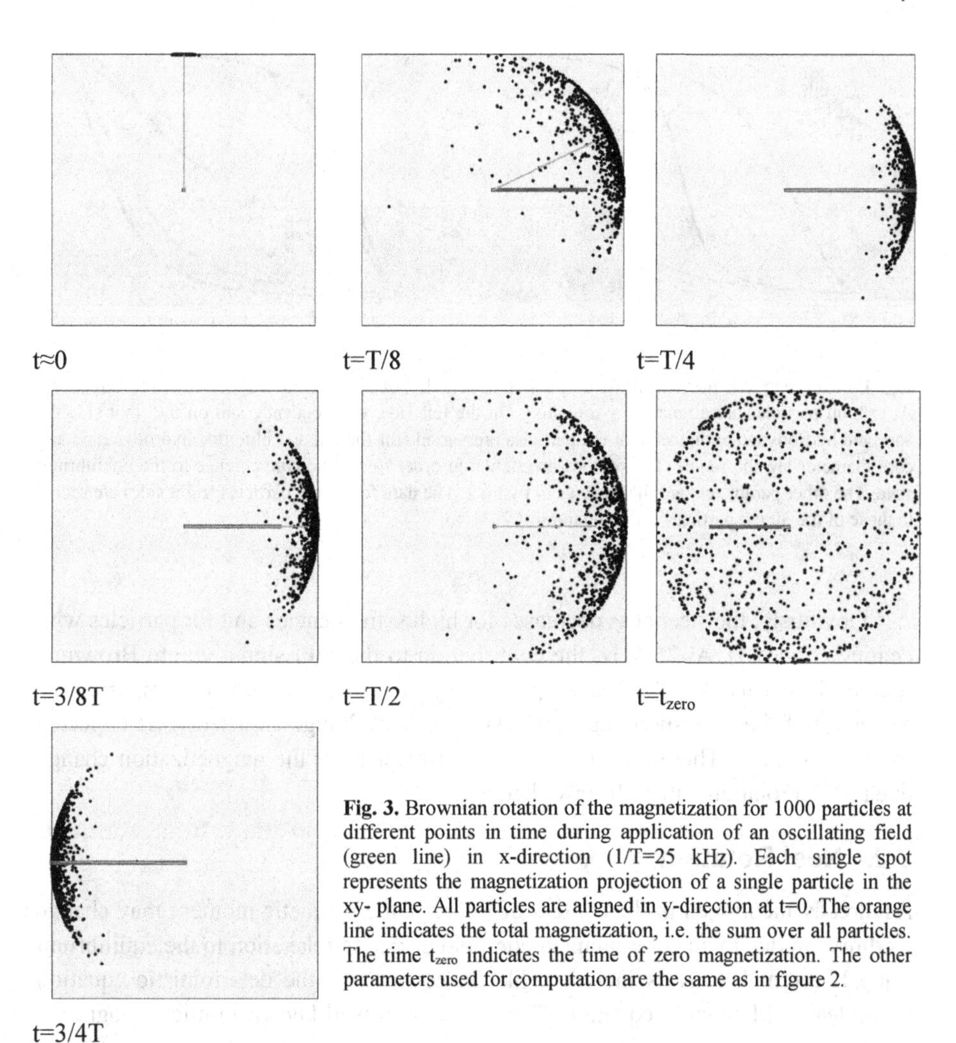

Fig. 3. Brownian rotation of the magnetization for 1000 particles at different points in time during application of an oscillating field (green line) in x-direction (1/T=25 kHz). Each single spot represents the magnetization projection of a single particle in the xy- plane. All particles are aligned in y-direction at t=0. The orange line indicates the total magnetization, i.e. the sum over all particles. The time t_{zero} indicates the time of zero magnetization. The other parameters used for computation are the same as in figure 2.

For sufficiently low frequencies, the hysteresis loop will collapse into the Langevin-Theory, as the thermodynamic equilibrium is maintained at each point in time. Figure 4 shows the hysteresis loops for different cases. Obviously, the magnetization behaviour depends sensitively on the particle diameter and the ratio of frequency and viscosity. As the steepness of the magnetization curve determines the spatial resolution for MPI, the hysteresis loop is of particular interest.

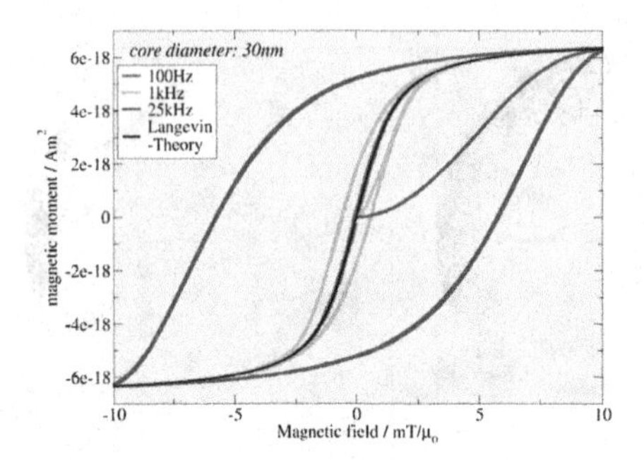

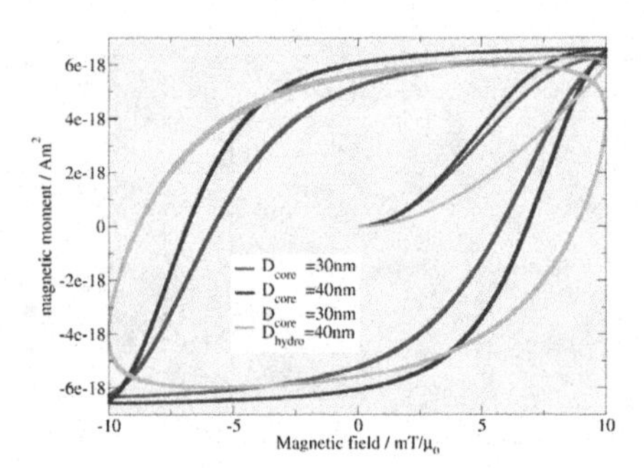

Fig. 4. Mean magnetic moment in field direction as function of the external magnetic field (x-direction). At t=0, all particles are aligned in y-direction. On the left side, the frequency and on the right side the core and hydrodynamic diameter of the particles are varied (for the red and blue line hydrodynamic and core diameter are the same). Ten periods are shown in order to see the convergence to the equilibrium state. The other parameters are the same as in figure 2. The data for 40 nm particles (right side) are scaled to those of the 30 nm particles for comparability.

Obviously, the steepness decreases for higher frequencies and for particles with coating (figure 4). At 25 kHz, the contribution to the MPI signal due to Brownian rotation is restricted to the low frequency regime, as can be seen by comparing the steepness of the corresponding hysteresis loop with Langevin-Theory, as expected for Néel rotation. Therefore, the theoretical treatment of the magnetization change due to Néel rotation will be briefly sketched.

2.2. Néel Rotation

As already mentioned in the context of figure 1, the magnetic moment may change its direction due to an external magnetic field or due to relaxation to the equilibrium state. If thermal noise is included, like in equation 1, the deterministic equation translates to a Langevin equation. This equation is well known in micro-magnetics and called Landau-Lifschitz-equation. The time evolution of the magnetization $\vec{M}$ for a single particle is given by[2].

$$\frac{d\vec{M}}{dt} = -\frac{\gamma}{(1+\alpha^2)}\left\{\vec{M}\times\left(\vec{B}_{total}(t)+\vec{\mathscr{B}}(t)\right)-\frac{\alpha}{M_s}\vec{M}\times\left[\vec{M}\times\left(\vec{B}_{total}(t)+\vec{\mathscr{B}}(t)\right)\right]\right\}$$

Here, $\vec{B}_{total}$ is the deterministic magnetic field the particle is exposed to, γ is the gyromagnetic ratio of the particle, α is a damping constant, and M_s is the saturation magnetization of the particle. Thermal noise is taken into account via a fluctuating magnetic field $\vec{\mathcal{B}}$. The properties of this stochastic field are according to the dissipation-fluctuation theorem

$$\langle \mathrm{B}_i(t) \rangle = 0 \qquad \langle \mathrm{B}_i(t)\mathrm{B}_j(t') \rangle = \frac{2\alpha k_B T}{\gamma M_s V_{core}} \delta(t-t')\delta_{ij} \quad i,j = 1,2,3$$

As already mentioned, the numerical solution of these types of equation depends on the calculus used. Again, the Stratonovitch interpretation is chosen and a Heun[11] scheme for the numerical solution of the above equation is used. In this case, however, the additional diffusion term after transformation can be omitted[1,9].

In $\vec{B}_{total}$, all contributions to the magnetic field, like external magnetic field, crystal field or demagnetization field, are included. In this paper, only an external magnetic field and axial field anisotropy due to the shape of the particle are taken into account. Already a small change of the large magnetic core diameter preferred in MPI in one direction induces an anisotropy comparable to the drive fields, as will be seen shortly. Hence, the total magnetic field can be written as

$$\vec{B}_{total}(t) = \vec{B}_{ext.}(t) - \mathbf{D} \cdot \vec{M}$$

The Matrix **D** represents the demagnetization tensor and contains the demagnetizations factors N_x, N_y, N_z on its diagonal if written in the principal axis system[10]. If the total magnetic field is substituted into equation (2), its numerical solution is comparable to the case of Brownian rotation. The respective analysis of the magnetization of 1000 single ellipsoidal particles with aspect ratio 31/30 is shown in figure 5.

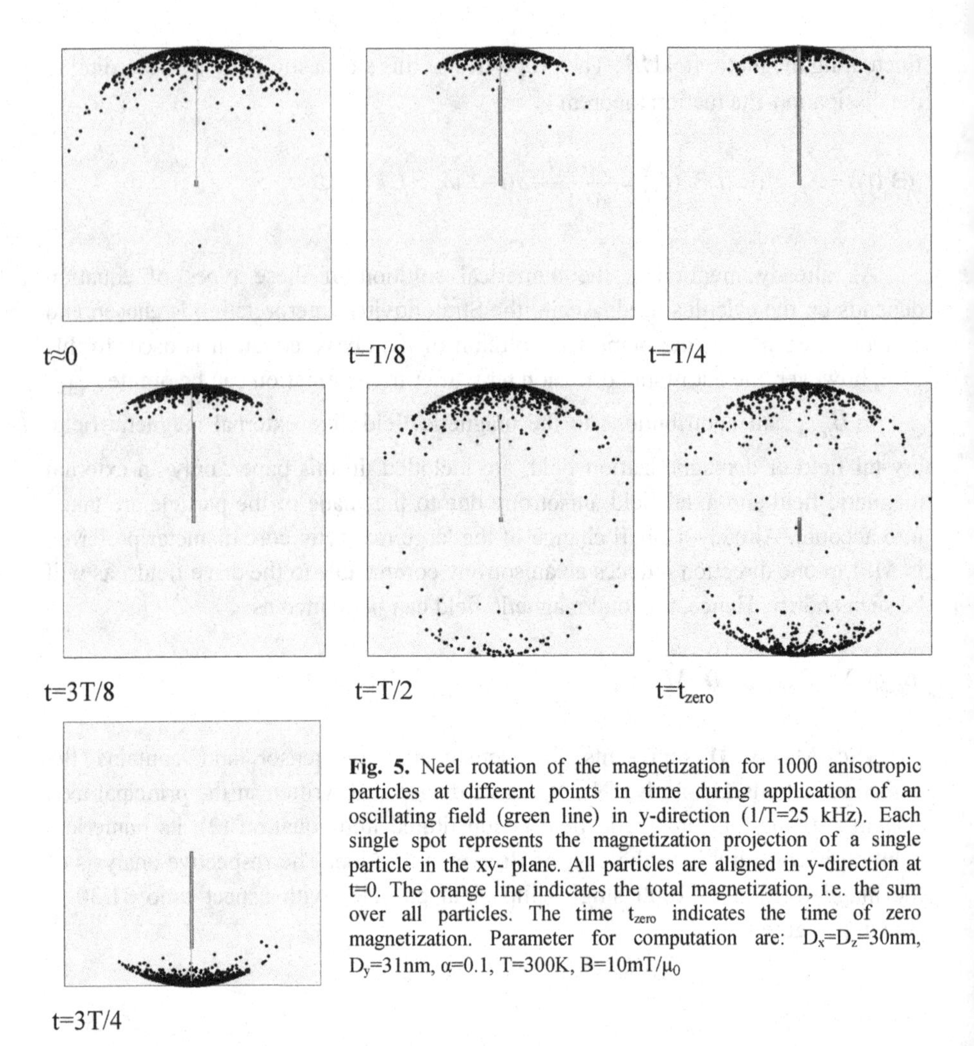

Fig. 5. Neel rotation of the magnetization for 1000 anisotropic particles at different points in time during application of an oscillating field (green line) in y-direction (1/T=25 kHz). Each single spot represents the magnetization projection of a single particle in the xy- plane. All particles are aligned in y-direction at t=0. The orange line indicates the total magnetization, i.e. the sum over all particles. The time t_{zero} indicates the time of zero magnetization. Parameter for computation are: $D_x=D_z=30$nm, $D_y=31$nm, $\alpha=0.1$, T=300K, B=10mT/μ_0

After a short decay, the magnetization is pinned in the direction of the anisotropy axis (vertical). At zero external magnetic field, the total magnetization remains aligned in that direction. After t=T/2, the magnetic field is reversed and the amount of particles overcoming the energy barrier with thermal assistance increases. The height of the energy barrier depends on the anisotropy of the particles. At a certain field the magnetization passes zero and the particles are equally distributed in both directions. Finally, the magnetization is again aligned vertically, but now in the opposite direction. Figure 6 shows the same process as in figure 5 for a single particle and different field directions. The thermal noise was suppressed by choosing T=1 K for better illustration. On the left side, the situation is similar to figure 5. For comparison, the single particle mean value at 300 K is also plotted. For a single particle, the magnetization reverses at the anisotropy field B_{aniso}, i.e. at about 7.8 mT/μ_0, which is for axial symmetry $M_s(N_y-N_x)$[14].Obviously, the mean magnetization at elevated temperatures flips at lower fields (~1.4mT/μ_0) due to thermally assisted barrier hopping (see also figure 5). If the field is aligned in horizontal direction (central graph, figure 6), the magnetic moment rotates from the axial (vertical) direction into the horizontal field direction. At the anisotropy field, the magnetization is aligned and rests in horizontal direction. If the field is lowered, both states, magnetization up or down, are equally likely (see non-periodically flips in blue line), so the magnetization will show no hysteresis effects in that direction. The right graph in figure 6 shows the magnetization dynamics if the field is aligned at 50° with respect to the vertical (axial) direction. So, again, the magnetization rotates in field direction. There remains, however, a certain angle between field and magnetization direction (see orange line).

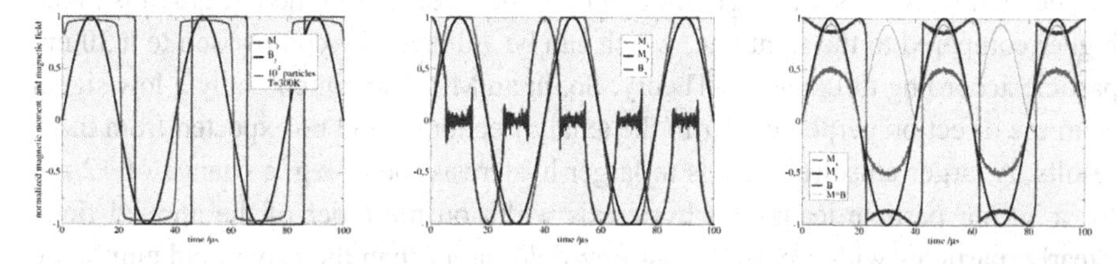

Fig. 6. Single particle dynamics for ellipsoidal particles with aspect ratio of 31nm to 30nm at low temperatures (1 K). On the left side, the field is directed into the vertical (axial) direction. The red line represents the mean value for 10^4 particles at 300 K. In the central graph, the field is perpendicular to the anisotropy (axial) axis. On the right side, the field is applied at an angle of 50° to the axial direction. The orange line represents the cosine of the angle between magnetization and magnetic field.

For the resolution in MPI the steepness of the magnetization curve is important, so the mean particle magnetization can also be plotted as a function of the magnetic field. This is shown for 10^4 particles for vertical (axial) and horizontal field directions in figure 7, beginning at t=0.

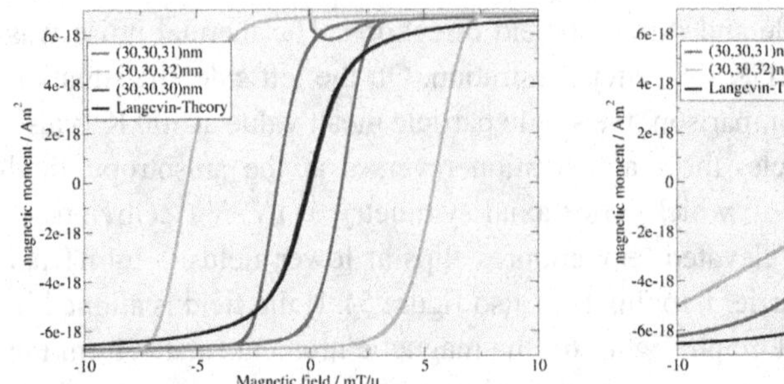

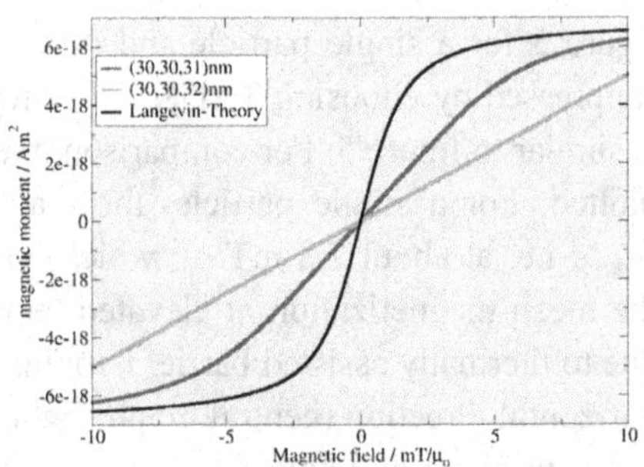

Fig. 7. Mean magnetic moment in field direction as function of external magnetic field for parallel (left) and perpendicular field direction with respect to the axial direction. At t=0 the magnetization is aligned in axial direction The calculated anisotropy fields are 7.8 mT/μ_0 and 15.3 mT/μ_0 for aspect ratios of 31/30 and 32/30, respectively. For 300 K, the width of the loops is lower than the anisotropy fields (2.8 mT/μ_0 and 10.8mT $/\mu_0$, respectively) .

As anticipated, for field variations in the direction of the anisotropy, a hysteresis loop is present, whereas for the direction perpendicular to this axis, the magnetization crosses the origin. In addition, the steepness in the left graph is much higher compared to the right one, which can be validated by comparison to a 30 nm particle according to Langevin-Theory. So, in an MPI experiment, only a low signal from the direction perpendicular to the axial direction would be expected from these results. A larger anisotropy leads to larger hysteresis loops, e.g. a change of +2 nm for a 30 nm particle leads to a hysteresis width on the order of the applied field. Clearly, particles with a mean anisotropy field larger than the drive field amplitude will not contribute to an MPI signal. Finally, comparing figure 7 and figure 4 indicates, that for axial alignment only the Néel process contributes to the MPI signal.

2.3. Combined Rotation

The combination of both causes of magnetization change is described by solving equation (1) and (2) simultaneously. The coupling between both equations is due to the magnetic torque in the first equation and the non-diagonal demagnetization tensor in the second equation. In the following the vector $\vec{n}$ points always in the direction of the easy axis (axial direction), which will in general be different from the direction of the magnetization. Therefore, a substitution according to

$(M_s\vec{n}\times\vec{B})\times\vec{n} \rightarrow (\vec{M}\times\vec{B})\times\vec{n}$ and $\mathbf{D} \rightarrow \mathbf{D}(\vec{n})$

is performed and a numerical solution is obtained as already described.

Figure 8 illustrates the dynamics of a single particle at T=1 K. The left graph shows the magnetization vector and the vector $\vec{n}$ (axial direction) as a function of time, after an oscillating magnetic field in horizontal direction has been applied.

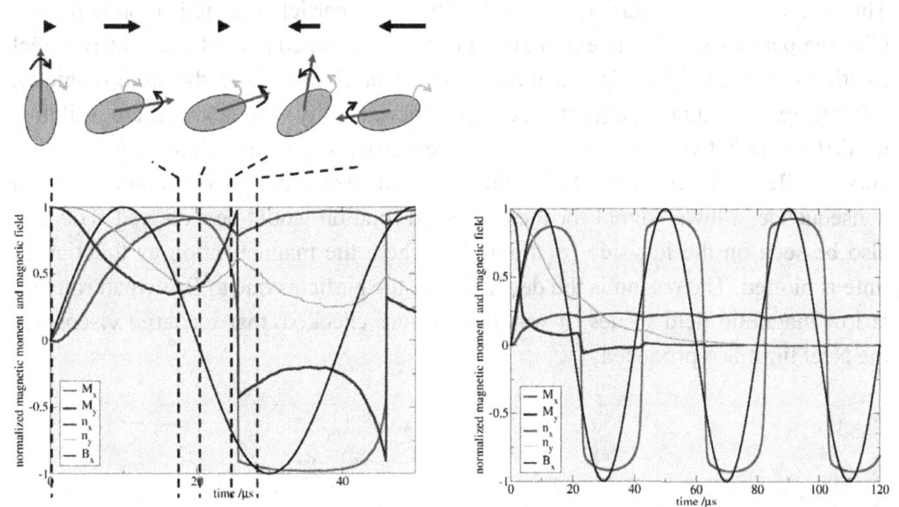

Fig. 8. Magnetization and rotational dynamics of a single particle at T=1 K (left side). On the right side, the mean value over 10^4 particles at 300 K is plotted. The axial anisotropy is represented by a diameter deviation of +2 nm for a 30 nm particle. The viscosity is 5 mPa s, the amplitude of the oscillating magnetic field is 10 mT/μ_0 at 25 kHz .The green ellipses and red arrows above the left graph indicate the direction of rotation of the particle and the magnetization. The black arrows indicate the direction and field strength.

The magnetization as well as the axial direction at t=0 was directed in positive y-direction (vertical). The green ellipses (particle) and the red arrows (magnetization) above the graph illustrate the dynamics of the rotation at different points in time, indicated by the dashed lines. At the very beginning, the magnetization as well as the particle rotates into the field direction, until a minimum vertical magnetization is reached. At that point, the external field is too low to further rotate the particle, so it starts rotating back into axial direction. At B_{ext}=0, the magnetization is aligned in axial direction $(\vec{n} \parallel \vec{M})$, which is the state of lowest energy and, thus, n_y reaches its minimum value. Afterwards, the field amplitude increases in negative x-direction, so the single particle magnetization further rotates in positive y-direction, as does n_y. If, finally, the magnetization exhibits a negative x-direction component due to the external magnetic field, the vector $\vec{n}$ will again change direction, to align itself in magnetization direction. This process will continue until all particles are aligned horizontally. This can be seen from the right side of figure 8. Again, 10^4 particles at 300K have been averaged. As expected, the magnetization does not flip at zero field, and again, a hysteresis loop is expected. This is confirmed in figure 9, right side. The mean particle magnetization is plotted after ten periods versus the external magnetic field and compared to exclusive Néel rotation (see also figure 7) and the case of an additional hydrodynamic diameter. After the equilibrium state (particles aligned horizontally) is reached, there is almost no difference between coated and uncoated particles. However, the magnetization curve differs significantly from the case of exclusive Néel rotation. As a consequence, a lower signal for the combined rotation would be expected. This can also be seen on the left side (of figure 9), where the magnetization as function of time is plotted. The reason is the dephasing of the particles due to Brownian rotation at low magnetic field values. It was furthermore checked, that for large viscosities the Néel limit is reproduced.

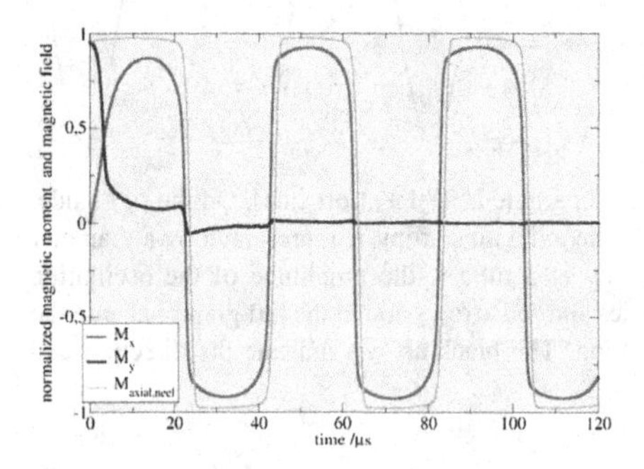

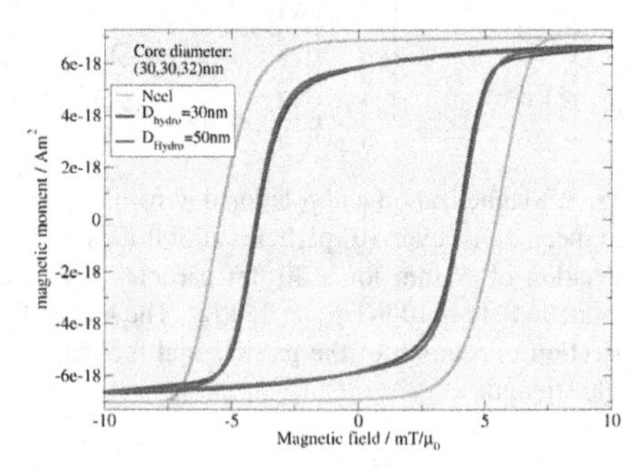

Fig. 9. The mean magnetic moment of 10^4 particles at T=300 K for the combined rotation. Left side: time evolution compared to exclusive Néel rotation; right side: the subsequent hysteresis loop. Additionally, the case for coated particles is also shown. In equilibrium there is only little difference, whereas the transient response (not shown) clearly differs due to different Brownian rotational time constants

3. CONCLUSION

In this paper, a detailed theory of Brownian, Néel and combined rotation of magnetic monodomain particles in the context of MPI was presented. A Langevin equation for the Brownian and Néel rotation was numerically solved. The relevant parameters like frequency, viscosity, particle diameter and anisotropy were chosen to apply to Magnetic Particle Imaging. It turned out, that the Néel process provides the main contribution to the MPI signal. The Brownian rotation, however, significantly influences the signal strength, even for magnetic fields directed permanently in axial direction. A small but defined anisotropy is acceptable, as the magnetization can be flipped with the external field. However, small diameter deviations induce substantial anisotropy fields.

REFERENCES

1 Gleich B, Weizenecker J, *Nature* 2005, **435**, p. 1214

2 Weizenecker J, Borgert J, Gleich B, *Phys Med Biol* 2007, **52,** p. 6363-6374

3 Knopp T, Biederer S, Sattel T F, Weizenecker J, Gleich B, Borgert J, Buzug TM, *Physics in Medicine and Biology*, 2009, **54**/2, p 385

4 Knopp T, Biederer S, Sattel TF, Weizenecker J, Gleich B, Borgert J, Buzug TM, *Bildverarbeitung für die Medizin*, 2010, Springer, 1-5.

5 Engel A, Reimann P, *Phys. Rev. E,* 2004, **70**, 051107

6 Coffey WT, Kalmykov YP, Waldron JT, *The Langevin Equation*, World Scientific (2004).

7 Kloeden PE, Platen E, *Numerical Solution of Stochastic Differential Equations,* Springer-Verlag (1999)

8 Scholz W, Schrefl T, Fidler J, *J. Magn. Magn. Mater.,* 2001, **233,** p. 296

9 Valberg PA, Butler JP, *Biophys. J.* 1987, **52** p. 537

10 Brown WF Jr, *Phys. Rev.,* 1963, **130,** p. 1677

11 Berkov DV, Gorn NL, *J. Condens. Matter,* 2002, **14,** p. L281

12 Martinez E, Lopez-Diaz L, Torres L, Alejos O, *Physica B,* 2004, **343,** p. 252

13 Osborn JA, *Phys. Rev.,* 1945, **67/11,** p. 12

14 $E_{demag} = -\vec{M}^T \mathbf{D} \vec{M} = M_s \sin^2(\theta)\, M_s(N_z - N_x) + \frac{1-N_z}{2} M_s^2 = M_s \sin^2(\theta) B_{aniso} + E_0$

[illegible] magnetic [illegible] strength [illegible] magnetic field [illegible] commercially [illegible] However, small diameter [illegible] anisotropy fields.

REFERENCES

1. [illegible] *Nature* [illegible] 425 [illegible]
2. [illegible] *Phys. Med. Biol.* 2006, 52 [illegible]
3. [illegible] Weber [illegible] *Biomedizinische Technik* 2000, 52 [illegible]
4. [illegible]
5. [illegible] *Phys. Rev.* [illegible]
6. [illegible] *Magnetic Materials* [illegible]
7. [illegible]
8. [illegible]
9. [illegible]
10. [illegible]
11. [illegible]
12. [illegible]
13. [illegible]
14. [illegible]

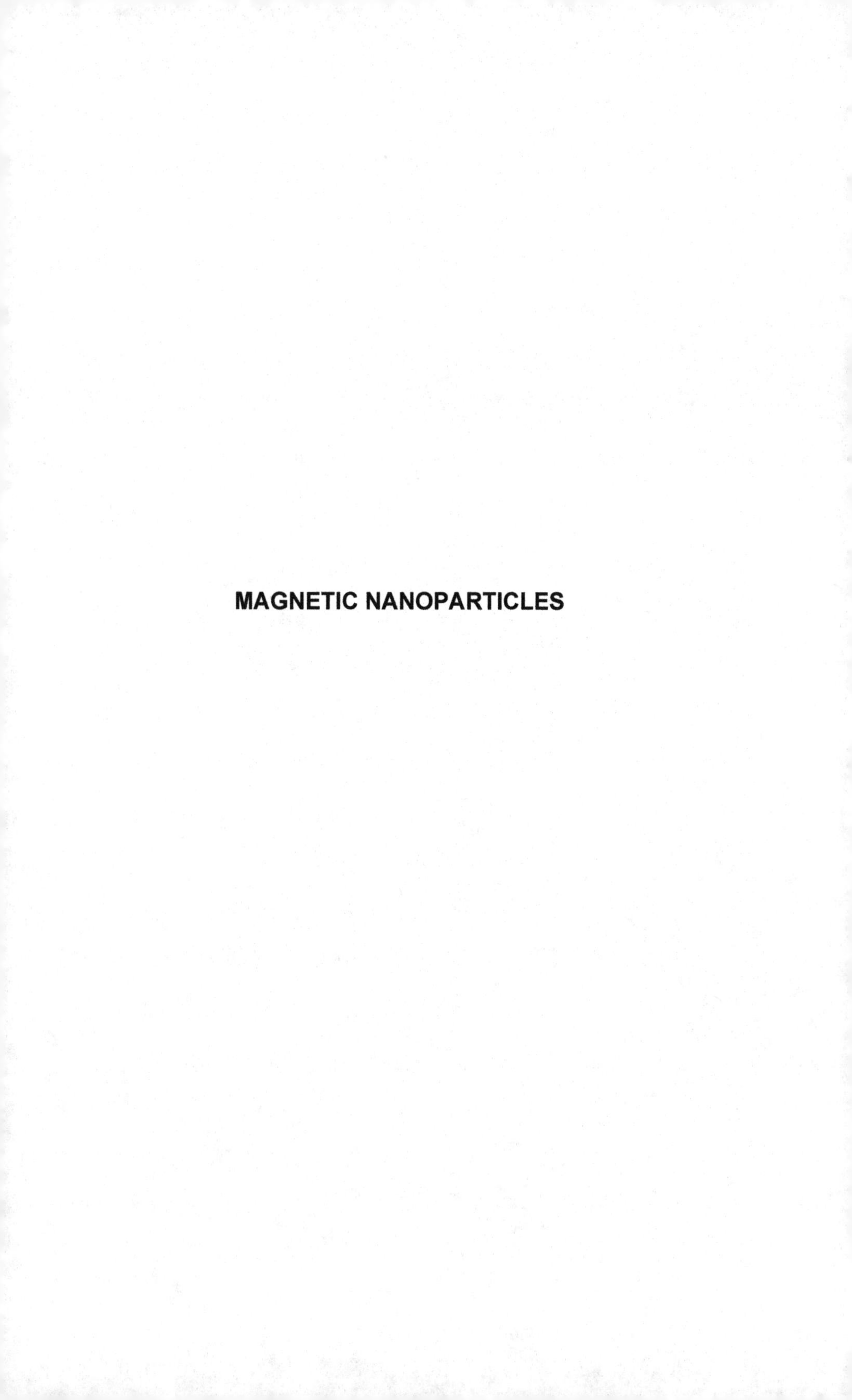

MAGNETIC NANOPARTICLES

THE EFFECTS OF MOLECULAR BINDING ON THE PHASE OF MSB MEASUREMENTS*

JOHN B. WEAVER

Department of Radiology, Dartmouth Medical School, Dartmouth-Hitchcock Medical Center
Lebanon, New Hampshire 03756, US
Email: john.b.weaver@hitchcock.org

ADAM M. RAUWERDINK

Thayer School of Engineering, Dartmouth College
Hanover, New Hampshire 03755, US
Email: Adam.M.Rauwerdink@Dartmouth.edu

Molecular binding effects the signal used in magnetic spectroscopy of nanoparticle Brownian motion (MSB). MSB uses the harmonics induced in magnetic nanoparticles by a sinusoidal applied magnetic field to estimate the Brownian motion of the nanoparticles. The harmonics reflect the balance between Lorentz forces and thermal effects on the alignment of the nanoparticles. Changes in the size of the harmonics caused by binding cannot be distinguished from changes in nanoparticle concentrations. We demonstrate that chemical binding also changes the phases of the harmonics. The change in phase observed for bound and free nanoparticles are different functions of frequency so sweeping the frequency should provide an internal control for other effects. The relative phase of the harmonics provides a concentration independent measure of chemical binding. The harmonics from very low nanoparticle concentrations can be measured *in vivo* so it should be possible to monitor chemical binding *in vivo* as well.

1. APPLICATIONS AND MEASUREMENT OF CHEMICAL BINDING

Chemical binding is important in a wide variety of biomedical applications. The most obvious example is antibody binding of targeted diagnostic and therapeutic agents[1,2]. Another important application is chemical binding of drugs to cell surface molecules, which is of central importance to pharmaceutical development.

---

* This work supported by the Norris Cotton Cancer Center, the Department of Radiology DHMC and the Innovation Program at Thayer School of Engineering.

Methods of measuring chemical binding *in vitro* have been very important. They include x-ray crystallography and NMR[3] and Raman scattering[4]. As important as those methods are, the applications are so pervasive that alternative methods are being actively explored. Recent work with colloid phase transitions[5] has shown promise in drug development. Simple residence times can be used to estimate binding if the proper models are used. Radioactive and optical tags are able to provide residence times for agents *in vivo*. But even the correct model cannot be used to distinguish binding energy from the number of binding sites[6]. A more sophisticated method, Fluorescence recovery after photobleaching (FRAP), can measure how fast molecular exchange between bound and unbound states repopulates fluorescent tags following bleaching[7] but again models are required and like all optical methods it can only function on tissue or cells near the surface. AC susceptibility, is being developed to measure binding of molecules tagged with a magnetic nanoparticles[8] but it requires long measurement times and a low noise background that are not feasible in *in vivo* applications. No current methods are capable of in vivo application.

2. SPECTROSCOPY OF NANOPARTICLE BROWNIAN MOTION (MSB)

A new technique capable of *in vivo* application measures the rotational Brownian motion of magnetic nanoparticles (NPs), magnetic spectroscopy of nanoparticle Brownian motion, MSB[9]. With appropriate controls and experimental design, MSB is capable of measuring any phenomenon that affects the rotational Brownian motion. For example, MSB has been used to measure temperature[10,11] and viscosity[12]. MSB employs the shape of the NP magnetization to characterize rotational Brownian motion. The magnetization induced by magnetic NPs in a pure sinusoidal magnetic field is a slightly distorted sinusoid. The magnetization produced by the NPs is limited by thermal effects and reflects a balance between the Lorentz forces tending to align the NPs and Brownian motion tending to randomize their directions. The distortion in the magnetization results in harmonics that can be detected independently and can be used to estimate Brownian motion. The ratio of the fifth over the third harmonics as a concentration independent measure of rotational Brownian motion. Because there are no other signals at the frequencies of the harmonics, they can be measured with very high sensitivity. It has been shown in imaging venues[13-16] that the harmonics can be measured *in vivo* at nanogram NP concentrations[13-15] so MSB could function *in vivo* as well.

2.1. The Effects of Chemical Binding on MSB

Chemical binding also impacts the Brownian motion of NPs. Indeed monitoring viscosity[12] is monitoring hydrogen bonding. But MSB has also been used to monitor antibody binding as well[16]. Modeling binding is more difficult. There are probably both static effects and dynamic effects. Static effects modeling bond bending can be described using Hookes Law. For low frequencies where the NPs are in equilibrium, the Hookes Law force simply adds to the potential in the Boltzmann distribution of the NP magnetic alignment. The potential energy, $E_p = -\mu H \cos\phi$, is a function of the angle the particle makes with the applied field ϕ, the moment of the particle, μ, and applied field, H. The magnetization integrated over ϕ provides the macroscopic magnetization in equilibrium:

$$M = \frac{n\mu}{\int_0^{\pi} e^{\alpha cos\phi} sin\phi d\phi} \int_0^{\pi} e^{\alpha cos\phi} sin\phi cos\phi d\phi \qquad (1)$$

where n is the number of particles and $\alpha=\mu H/kT$, k is the Boltzmann constant and T is the temperature. The first term is the partition function. Evaluating the integrals results in the Langevin function solution for the equilibrium magnetization[9]:

$$M = n\mu\left(coth\left(\alpha\right) + \alpha^{-1}\right)$$

For bound particles, the potential energy becomes a function of both a) the angle between the magnetization and the applied field, ϕ, and b) the angle between the magnetization and the bond, ϕ_B: $E_p = -\mu H \cos\phi - \frac{1}{2} k_S \phi_B^2$, where k_S is the spring constant for the bond. Assuming the bonds are uniformly distributed and are not a function of ϕ, the energy for each ϕ can be obtained by integrating over ϕ_B producing a term that is constant with respect to ϕ: $E_p = -\mu H \cos\phi - \frac{1}{2} k_S(\pi\text{-}4)$. The extra term generates a multiplicative exponential term that appears in both integrals in the expression above for the magnetization so it has no effect on the harmonics. Although the static effects do not impact the shape of the harmonics, the dynamic effects will affect the harmonics through the exchange rate between the free and bound states. Dynamic effects of binding characterizing exchange limited rotational motion of the NPs can be modeled by an increased Debye relaxation time τ which is related to the magnetization by an ordinary differential equation[17]:

$$\frac{dM}{dt} = -2/\tau\left[M(t) - \frac{M(t)}{\alpha_M(t)}\left(\xi_o cos\omega t + 3CM(t)\right)\right] \qquad (2)$$

Where $\xi_o cos\omega t$ is the applied field, C is the interaction between the nanoparticles and α_M is related to the magnetization by the inverse Langevin function: $M(t) = n\mu\left(coth\left(\alpha_M\right) + \alpha_M^{-1}\right)$. Numerical solutions provided below show that as the relaxation time increases, the phase lag between the magnetization and the applied field increases. The phenomenon can be observed as a wider hysteresis curve as shown below.

When comparing the phase of harmonics it is important to normalize the angle with the frequency. So the phase difference between the fifth and third harmonics is: $\theta_5 - \theta_3 = \theta_5^m/5 - \theta_3^m/3$, where θ_5^m is the measured phase of the fifth harmonic and θ_5 is the corrected phase at the frequency of the first harmonic.

3. SIMULATION RESULTS

Simulations of the phase angle difference between the fifth and third harmonics are shown below in Fig. 1. The simulations used Equation 2 and assumed iron oxide magnetization. A forward Euler method was used to numerically integrate the differential equation providing the magnetization and its time derivative which is proportional to the signal detected. The normalized phase difference between the fifth and third harmonics is shown for several values of the relaxation time. Over this range of parameters the phase difference drops to a minima before increasing to a broad peak. The width of the minima widens for larger NPs. More tightly bound nanoparticles have longer relaxation times. The simulation has limitations including ignoring the effects of frequency and field amplitude on the relaxation time, size distribution and variations in anisotropy.

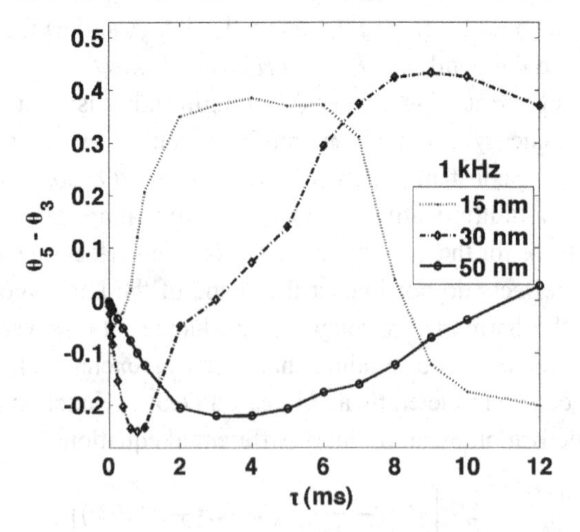

Fig. 1. The results of a simulation calculating the normalized phase angle difference between the fifth and third harmonics for different values of relaxation time, τ. The frequency is 1 kHz. The change in the normalized difference increases with frequency till they converge to the asymptotic value. This data implies the selection of frequency has a large impact on the contrast.

4. EXPERIMENTAL RESULTS

The normalized phase difference between the 5th and 3rd harmonics for bound and free NPs was measured using an apparatus previously described[9-11]. The NPs were 30 nm streptavidin functionalized iron oxide NPs. Some were allowed to bind to 2-micron polystyrene spheres. The free NPs were mixed with the same 2-micron polystyrene spheres that were previously coated with BSA to prevent binding as a control. The control NPs are labeled "Free" in Fig. 2. There is very little change in the phase difference with changes in frequency in the simulations which is congruent with the free NPs but not as closely with the bound NPs.

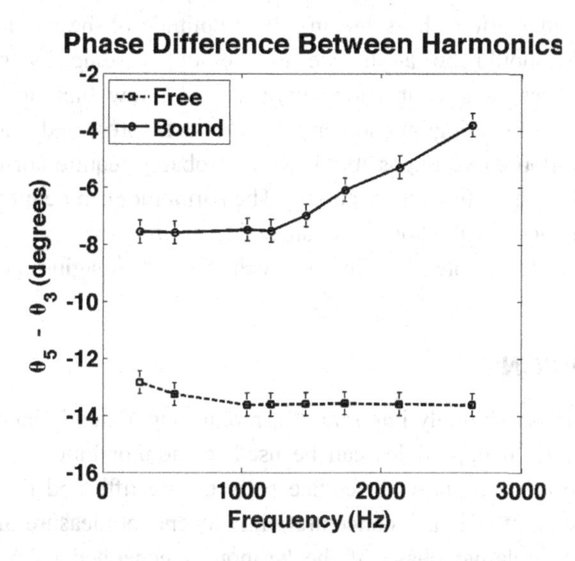

Fig. 2. The measured normalized phase angle difference between the fifth and third harmonics for bound and free NPs. The change in the normalized difference with frequency is much larger for bound NPs than for free NPs.

5. DISCUSSION

The experimental data fits the simulated data in general shape. The data fits into the ranges of simulated data curve well. The range of phase differences shown in Fig. 2 for free NPs is probably from the τ range from 2 to 4 on the 50nm curve. The phase difference is slightly decreasing over this range and is around -11°; only slightly higher than the measured values. The bound NPs are from farther to the right on the 50nm curve; in the τ range from 6 to 10 where the phase difference is increasing. The simulated data is -6° at τ of 8. The comparison of the simulation with experimental data is imperfect for several reasons including no size distribution. Estimates of the relaxation time for 30nm iron oxide nanoparticles are around 75 μs but there is strong dependence on anisotropy which is not well known for these NPs. In general, the shape of the simulated curve for 50nm NPs is very close to the shape of the measured data.

The data shows that the bound state to be monitored using the phase of the MSB signal. The binding energy can be identified if a calibration curve providing the MSB signal as a function of bound state is obtained independently. Alternatively, the bound fraction can be monitored in near real time if the MSB signal is known for each specific binding state present. Temperature can be separated from other effects by sweeping the amplitude of the applied field[10] and similar methods should be applicable to measure binding by sweeping the frequency. The resulting calibration curve should allow binding effects to be separated from confounding phenomenon. The data presented suggests that a frequency calibration curve is possible but will probably require correction factors not yet included to be sufficiently accurate. The harmonics can be measured *in vivo* so the methods described should be amenable to *in vivo* use as well. The phenomenon provides a potential contrast mechanism for imaging methods similar to MPI.

6. CONCLUSIONS

Chemical binding is extremely important for monitoring antibody binding and drug function. Magnetic nanoparticles can be used to monitor binding of conjugated agents using the relative phase difference between the fifth and third harmonics. The phase of the harmonics is a concentration independent measure of the mobility of the NPs. The relative phase of the harmonics generated using a sinusoidal applied field provides a mechanism to monitor the binding of those agents. Because the harmonics can be measured *in vivo*, it should be possible to monitor chemical binding *in vivo*.

REFERENCES

1 Mason DW, Williams AF. The kinetics of antibody binding to membrane antigens in solution and at the cell surface. *Biochem J.* 1980; 187(1): 1–20.

2 Pohlers D, Schmidt-Weber CB, Franch A, Kuhlmann J, Bräuer R, Emmrich F, Kinne RW. Differential clinical efficacy of anti-CD4 monoclonal antibodies in rat adjuvant arthritis is paralleled by differential influence on NF-κB binding activity and TNF-α secretion of T cells *Arthritis Res* 2002; 4:184-189.

3 Schwieters CD, Kuszewski JJ, Tjandra N, Clore GM. The Xplor-NIH NMR molecular structure determination package *J. of Mag. Reson.* 2003; 160:65–73.
4 Choo-Smith P, Edwards HGM, Endtz HP, Kros JM, Heule F, Barr H, Robinson JS, Bruining HA, Puppels GJ. Medical Applications of Raman Spectroscopy: From Proof of Principle to Clinical Implementation *Biopolymers* 2002; 67:1–9.
5 Baksh M, Jaros M, Groves J. Detection of molecular interactions at membrane surfaces through colloid phase transitions *Nature* 2004; 427(8):139-141.
6 Innis RB, et al. Consensus nomenclature for in vivo imaging of reversibly binding radioligands *J. of Cerebral Blood Flow & Meta.* 2007; 27:1533–1539.
7 Berk DA, Yuan F, Leunig M, Jain RK. Direct in vivo measurement of targeted binding in a human tumor xenograft *PNAS USA* 1997; 94:1785–1790.
8 Chung SH, Hoffmann A, Bader SD, Liu C, Kay B, Makowski L, Chen L. Biological sensors based on Brownian relaxation of magnetic nanoparticles *Applied Physics Letters* 2004; 85(14):2971-73.
9 Weaver J, Rauwerdink A, Sullivan C, Baker I. Spectral Distribution of MPI Signals in the Presence of a Static Magnetic Field *Med Phys* 2008; 35,1988-94.
10 Weaver JB, Rauwerdink AM, Hansen EW. Magnetic Nanoparticle Temperature Estimation *Medical Physics* 2009; 36(5): 1822-1829.
11 Rauwerdink AM, Hansen E, Weaver JB. Nanoparticle temperature estimation in combined ac and dc magnetic fields *Phys. Med. Biol.* 2009; 54:L51–L55.
12 Rauwerdink AM, Weaver JB. Viscous effects on nanoparticle magnetization harmonics" Journal of Magnetism and Magnetic Materials in press.
13 Gleich B, Weizenecker J. Tomographic imaging using the nonlinear response of magnetic particles *Nature* 2005; 435(30):1214-9.
14 Ferguson RM, Minard KR, Krishnan KM Optimization of nanoparticle core size for magnetic particle imaging *Journal of Magnetism and Magnetic Materials* 2009; 321:1548–1551.
15 Knopp T, Biederer S, Rahmer J, Weizenecker J, Gleich B. Model-Based Reconstruction for Magnetic Particle Imaging 2009.
16 Weizenecker J, Borgert J, Gleich B. A simulation study on the resolution and sensitivity of magnetic particle imaging *Phys. Med. Biol.* 52 (2007) 6363–6374.
17 Felderhof BU, Jones RB Mean field theory of the nonlinear response of an interacting dipolar system with rotational diffusion to an oscillating field *J. Phys.: Condens. Matter* 2003; 15:4011–4024.

SPIO NANOPARTICLES ENCAPSULATION INTO HUMAN ERYTHROCYTES FOR MPI APPLICATION

MARKOV D., BOEVE H.

Philips Research Europe, High Tech Campus 34
Eindhoven, 5656 AE, The Netherlands
Email: denis.markov@philips.com

GLEICH B., BORGERT J.

Philips Research Europe, Sector Medical Imaging Systems,
Röntgenstrasse 24-26, 22335 Hamburg, Germany
Email: bernhard.gleich@philips.com

ANTONELLI A., SFARA C., MAGNANI M.

Department of Biomolecular Sciences, University of Urbino, Via Saffi 2
Urbino, 61029, Italy
Email: mauro.magnani@uniurb.it

We report the first magnetic characterization of superparamagnetic iron oxide (SPIO) nanoparticles loaded red blood cell (RBC) constructs to serve as potential blood tracer agent in imaging of the circulatory system by Magnetic Particle Imaging (MPI). MPI is an emerging, quantitative medical imaging modality, which holds promise in terms of sensitivity in combination with spatial and temporal resolution. The results that have been obtained suggest that, while SPIO show a short in vivo half-life that limits MPI, the RBCs loaded with SPIO overcome this problem. Furthermore we show that the encapsulation of the tracer materials is affected by its size and by the size of pores on the RBC membrane generated during the encapsulation procedure.

1. INTRODUCTION

Erythrocyte (red blood cells, RBCs) constitute potential biocompatible carriers for different bioactive substances including therapeutic proteins (enzymes and vaccines), nucleotide analogues, cancer chemotherapeutics, nucleic acids, to be applied for several clinical purposes. They feature unique properties such as biodegradability, biocompatibility and large carrier volumes (the mean corpuscular volume, MCV, of RBC is 87 ± 5 fl) and thus are well suited to be used for drug encapsulation. Once inside the RBC the molecules can be protected from inactivation by endogenous factors and, at the same time, the encapsulation of drugs into autologous RBCs results in a protection of the organism against the toxic effects of the drug itself, thus avoiding immunological reactions. RBCs have a longer lifespan in circulation as compared to synthetic carriers that are currently available (soluble macromolecules as synthetic polymers or complex particulate structures such as microparticles and liposomes) and could act as bioreactors due to the presence of several enzymatic activities that can directly affect the loaded molecules and, in the case of loaded prodrugs, give rise to the active drug itself. Thus, erythrocyte-based drug delivery represents an attractive and versatile carrier system suitable for several clinical purposes, depending on the drug to be transported or on the cells to be targeted.

Recently, we have proposed a method of SPIO (Superparamagnetic Iron Oxide) nanoparticles encapsulation into RBCs that avoids fast uptake by the reticuloendothelial system (RES), thus prolonging blood half-life of these contrast agents enabling medical application in Magnetic Resonance Imaging (MRI), and more specifically in MRI imaging of the circulatory system. In fact, the advantage of these SPIO loaded erythrocytes is that they are stable constructs that are able to survive for a number of days without being eliminated, and often have a lifespan comparable to that of untreated erythrocytes [1]. Moreover, up to 25% of the total mouse blood was replaced by nanoparticles-loaded erythrocytes without any toxic effect. Here we report on the potential of RBCs loaded with iron oxide nanoparticles as tracer material for Magnetic Particle Imaging (MPI), a novel imaging modality introduced by Philips that hold great promise to comply with the requirements of a next generation imaging concept [2]. The MPI principle is based on the nonlinear magnetization response at low magnetic field which is typical for iron oxide based magnetic nanoparticles. The MPI concept is different from MRI. When subjected to an oscillating magnetic field with a frequency f_1 the nanomaterial generates an output signal at odd multiple harmonics $n{\cdot}f_1$ of this base frequency. Analysis of the spectral intensity of these higher harmonics results in highly sensitive method for detection of magnetic material. Spatial encoding is realized by using a coil arrangement that allows for a field-free point motion across the otherwise magnetically saturated field-of-view. This method results in images with high spatial and temporal resolution as well as the high contrast that scales linearly with the tracer concentration. Initial MPI experiments with the MRI-contrast agent Resovist from Bayer Schering Pharma, a water-based polydisperse colloid of carboxydextran coated iron oxide particles, have shown a high spatial resolution of

0.3 mm in tomographic imaging. It has further been found that the MPI signal is mainly generated by particles with 30 nm magnetic core diameter [3]. Coated with dextran derivatives for stabilization, these iron oxide particles have an average hydrodynamic size of 50 to 60 nm. This results in a short blood half-life of several minutes due to rapid excretion via the RES which limits the applicability of such compound in MPI. The use of longer blood half-time tracer materials would make MPI highly suitable for e.g. perfusion imaging, image guided drug delivery or interventional applications that require repeated imaging. In this way, the use of RBCs as SPIOs carriers can be an advantage because of the long in vivo survival of RBCs and a cell volume that theoretically could contain up to 100.000 particles per cell.

2. ENCAPSULATION OF MAGNETIC NANOPARTICLES INTO RBCS

The loading procedure has been essentially reported in Antonelli A. et al. [1]. Briefly, the encapsulation of magnetic nanomaterials into erythrocytes was attempted by a loading procedure consisting of a dialysis of red blood cells in the presence of nanomaterials against a hypotonic solution, in order to open pores of the red cell membrane, and successive resealing and reannealing of dialysed cells using isotonic buffer. Erythrocytes were loaded using two different amounts of Resovist (540 mg/ml of ferucarbotran, corresponding to 28 mg Fe/ml or 0.5 mmol/ml, by Bayer Schering Pharma) or Sinerem (20 mg Fe/ml or 0.357 mmol/ml, by Guerbet) contrast agents. 1 ml of RBC70% was dialysed both in presence of 5.6 mg Fe (corresponding to 200μl of Resovist or 280μl of Sinerem contrast agents) ($L1_R$-RBCs, $L1_S$-RBCs) and 22.4 mg Fe (corresponding to 800μl of Resovist or 1120 μl of Sinerem contrast agents) ($L2_R$-RBCs, $L2_S$-RBCs). Following the same procedure unloaded erythrocytes (UL-RBCs) were prepared using the same dialysis protocol in the absence of magnetic material. The total preparation procedure typically resulted in a cell recovery of loaded erythrocytes ranging from 60% to 70%, similar to that for unloaded cells. The loaded erythrocytes were slightly smaller on average than the untreated cells, with less haemoglobin per cell but with a near normal mean cellular haemoglobin concentration. It should be noted that the reduced mean cell volume (MCV) reported above is due to the dilution of RBCs applied in these loading procedure and not to the use of contrast agents, as similar values were observed when unloaded erythrocytes were prepared using identical conditions.

The electron microscope analyses of L1- and L2-RBCs confirm the cell integrity. Scanning Electron Microscopy (SEM) shows that loaded erythrocytes have normal cell morphology and no significant differences with respect to control cells (data not shown). Moreover, TEM analyses of Resovist and Sinerem loaded RBCs demonstrates a uniform non-aggregated distribution of the tracer material throughout the cell with no significant clustering or accumulation at the erythrocyte membrane (data not shown).

3. TRACER CHARACTERIZATION

The iron concentration of SPIOs loaded into erythrocytes was determined by NMR, VSM and ICP-OES analyses (Table 1). NMR measurements of the longitudinal (T1) and transverse (T2) relaxation times of the loaded samples were performed using an AC-200 NMR-Bruker spectrometer and Fe concentration content was calculated using r1 and r2 values obtained from a dose-response curve generated by adding known amounts of Resovist or Sinerem contrast agents to human blood samples. T1 and T2 relaxation times of Sinerem or Resovist L1-RBCs and L2-RBCs samples are significantly lower than values of control cells (data not shown). This decrease is attributed to the presence of magnetic nanomaterials in loaded RBCs. T1 measurements were used to derive the nanoparticle concentrations due to a higher signal-to-noise ratio of T1 compared to T2.

Table 1. Fe concentrations of loaded RBCs resulting from NMR, VSM, ICP analyses.

Sample	Tracer Fe (NMR) [mM]	Tracer Fe (VSM) [mM]	Tracer Fe (ICP) [mM]
Control RBCs	-	-	-
Resovist-L1-RBCs	6.33	8	6.036
Resovist-L2-RBCs	13.9	21	19.554
Sinerem-L1-RBCs	5	6.66	6.857
Sinerem-L2-RBCs	10	15	16.071
Bulk Resovist		-	500
Bulk Sinerem		-	357

To provide additional control values, the VSM was employed as a direct method to detect the magnetic content in the samples. A rather poor correlation between the NMR- and VSM- based tracer iron concentrations has been found, which can be attributed to the limited quantification potential of NMR. To further validate agent contents in the samples, ICP-OES was utilized providing an independent measure for iron concentrations, and corrected by control (unloaded RBCs) samples. The Fe concentrations of the Resovist and Sinerem-Loaded RBCs samples were derived from ICP analysis and corrected with a control sample (RBC with no tracer). VSM and ICP based values agreed in all loaded samples while NMR measurements generally underestimate the iron content (Table 1). This is particularly evident in erythrocyte samples loaded with a higher amount of contrast agents (L2-RBCs).

Due to the good match between the VSM and ICP-OES measurements, agent iron concentrations derived from DC magnetization measurements were further used in this study.

4. MPS ANALYSIS

All samples were characterized with Magnetic Particle Spectroscopy (MPS): bulk tracer materials and SPIO-loaded RBC samples have generated significant MPS signal in the high frequency range while the tracer-free RBC sample did not result in any considerable MPS spectral output (at the noise level). Sample magnetic moments normalized by tracer Fe content (as derived from VSM) are shown in Fig.1 as a function of output frequency. The MPS signal generated by Resovist reduces by about a factor 8 and by a factor 4 in the case of Sinerem upon RBC encapsulation.

The discrepancies in the MPS signals between bulk tracer materials and tracer loaded RBCs can be attributed to size-selection during the RBC loading protocol, which would result in encapsulated particles with a different size distribution compared to bulk and therefore generates a modified MPI spectral response. Although the different distribution of magnetic core diameters, the peak is around 5 to 7 nm for bulk and tracer-loaded RBCs samples corresponding to a mean hydrodynamic particles size of 50-60 nm (data not shown).

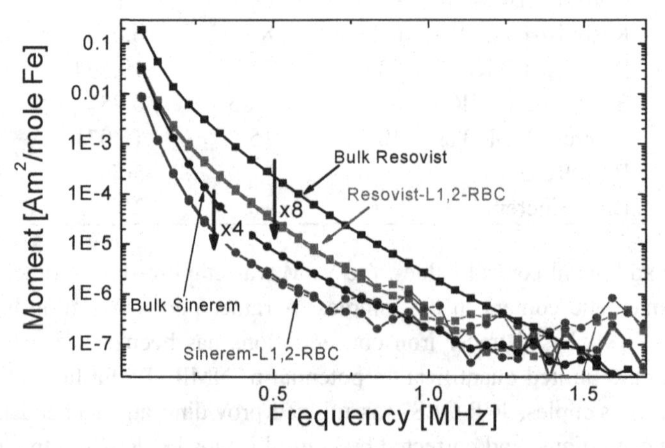

Fig. 1. MPS experimental data (symbols), lines are guides to the eye. Magnetic moment normalized by Fe content vs. frequency

5. CONCLUSIONS

The results reported in this paper have demonstrated the potential of RBCs as nanoparticle carriers in MPI and have further refined some of the requirements for optimal signal generation using RBCs. Despite the fact that Resovist or Sinerem-loaded erythrocytes have shown a reduced performance in MPI compared to their respective bulk materials, the data obtained from NMR and VSM characterization confirms the attractiveness of RBCs in MPI using an optimal nanoparticle-based contrast material, i.e. starting from monodisperse colloids with a core diameter of about 30 nm and a hydrodynamic size of 50-60 nm. Moreover, preliminary *in vivo* experiments have shown that MPI using nanoparticles-loaded erythrocytes is possible at least in the mouse. It is to be noted that the loading protocol of magnetic nanoparticles into human RBCs has now been shown to be optimal for a hydrodynamic diameter of about 60 nm. Therefore one of the challenges will be to find new synthesis protocols and optimize next generation nanoparticle tracer materials.

ACKNOWLEDGMENTS

This work was partially supported by EU NACBO Project 500804-2 and FIRB-NANOMED project RBLA03WK4R-005.

REFERENCES

1 Antonelli A, Sfara C, Mosca L, Manuali E, Magnani M. New biomimetic constructs for improved in vivo circulation of superparamagnetic nanoparticles. *J Nanosci. Nanotechnol.* 2008; **8**: 1–9.

2 Gleich B, Weizenecker J. Tomographic imaging using the nonlinear response of magnetic particles. *Nature* 2005; **435**: 1214–1217.

3 Weizenecker J, Borgert J, Gleich B. A simulation study on the resolution and sensitivity of magnetic particles imaging. *Physics in Medicine and Biology* 2007; **52**: 6363–6374.

USE OF RESOVIST IN MAGNETIC PARTICLE IMAGING

GUNNAR SCHÜTZ*

Bayer Schering Pharma AG, Cardiovascular Imaging & Contrast Media Research
Müllerstrasse 178,13353 Berlin, Germany
Email: gunnar.schuetz@bayerhealthcare.com

JESSICA LOHRKE

Bayer Schering Pharma AG, Cardiovascular Imaging & Contrast Media Research
Müllerstrasse 178, 13353 Berlin, Germany
Email: jessica.lohrke@bayerhealthcare.com

JOACHIM HÜTTER

Bayer Schering Pharma AG, Cardiovascular Imaging & Contrast Media Research,
Muellerstrasse 178, Berlin, 13353, Germany
Email: joachim.huetter@bayerhealthcare.com

Magnetic particle imaging (MPI) is a novel tomographic imaging technique visualizing colloidal magnetic material. Experimental data of several research groups indicate that Resovist, a clinically approved MRI contrast agent consisting of superparamagnetic iron oxide (SPIO) nanoparticles, is superior to a number of other experimental as well as clinically approved SPIO in its performance as MPI tracer. Nevertheless, the dose of Resovist needed to achieve a good spatial and temporal resolution in simulation studies and initial animal experiments is rather high. Therefore, novel tracer materials are needed in order to foster further improvement of this new imaging modality. This contribution summarizes data for Resovist in MPI and ideas for tracer optimization.

1. USE OF RESOVIST IN MPI STUDIES

Resovist was first launched as MRI contrast agent for early liver diagnosis in 2001. It contains a suspension of carboxydextran coated superparamagnetic iron oxide (SPIO) nanoparticles. In their initial experiments to establish the magnetic particle imaging (MPI) technology B. Gleich and J. Weizenecker used Resovist as magnetic particle formulation to acquire first phantom images[1]. In a prototype MPI scanner

* Corresponding author: Gunnar Schütz, gunnar.schuetz@bayerhealthcare.com

use of undiluted Resovist containing 0.5 M iron resulted in a sub-millimeter spatial resolution at 1 minute data acquisition time. In 2007 Philips Research Hamburg together with Bayer Schering Pharma performed initial animal experiments indicating that a Resovist dose of 4,5 mg Fe/kg bodyweight (7 times of the recommended human dose) is sufficient to visualize the imaging agent bolus by MPI in mice in a time-resolved fashion (unpublished results).

In early 2009 Weizenecker and co-workers published an animal study nicely exploiting the high temporal resolution of MPI [2]. They injected Resovist at a dose of 2,5 mg Fe/kg (3,8 fold max. recommended human dose) and could acquire signal in 3 dimensions from heart and large vessels. Left and right ventricle as well as the vena cava could be differentiated albeit at a voxel size greater than the actual object of interest. The temporal resolution, however, is good enough to resolve the heart beat frequency of the mouse. As the method is quantitative, iron concentration is given at any time point after Resovist injection. The bolus is nicely time resolved at a concentration of about 3.8 mM and passage of the tracer can be tracked through vena cava, right atrium and right ventricle followed by left atrium and left ventricle. At equal distribution of the tracer in blood which is almost reached after 20 seconds post injection iron concentration has declined to 250 µM and will be further reduced at a half life of approximately 15 minutes. According to a simulation study published by Weizenecker et al. in 2007[3] spatial resolution drops with decline of tracer concentration. It thus remains to be elucidated, whether feasible imaging results can just be obtained during bolus passage within a couple of seconds or whether tracer concentrations at later time points will also allow acquisition of diagnostically useful images.

At the world molecular imaging congress 2009 in Montreal, Canada, Rahmer and colleagues presented results on an in vivo organ perfusion study in mice[4]. A 3D real-time mouse brain perfusion study using Resovist was shown at a spatial resolution of 1.5x3x3 mm. The Resovist dose in this study was reported to be between 1,5 and 5,8 mg Fe/kg bodyweight. As the max. dose for Resovist tested as safe in clinical studies is 2.2 mg Fe/kg. Some application doses used by Rahmer et al. and others would thus exceed the clinically acceptable range.

At the 2008 ISMRM in Toronto J. Bulte and collegues reported cell labelling studies indicating that Resovist has a 4-fold higher imaging efficacy per unit of iron than Ferridex has[5]. They found that MPI has in fact a potential for non-invasive quantitative cell tracking.

The articles cited above describe Resovist as an imaging tracer suitable for magnetic particle imaging, although the doses used to acquire sufficiently well resolved images are close to or even exceed the maximum tolerable dose for humans. By increasing magnetic properties of the tracer material and by separating the optimal particle fraction of a synthesis approach signal and therefore spatial resolution might be increased substantially.

2. OPTIONS FOR TRACER OPTIMIZATION

In the literature some options to generate a tracer performing better than Resovist are discussed. B. Gleich suggests that only a 3 % fraction of Resovist contributes to its overall signal in MPI[1] implicating that separation of this particular colloidal fraction would lead to significant signal enhancement. Resovist contains superparamagnetic iron oxide particles in a rather broad size distribution as shown in figure 1. Magnetic separation of this suspension into 7 fractions ranging from 20 nm to 80 nm mean hydrodynamic diameter with narrow size distributions (corresponding iron oxide core sizes range from approx. 5 nm to 25 nm as determined by SAXS) did, however, not result in a marked signal increase in magnetic particle spectroscopy (our unpublished observations). These results suggest that neither mean diameter nor particle size distribution are the main parameters accounting for signal determination. It though has to be mentioned that Resovist cores consist of aggregates of approx. 5 nm iron oxide crystallites. Whereas the smallest separated fraction contains single crystallite cores the larger fractions contain multiple such crystallites as core. This may result in magnetic properties differing from those calculated for "solid" magnetite core structures.

Ferguson and colleagues published some mathematical considerations on optimizing size and size distribution of magnetite nanoparticles in order to improve their harmonic response in MPI [7]. The authors simulate magnetite particles ranging from 10 to 16 nm coated by a 23 nm surfactant layer. They conclude that signal increases with particle size before decreasing steeply due to increased relaxation time. A particle core diameter of 14 nm results in the highest magnetization and third harmonic amplitude at the conditions chosen. According to their calculations the partical size distribution influences harmonic response significantly. The broader the size distribution the lower the signal amplitude will be. This contrasts to our findings for Resovist fractions, may, however, be explained by the Resovist core structure as mentioned above.

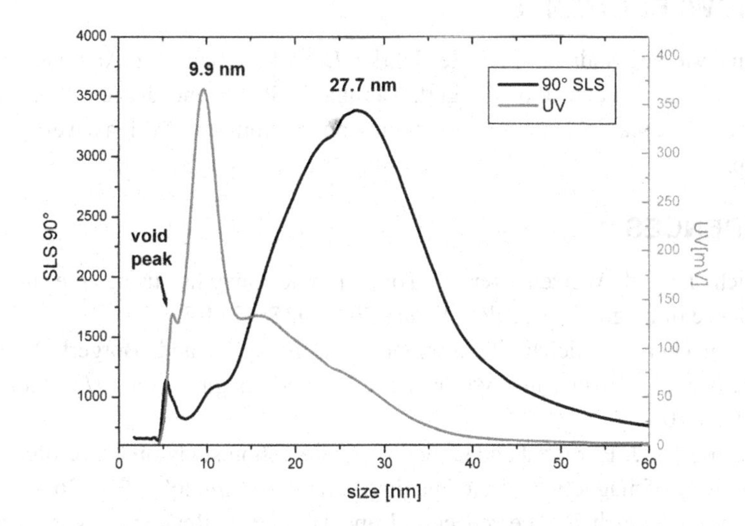

Fig. 1 Fractogram of the asymmetrical flow–field–flow–fractionation (A4F) of the particle size distribution of Resovist (Lot# 43042T). Two detections methods were used to account for signal weighting differences of different particle sizes in the same sample; black curve: 90° static light scattering (SLS) detecting primarily larger particles, grey curve UV detector (wavelength: 254 nm) detecting predominantly smaller particles. The signal amplitude therefore is not a measure of relative content of a particular particle size in the sample. The A4F characterization method and the equipment used were described before[6]. Here the channel thickness was 500µm, the detector flow rate was 0.5 ml/min and the cross–flow rate decreased linearly with time, starting with a cross–flow rate of 2.5 ml/min.

The same was principally found by S. Biederer and his colleagues when describing the construction of a magnetic particle spectrometer and its use in characterizing Resovist[8]. Simulated particles of identical size do result in higher harmonic response compared to a simulated size distribution. The presented magnetic particle spectrometer will have impact on future particle synthesis approaches as it allows quick and precise analysis of harmonic response and thus provides an important tool for particle lead structure optimization.

In contrast to particle size and size distribution little if any data is available addressing additional particle parameters like material variations and particle shape. In practice synthesized particles might not consist of pure magnetite but may also contain to some extent maghemite or iron hydroxide. The introduction of other metals in addition to iron may also influence the magnetization and therefore harmonic response. The shape of magnetic particles is mostly considered as sphere. It remains to be elucidated, however, whether other shapes like egg-shape, cubes or octahedrons will offer improved performance in MPI.

ACKNOWLEDGMENTS

We thank Violetta Sudmann, Nicole Gehrke, Danielle Franke and Andreas Briel for initial experiments and Jörn Borgert, Bernhard Gleich and Jürgen Weizenecker from Philips research Hamburg for their cooperation and MPI as well as MPS measurements.

REFERENCES

1 Gleich B and Weizenecker J. Tomographic imaging using the nonlinear response of magnetic particles. *Nature* 2005; **435**: 1214-7.
2 Weizenecker J, Gleich B, Rahmer J, Dahnke H and Borgert J. Three-dimensional real-time in vivo magnetic particle imaging. *Phys Med Biol* 2009; **54**: L1-L10.
3 Weizenecker J, Borgert J and Gleich B. A simulation study on the resolution and sensitivity of magnetic particle imaging. *Phys Med Biol* 2007; **52**: 6363-74.
4 Rahmer J, Gleich B, Weizenecker J and Borgert J. Real-Time Volumetric in vivo Magnetic Particle Imaging of Cerebral Perfusion. *WMIC 2009* 2009; **Poster Abstract 0529**:
5 Bulte JWM, Gleich B, Weizenecker J, Bernard S, Walczak P, Markov DE, Aerts HCJ, Borgert J and Boeve H. Developing Cellular MPI: Initial Experience. *ISMRM 2008* 2008; **Poster Abstract 1675**:
6 Lohrke J, Briel A and Mader K. Characterization of superparamagnetic iron oxide nanoparticles by asymmetrical flow-field-flow-fractionation. *Nanomed* 2008; **3**: 437-52.
7 Ferguson RM, Minard KR and Krishnan KM. Optimization of nanoparticle core size for magnetic particle imaging. *J Magn Magn Mater* 2009; **321**: 1548-1551.
8 Biederer S, Knopp T, Sattel T, Luedtk-Buzug K, Gleich B, Weizenecker J, Borgert J and Buzug TM. Magnetization response spectroscopy of superparamagnetic nanoparticles for magnetic particle imaging. *J. Phys. D: Appl. Phys.* 2009; **42**: 7-4.

LARGER SINGLE DOMAIN IRON OXIDE NANOPARTICLES FOR MAGNETIC PARTICLE IMAGING

SILVIO DUTZ

Department of Bio NanoPhotonics, Institute of Photonic Technologies,
Albert-Einstein-Straße 9, Jena, 07745, Germany
Email: silvio.dutz@ipht-jena.de

ROBERT MÜLLER

Department of Bio NanoPhotonics, Institute of Photonic Technologies,
Albert-Einstein-Straße 9, Jena, 07745, Germany

MATTHIAS ZEISBERGER

Department of Spectroscopy and Imaging, Institute of Photonic Technologies,
Albert-Einstein-Straße 9, Jena, 07745, Germany

In the last years of research in magnetic particle imaging it was posited that the best spatial resolution will be achieved by use of iron oxide single domain nanoparticles in the size range from 20 to 30 nm. The present article gives a short review about the experiences of our group concerning the preparation and the characterisation of particles in this size range. A further increase of the spatial resolution of magnetic particle imaging can be expected for the use of mono sized particles. For this reason two fractionation methods for the narrowing of the size distribution width are mentioned.

1. INTRODUCTION

Magnetic nanoparticles (MNP) are very interesting for a lot of biomedical applications. The magnetic particle imaging (MPI) is a relatively new approach of imaging which utilize the fact that magnetically saturated particles do not show a change in their magnetic behavior when exposed to an additional alternating magnetic field, whereas the unsaturated particles show a strong change in their magnetization[1]. Therefore it is possible to detect very small amounts of magnetic material serving as magnetic marker by moving a zero field of very small dimensions through the body and measuring the magnetic response of MNP bound to the tissue in the zero field to the additional alternating field. Biederer et al. stated that magnetic particles with a diameter in the range between 20 and 30 nm and a narrow size distribution have the largest contribution to the MPI signal[2].

To meet the requirements of the particles for MPI in the present article different routes to prepare larger single domain particles (LSDP) in the interesting size range are described. The resulting particles are characterized and the most interesting properties for MPI are compared. For the narrowing of the size distribution width magnetic fractionation methods seems to be interesting. Here are two methods mentioned which achieved good results during our studies concerning the increase of the specific heating power of MNP for magnetic particle hyperthermia.

2. PARTICLE PREPARATION

The most popular methods for the preparation of iron oxide nanoparticles are wet precipitation procedures as described by Khallafalla[3]. In principle, to an aqueous solution of mixed Fe^{2+}- und Fe^{3+}-salts an alkaline medium is added which leads to the precipitation of iron oxide nanoparticles. Typically the resulting particles show a mean size of about 10 nm and a broad particle size distribution. By changing the synthesis conditions (e.g. drop time, temperature, concentrations) the particle diameter can be increased up to 100 nm[4].

Another variation of this method is the so called cyclic precipitation[5]. During the first cycle a standard wet precipitation is carried out. Following this, the mixed iron salts are added again and a second precipitation takes place after addition of the alkaline medium. By controlling the reaction kinetics it can be reached that the second precipitate grows on the particles from the first step without any further formation of new particles. Up to now 4 consecutive cycles were successfully carried out which lead to particles up to 26 nm and a narrower size distribution in comparison to the larger particles from Dutz et al.[4].

For comparison another type of MNP will be described here – the so called magnetic multi-core nanoparticles. These particles are prepared by a similar method to the method of Khallafalla but the processing of the synthesis is changed in a way that the resulting particles are clusters in the size of 50 to 80 nm consisting of single domain cores of 13 nm[6,7]. By coating these particles with carboxymethyldextrane, sedimentation stable suspensions of larger particles can be prepared.

Beside the classical wet precipitation of MNP there are some other ways to prepare LSDP. A very simple method is the milling of larger particles. But due to the strong forces during the grinding process of the particles the crystal lattice is damaged which leads to a higher coercivity of the particles which is not so advantageous for the application in MPI[4,8].

A more suitable method is the controlled growth of particles in a glass matrix – the so called glass crystallization method[9]. For this method hematite is dissolved in a borate glass and heated above the melting point. Then the melt is cooled down rapidly between two water cooled rollers. The resulting flakes show an amorphous structure. The first annealing step of the flakes leads to the nucleation of magnetite cores and during the second step the particles grow without further nucleation. After dissolution of the glass matrix by means of acetic acid the obtained particles can be coated and transferred to a suspension. The resulting particles show a diameter of about 14 nm and a much narrower size distribution than the precipitated MNP.

A completely different method for the preparation of large single domain MNP is the laser evaporation method. For this a coarse hematite powder (µm size) is evaporated by means of a CO_2 laser. Due to the relatively steep temperature gradient outside of the evaporation zone a very fast condensation of particles from the gas phase takes place. The resulting particles are in the mean size range from 20 to 70 nm and show a relative small size distribution. Unfortunately, up to now only the preparation of dry powders is possible but by an in situ coating it could be possible to form a shell around the particles which enables the suspension of the MNPs. This preparation route is being carried out in collaboration with the group of Dr. Kurland from the University of Jena[10].

3. PARTICLE CHARACTERISATION

Typically the particles were characterized by X-ray diffraction (XRD). This investigation gives information about the phase composition of the particles as well as the mean crystallite size of the particles. Additionally TEM imaging is carried out to verify the results of XRD and to get information about the agglomeration behaviour of the MNP as well as the shape of the particles (Figure 1).

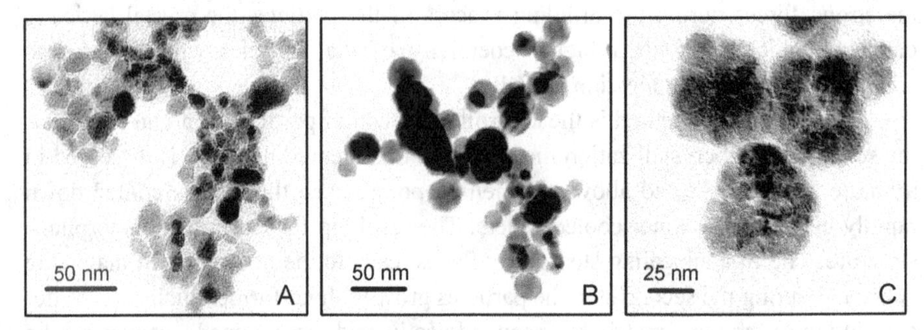

Fig. 1. Typical TEM images of particles prepared by glass crystallisation (A) and laser evaporation (B) as well as multi-core particles (C).

The magnetic properties are determined by vibrating sample magnetometry (VSM) measurements. For the application of the particles in MPI the most interesting properties are the saturation magnetization (M_s), the coercivity (H_c), and also especially the initial susceptibility (χ_0). All these parameters can be derived from the saturation loop of the particles.

In table 1 typical values of the above mentioned MNP properties for particles prepared by the described methods are shown. It is clearly seen that the standard wet precipitated particles show a very small coercivity but also a relatively small initial susceptibility which should result in weak signals in MPI.

An increase of the single domain core size leads to an unavoidable increase of the coercivity as established before[4]. But the particles with a larger coercivity than the standard particles do not show a higher χ_0 automatically. In general the χ_0 for superparamagnetic MNP is obtained from

$$\chi_0 = \mu_0 M_s^2 / 3kT$$

with the permeability μ_0, the Boltzmann constant k, and the Temperature T. The particles in table 1 show an M_s varying from 60 to 80 Am^2/kg which does not explain the differences in the χ_0. For particles showing a hysteresis χ_0 is not defined exactly. In the case of this article the coercivity was neglected and χ_0 is given by the slope of the initial magnetization curve.

Table 1: Typical values for the mean diameter (d), saturation magnetisation (M_s), coercivity (H_c), and the initial susceptibility (χ_0) of the prepared particles.

preparation method	d (XRD) [nm]	M_s [Am^2/kg]	H_c [kA/m]	χ_0 [10^{-3} m^3/kg]
precipitated, standard	12	66.7	1.0	1.44
precipitated, larger	28	80.1	7.5	1.58
cyclic	26	60.0	7.2	1.10
multi-core	60 (TEM)	69.3	1.8	2.46
milled	28	74.9	12.9	1.09
glass crystallization	14	63.0	1.0	1.15
laser evaporation	28	69.2	10.6	2.06

The MNP with the highest χ_0 of 2.06 and 2.46 10^{-3} m^3/kg show a comparable M_s and a coercivity of 10.6 and 1.8 kA/m, respectively. Because a strong coercivity requires a high gradient from the zero field to the saturation field as well as high amplitude of the alternating field the particles from the laser evaporation seems to be not so suitable for MPI. The most promising of our prepared particles are the multi-core MNP – they combine a high χ_0 with a relatively low coercivity.

4. PARTICLE FRACTIONATION

Because the task to prepare monosized particles was not satisfactorily solved till now we are working on another method to obtain particles with a narrow size distribution which is the size dependent fractionation of the existing particle ensembles.

An easy method based on centrifugal forces acting upon the MNP. In a few consecutive centrifugal runs the unwanted particles which are too large or too small can be removed by applying different acceleration forces to the particles. By using this method good results concerning the increase of the specific heating power of particles for magnetic hyperthermia were obtained[7].

More complicated is the fractionation of the particles in a magnetic quadrupol separator. A glass column is placed between permanent magnets in a manner that in the centre of the column there is a zero field which shows an increase of the field in direction to the column wall with a high magnetic field gradient. The magnetic force to the smaller particles is very weak and they move very slowly to the wall when passing the column. In contrast the force to the lager particles is much stronger and they move to the wall of the column. By this way size dependent separation can be achieved[11].

Up to now none of both methods was used to prepare fractions of different particle sizes from a broad size distributed ferrofluid for the investigation of the initial susceptibility. An influence of the particle size in the different fractions on its coercivity was shown before[7].

5. SUMMARY / DISCUSSION

In this article we show different ways to prepare large single domain nanoparticles. For our particles no direct correlation between mean particle size and initial susceptibility was found. This means, that the initial susceptibility is affected by a lot of different parameters beside the particle size, e.g. particle size distribution in the ensemble, the quality of the crystal lattice, or changes in the magnetic interactions between the single particles caused by the coating.

The saturation magnetization of the prepared particles varies from 60 to 80 Am^2/kg. The first reason for this is the different phase composition of the resulting particles depending on the preparation method. In general, the particles consist of a mix of magnetite and maghemite or a solid solution of both phases[8]. Additionally, the saturation magnetization is affected by the particle size due to the surface-to-volume ratio. The stronger oxidation of smaller particles to maghemite because of the relatively large surface leads to a lower saturation magnetisation[8].

Up to now none of our particles was tested for the suitability for MPI. As a result of this comparison the multi-core MNP seems to be interesting for MPI. Although or even because these particles are not single domain they show a high initial susceptibility but only a relatively small coercivity.

ACKNOWLEDGMENTS

The authors thank the groups of H.-D. Kurland (University of Jena) and J. Töpfer (University of Applied Sciences Jena) for the cooperation in the field of nanoparticle preparation. The work was founded by the "Deutsche Forschungsgemeinschaft" (ZE825/1-1).

REFERENCES

1 Gleich B, Weizenecker J. Tomographic imaging using the nonlinear response of magnetic particles. *nature* 2005; **435:** 1214–1217.

2 Biederer S, Knopp T, Sattel TF, Lüdtke-Buzug K, Gleich B, Weizenecker J, Borgert J, Buzug TM. Magnetization response spectroscopy of

superparamagnetic nanoparticles for magnetic particle imaging. *J Phys D: Appl Phys* 2009; **42:** 205007.

3 Khallafalla SE, Reimers GW. Preparation of dilution-stable aqueous magnetic fluids. IEEE Trans. Magn 1980; **16/2:** 178–183.

4 Dutz S, Hergt R, Mürbe J, Müller R, Zeisberger M, Andrä W, Töpfer J, Bellemann ME. Hysteresis losses of magnetic nanoparticle powders in the single domain size range. *J Magn Magn Mater* 2007; **308/2:** 305–312.

5 Müller R, Hergt R, Dutz S, Zeisberger M, Gawalek W. Nanocrystalline iron oxide and Ba ferrite particles in the superparamagnetism–ferromagnetism transition range with ferrofluid applications. *J Phys: Condens Matter* 2006; **18/38:** 2527–2542.

6 Dutz S, Andrä W, Hergt R, Müller R, Oestreich Ch, Schmidt Ch, Töpfer J, Zeisberger M, Bellemann ME. Influence of dextran coating on the magnetic behaviour of iron oxide nanoparticles. *J Magn Magn Mater* 2007; **311/1:** 51–54.

7 Dutz S, Clement JH, Eberbeck D, Gelbrich Th, Hergt R, Müller R, Wotschadlo J, Zeisberger M. Ferrofluids of magnetic multicore nanoparticles for biomedical applications. *J Magn Magn Mater* 2009; **321/10:** 1501–1504.

8 Dutz S. *Nanopartikel in der Medizin.* Hamburg: Verlag Dr. Kovač, 2008.

9 Müller R, Steinmetz H, Hiergeist R, Gawalek W. Magnetic particles for medical applications by glass crystallisation. *J Magn Magn Mater* 2004; **272-276, Part 2:** 1539–1541.

10 Kurland HD, Grabow J, Staupendahl G, Andrä W, Dutz S, Bellemann ME. Magnetic iron oxide nanopowders produced by CO_2 laser evaporation. *J Magn Magn Mater* 2007; **311/1:** 73–77.

11 Zeisberger M, Dutz S, Lehnert J, Müller R. Measurement of the distribution parameters of size and magnetic properties of magnetic nanoparticles for medical applications. *J Phys: Conf Ser* 2009; **149:** 012115.

SUPERPARAMAGNETIC IRON OXIDE NANOPARTICLES FOR MAGNETIC PARTICLE IMAGING

KERSTIN LÜDTKE-BUZUG

Institute of Medical Engineering, University of Lübeck, Lübeck, Germany
Email: luedtke-buzug@imt.uni-luebeck.de

SVEN BIEDERER, MARLITT ERBE, TOBIAS KNOPP, TIMO F. SATTEL, THORSTEN M. BUZUG

Institute of Medical Engineering, University of Lübeck, Lübeck, Germany
Email: buzug@imt.uni-luebeck.de

In the last few years, nanomaterials have emerged with interesting properties for new applications in nearly all areas of life. Particularly, SPIONs, i.e. nanosized superparamagnetic particles based on iron oxide, became more and more interesting in medicine. For instance, SPIONs have successfully been used in cancer therapy and for contrast enhancement in magnetic resonance imaging (MRI). Recently, SPIONs have shown viability as tracer in magnetic particle imaging (MPI), a method for visualization of the spatial distribution of iron oxide nanoparticles. In this paper, a simple synthesis strategy for SPIONs is presented. It has been shown that the image quality of MPI is highly dependent on the particle core diameter. Therefore, the particles must be optimized to improve imaging quality. It is explained how the raw synthesized particles are subjected to a separation and purification chain. Finally, the results of the separation efforts are validated by spectral analysis.

1. INTRODUCTION

During the last years, nanoparticles have been advanced to one of the most versatile materials.[1-3] Hence, nanoparticles are in the focus of many research activities due to their rather attractive properties, which may have potential use in fields like biomedicine[4], MRI[5] or even in environmental rehabilitation.[6] Especially in medicine, these particles are in the center stage of research for novel carrier agents that may transport therapeutic substances[7]. In this paper, nanoparticles are described that may act as tracer material for imaging purposes.[8] Particularly, magnetic nanoparticles play a key role in MRI, where they are used as contrast media leading to improved diagnostics in a broad spectrum of applications ranging from liver diagnostics (e.g. detection of malignant liver lesions[9]) to bone marrow imaging (differentiating metastasis and osteomyelitis[10]).

A well established nanoparticle-based contrast agent in MRI is Resovist™ (Bayer Schering Pharma).[11] This agent falls into the category of SPIONs, i.e. superparamagnetic iron oxide nanoparticles. It consists of a magnetite (Fe_3O_4) core coated with carboxydextran, which prevents the particles from agglomeration. Due to structure and size of these particles, Resovist™ is a reticuloendothelial system (RES) specific MRI contrast media, originally used for imaging of liver lesions since the early 1990s.[12]

Recently, Resovist™ has been used to demonstrate the feasibility of magnetic particle imaging (MPI).[13-15] MPI is a new imaging modality, which is directly based on the nonlinearity of the magnetization curve of the respective nanoparticles. However, Resovist™ does not meet all expectations for MPI and, unfortunately, it has been withdrawn by Bayer Schering Pharma in the end of 2008. In this paper, a simple synthesis and separation process design is presented for producing suitable tracer particles for MPI. The particles are characterized by their diameter distribution.

2. DEXTRAN-COATED IRON OXIDE NANOPARTICLES

2.1. Synthesis

For synthesis of iron oxide nanoparticles, different methods can be used. Very common procedures of SPION preparation work with micro-emulsions, sol-gels, thermal decomposition, or gas deposition.[16,17] The strategy proposed here consists of the classical co-precipitation of iron oxide in an alkaline solution

$$2Fe^{3+} + Fe^{2+} + 8OH^- \xrightarrow[\text{temperature}]{\text{at room}} Fe(OH)_2 + 2Fe(OH)_3$$

$$Fe(OH)_2 + 2Fe(OH)_3 \xrightarrow[\text{for 30-60 minutes}]{\text{heating (~70 °C)}} Fe_3O_4 + 4H_2O$$

in presence of dextran under accurately defined conditions. The molecular weight of dextran used for the particles analyzed here is 70 kDa. However, even under defined conditions[18], a narrow mono-modal particle size distribution requires a consecutive chain of separation and purification steps. Mono-dispersed particles are a crucial prerequisite to improve the sensitivity for MPI.[13]

2.2. Coating

Dextran, a polysaccharide based on glucose molecules, can be composed of chains of varying lengths (from 10 to 150 kDa). The main chain consists of α-1,6 glycosidic linkages between glucose molecules, while branches begin from α-1,4 linkages and, in some cases, α-1,2 and α-1,3 linkages as well (see Fig. 1).

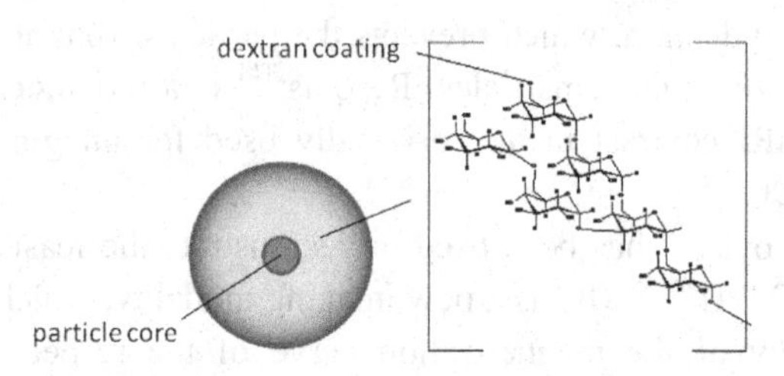

Fig. 1. Structure of dextran, build on α-1,6 glycosidic linked glucose molecules and α-1,3 linkages.

Dextran can be synthesized from sucrose by lactic-acid bacteria. Over the past decades, the clinical use of dextran shows evidence of quality and safety. The key advantages of dextran as coating material are that it is water soluble, biocompatible and biodegradable. In addition to these positive biochemical characteristics, dextran has proven stability for a period of several years. Most of the safety studies have been carried out with parenterally administered dextran solutions. However, dextran may be administered orally as well. It is well tolerated and shows a reductive effect on blood viscosity or acts as a volume expander in anemia.[19,20] In general, after many years of observation, it can be concluded that dextran shows excellent biocompatibility.

2.3. Separation

In simulations, it has been shown that SPIONs of 30 nm in iron-core diameter are expected to perform optimal in MPI.[13] Unfortunately, the dark-brown magnetic fluid, obtained from the synthesis described above, consists of a poly-disperse particle size distribution. Therefore, efforts are necessary to separate the undesired particles of larger and smaller diameter.

After cooling the fluid to room temperature, the solution is treated with a permanent magnet over night to remove large particles. Then, to isolate the medium sized particles, the solution is centrifuged. The next step is to dialyze the solution of the particles. To get an acceptable concentration of iron, in a final step, the fluid has to be centrifuged in tubes with a special filter system. The resultant particles exhibit a hydrodynamic diameter in the range between 80 nm and 90 nm as measured with a photon cross-correlation spectrometer.[21]

3. PARTICLE CHARACTERIZATION

Today, different methods are used to obtain an estimate of the mean particle core diameter. Typically, transmission electron microscope (TEM) images are analyzed or relaxation experiments are carried out. However, image analysis of TEM leads to poor statistics and relaxation is a rather indirect method to obtain an estimate of the paramagnetic core diameter, d_c.

To characterize the nanoparticle size distribution, in this paper, two spectral methods are compared. The first spectrometer is based on photon-correlation spectroscopy (PCS) and photon cross-correlation spectroscopy (PCCS). PCCS allows the determination of the hydrodynamic particle size and the stability of the suspension.[21] Both parameters are of particular interest for medical imaging. The second particle spectrometer, a magnetic particle spectrometer (MPS), is directly based on the MPI principle.[13] The decay of the harmonics in the nonlinear magnetization response mentioned above can be used to identify the iron-core size.

3.1. Photon Cross-Correlation Spectroscopy (PCCS)

Dynamic light scattering can be used for spectroscopy of a particle size distribution. Spectrometers that are commercially available (Nanophox, Sympatec, Clausthal-Zellerfeld, Germany) are either based on photon-correlation spectroscopy (PCS) or photon cross-correlation spectroscopy (PCCS).

For the results presented here, PCCS is used. PCCS allows for simultaneous measurement of particle size distribution and stability in the range of $d_h = 1$ nm to some micrometers in suspensions, where d_h is the hydrodynamic diameter.

3.2. Magnetic Particle Spectroscopy (MPS)

Magnetic particle spectroscopy (MPS) can be understood as measurement of the magnetization response, $M(t)$, when applying a sinusoidally oscillating magnetic field, $H(t)$. The dynamics can be modeled by Langevin's theory of paramagnetism,

$$M(t) = m_s c\left(\coth\left[\frac{m_s\mu_0 H(t)}{k_B T}\right] - \frac{k_B T}{m_s\mu_0 H(t)}\right)$$

where μ_0 is the permeability of vacuum, k_B the *Boltzmann* constant, T the temperature in Kelvin and, c the particle concentration. The magnetic moment at saturation, m_s, of the particles is given by $m_s = 1/6\pi d_c^3 M_s$, with M_s being the saturation magnetization, i.e. 0.6 T/μ_0 for magnetite. Biederer et al.[22] have shown that an estimate of the iron-core diameter d_c, named apparent core diameter, can be obtained by solving an inverse problem based on the measured decay of the harmonics.

4. RESULTS AND DISCUSSION

The tracer material synthesized with the method described in this paper shows excellent results in PCCS and MPS. Actually, it is competitive to Resovist, a carboxy-dextran coated SPION, with respect to particle size and magnetization response.

With the proposed technique to separate dextran-coated iron-oxide nanoparticles, an improvement in standard deviation of the particles can be obtained. The mean and the variation of the particle's hydrodynamic diameter is concluded from measurements of independent water-based suspensions. The particles show sufficient uniformity.

In PCCS measurements, a variation of the mean hydrodynamic diameter was found from d_h = 83 nm to 86 nm. Recently, it has been published that different – arbitrarily chosen – lots of Resovist™, show a variation of the mean hydrodynamic diameter from 56 nm to 86 nm.[18,23] For the dextran-coated particles, the estimated apparent mean core diameter was d_c = 21.13 nm with a standard deviation of 1.93 nm. The standard deviation depends highly on the parameters of the separation and purification strategy. For different lots of Resovist™, the estimated particle core diameter was d_c = 13.57 nm with a standard deviation of 3.69 nm.

As a general conclusion, it can be stated that the synthesized dextran-coated SPIONs do not meet the ideal parameters for MPI. However, with respect to the apparent iron-core diameter, the SPIONs synthesized here are superior to the commercially available carboxy-dextran nanoparticles.

ACKNOWLEDGMENTS

Parts of this work have been supported by the Innovation Foundation Schleswig-Holstein (Grant Number 2007-60).

REFERENCES

1 Paschen H, Coenen C, Fleischer T, Grünwald R, Oertel D, Revermann C, *Nanotechnologie – Forschung, Entwicklung, Anwendung*. Springer-Verlag, Berlin, Heidelberg, New York 2004.

2 Leyendecker S, *Nanomaterialien in Architektur*, Innenarchitektur und Design. Birkhäuser, Basel 2008.
3 Bönnemann H, Brijour W, Brinkmann R. *Angew. Chemie* 1991; **103**(10): 1344-1346.
4 Gupta AK, Gupta M Synthesis and surface engineering of iron oxide nanoparticles for biomedical applications. *Biomaterials* 2005; **26** (18): 3995–4021.
5 Mornet S, Vasseur S, Grasset F, Verveka P, Goglio G, Demourgues A, Portier J, Pollert E, Duguet E, *Prog. Solid State Chem.* 2006; **34**: 237.
6 Elliott DW, Zhang WX, *Environ. Sci. Technol.* 2001; **35:** 4922.
7 Gulyaev AE et al. Significant transport of doxorubicin into brain with polysorbate 80-coated nanoparticles. *Pharm. Res.* 1999; 16(10): 1564-1569.
8 Lanza GM, Lamerichs R, Caruthers S, Wickline AS. Molekulare Bildgebung in der MRT mit paramagnetischen Nanopartikeln. *MEDICAMUNDI* 2004; 6:11-17.
9 Savranoglu P, Obuz F, Karasu S, Coker A, Secil M, Sagol O, Igci E, Dicle O, and Astarcioglu I, The role of SPIO-enhanced MRI in the detection of malignant liver lesions, *Clinical Imaging*, 30(6), 2006, pp. 377-381.
10 Fukuda Y, Ando K, Ishikura R, Kotoura N, Tsuda N, Kato N, Yoshiya S, and Nakao N, Superparamagnetic Iron Oxide (SPIO) MRI Contrast Agent for Bone Marrow Imaging: Differentiating Bone Metastasis and Osteomyelitis, *Magn. Resn. Med. Sci.*, 5(4), 2006, pp. 191-196.
11 Reimer P et al., Neue MR-Kontrastmittel in der Leberdiagnostik. Erste klinische Ergebnisse mit hepatobiliärem Eovist (Gadolinium-EOB-DTPA) und RES-spezifischem Resovist. *Der Radiologe* 1996; **36**(2):124-133.
12 Hamm B, Reichel M, Vogl T, Taupitz M, Wolf K J, Superparamagnetische Eisenpartikel. Klinische Ergebnisse in der MR-Diagnostik von Lebermetastasen. *Fortschr Röntgenstr* 1994; **160**: 52-58.
13 Gleich B, Weizenecker J, Tomographic imaging using the nonlinear response of magnetic particles. *Nature* 2005; **435**: 1214-1217.
14 Knopp T, Biederer S, Sattel T, Weizenecker J, Gleich B, Borgert J, Buzug T M, Trajectory Analysis for Magnetic Particle Imaging. *Physics in Medicine and Biology* 2009, **56**(2): 385-397.
15 Sattel T, Knopp T, Biederer S, Gleich B, Weizenecker J, Borgert J, Buzug T M, Single-Sided Device for Magnetic Particle Imaging. *Journal of Physics D: Applied Physics* 2009; **42**(2): 1-5.
16 Demirer M, Controlled synthesis of superparamagnetic iron oxide nanoparticles in the presence of poly(acrylic acid). Master thesis 2006, Koc University.

17 Gupta A K, Gupta A, Synthesis and surface engineering or iron oxide nanoparticles for biomedical applications. *Biomaterials* 2005 26:3995-4021.

18 Lüdtke-Buzug K, Biederer S, Sattel T, Knopp T, Buzug T M, Preparation and Characterization of Dextran-Covered Fe_3O_4 Nanoparticles for Magnetic Particle Imaging. Proc. 4th European Congress for Medical and Biomedical Engineering, Springer IFMBE Series 2008, **22**: 2343-2346.

19 Lewis SL, Virtual clinical excursion for medical-surgical nursing, 2008.

20 Scheel v J, Laubenthal H, Meßmer K, Prevention of Dextran-induced Anaphylactic Reactions in the Treatment of ENT Disesases, *European Archieves of Oto-Rhino-Laryngology*, 1982, Vol. 235, No.2-3, 644-646.

21 Witt W, Aberle L, Geers H, Measurement of particle size and stability of nanoparticels in opaque suspensions and emulsions with photon cross correlation spectroscopy. *Particulate Systems Analysis* 2003 Harrogate, UK.

22 Biederer S, Knopp T, Sattel T F, Lüdtke-Buzug K, Gleich B, Weizenecker J, Borgert J, Buzug T M: Magnetization Response Spectroscopy of Superparamagnetic Nanoparticles for Magnetic Particle Imaging, *Journal of Physics D: Applied Physics*, 2009, **42(20)**: 1-7.

23 Lüdtke-Buzug K, Biederer S, Sattel T, Knopp T, Buzug T M, Particle-Size Distribution of Dextran- and Carboxydextran-Coated Superparamagnetic Nanoparticles for Magnetic Particle Imaging *World Congress on Medical Physics and Biomedical Engineering, Springer IFMBE Series*, 2009, **25/VIII**: 226-229.

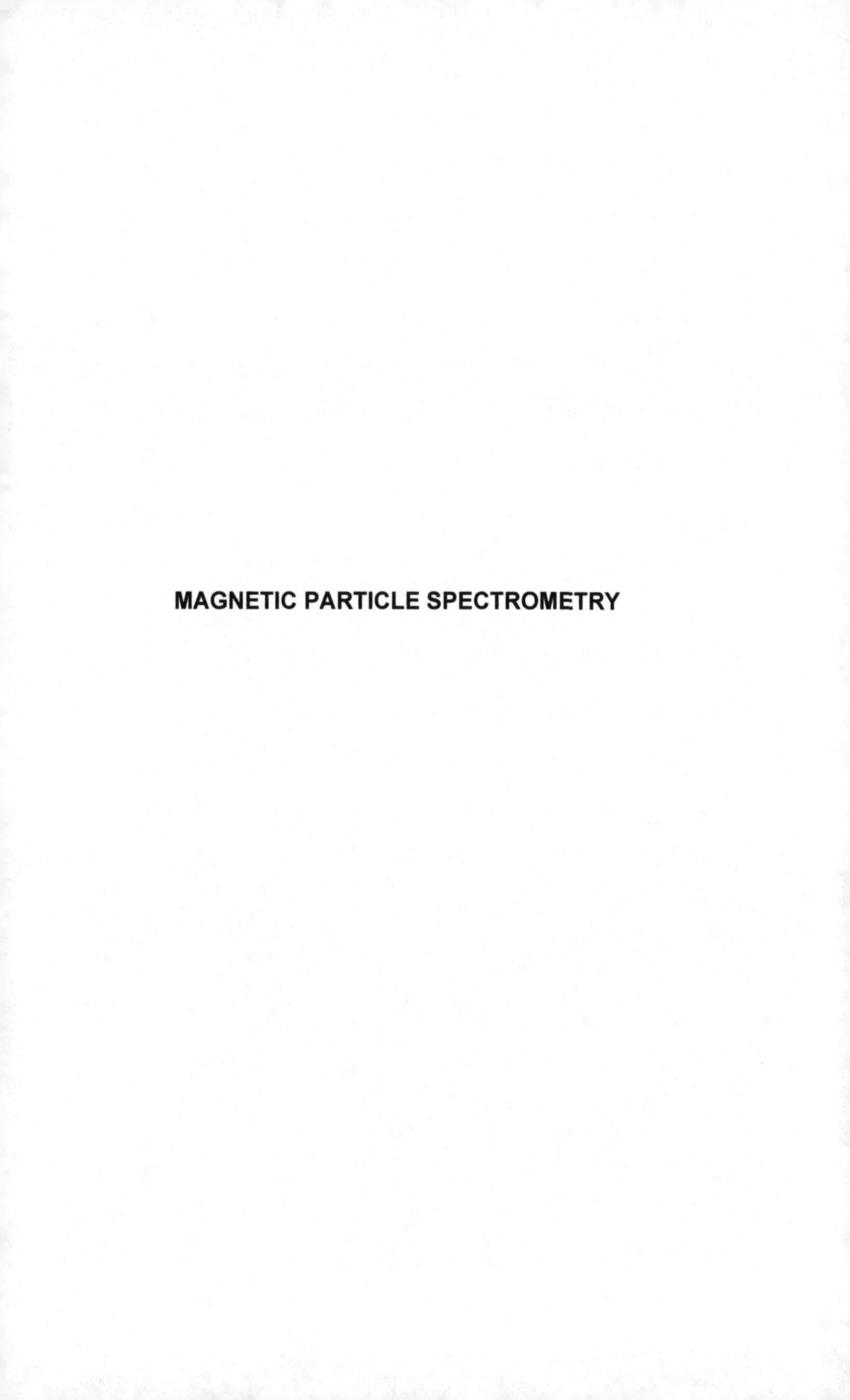

MAGNETIC PARTICLE SPECTROMETRY

SIZE-OPTIMIZED MAGNETITE NANOPARTICLES FOR MAGNETIC PARTICLE IMAGING

R. MATTHEW FERGUSON

Materials Science & Engineering Dept., University of Washington, Box 352120
Seattle, WA, 98195-2120, USA

AMIT P. KHANDHAR

Materials Science & Engineering Dept., University of Washington, Box 352120
Seattle, WA, 98195-2120, USA

KEVIN R. MINARD

Biological Monitoring & Modeling, Pacific Northwest National Labs
902 Battelle Blvd, P.O. Box 999; MSIN P7-58 Richland, WA 99352, USA
Email: kevin.minard@pnl.gov

KANNAN M. KRISHNAN

Materials Science & Engineering Dept., University of Washington, Box 352120
Seattle, WA, 98195-2120, USA
Email: kannanmk@u.washington.edu

We present experimental results to demonstrate that there is an optimum size for magnetite nanoparticles that are used to generate MPI signal, where the signal is detected as the third harmonic of nanoparticle magnetization, M, for any driving field frequency, ν. Our experimental results, for an arbitrarily chosen ν = 250 kHz, agree with predictions for a nanoparticle magnetization model based on the Langevin theory of superparamagnetism.

1. INTRODUCTION

For MPI to successfully move beyond proof-of-principle experiments into the clinic or research laboratory, it is critical to develop efficient tracer materials. This is especially true for potential applications that depend on active targeting, where for the highest sensitivity, each unit of tracer must generate the maximum achievable MPI signal voltage. For the pioneering MPI scheme developed by Gleich et al.,[1] signal is generated by harmonics in superparamagnetic nanoparticle magnetization, and the critical metric is harmonic amplitude per unit mass of magnetic material.

After many recent advances in chemical synthesis techniques, it is possible to produce highly uniform magnetic nanocrystals with fine control of particle size and shape.[2] By carefully controlling size, we show that it is possible to engineer *biocompatible* magnetite nanoparticles with optimum physical dimensions that maximize MPI's mass sensitivity. This result is explained using the Langevin theory, is demonstrated experimentally, and provides a basis for synthesizing optimal materials with dramatically increased performance relative to commercial options.

2. METHODS

2.1. Magnetite Nanoparticle Synthesis

For this work, magnetite nanoparticles were synthesized by the pyrolysis of Iron (III) oleate in 1-Octadecene (technical grade, 90%, Aldrich). Iron (III) oleate synthesis was based on the method described by Jana, et al.[3] In a typical reaction to produce 15 nm magnetite nanoparticles, 12 mmol of oleic acid (technical grade, 90% Aldrich) was added to 0.5 mmol of the iron (III) oleate complex dissolved in 2.5 g of 1-Octadecene. After purging under argon for 30 minutes, the mixture was heated, also under argon atmosphere, and refluxed for 24 hours. Finally, the reaction mixture was cooled to room temperature and the nanoparticles were collected and washed in a 1:1 mixture of chloroform and methanol.

To prepare for MPI signal testing, each sample was transferred from the organic to water phase for biocompatibility using the amphiphyllic polymer poly(maleic anhydride-alt-1-octadecene) – poly(ethelene glycol) (PMAO-PEG), and dissolved in 1x Phosphate Buffered Saline (PBS) solution. General guidelines for determining iron oxide nanoparticle toxicity are well established,[4] and we have previously studied the toxicity of iron oxide nanoparticles made in our laboratory.[5] Following phase transfer, iron concentration was measured using an Inductively Coupled Plasma – Atomic Emission Spectrophotometer (Jarrel Ash 955). The iron concentration in synthesized samples generally ranged from 0.5 to 3.6 mgFe/mL. The median diameter and size distribution of each was measured by fitting magnetization vs. field data according to the Chantrell method.[6]

2.2. MPI Signal Testing

MPI signal performance was measured using a custom-built transceiver that was specially designed for detecting the 3rd harmonic of nanoparticle magnetization.

During its operation sample harmonics are excited using an air-cooled solenoid that is driven at 250 kHz using a commercial radio-frequency (RF) amplifier (Hotek Technologies, Model AG1017L). Harmonics are then detected using a smaller receiver coil and counter-windings that both reside coaxially inside. To narrow receiver bandwidth and provide optimal power transfer for harmonic detection, the receiver coil is tuned and matched to 50 Ω at 750 kHz. Induced harmonics are also amplified using ~ 24 dB of gain before detection with a commercial spectrum analyzer (Rohde & Schwarz, Model FSL303).

During testing, the transceiver transmitter coil was driven with 10 Watts of RF power to produce an excitation field of 10 $mT\mu_0^{-1}$. To assess measurement variability, MPI signal testing was performed in triplicate. For each triplicate, 3 small cuvettes were filled with 100 µl of sample at the measured concentration listed in Table 1. Sample cuvettes were then inserted into the transceiver coils.

2.3. Langevin Model of Nanoparticle Magnetization

In previous work, we developed a Langevin model of superparamagnetism to predict how efficiently a system of nanoparticles will respond to an ac field, generate harmonics, and therefore a MPI signal.[7] For a sample of nanoparticles, we model the time dependent magnetization M, as a function of median nanoparticle diameter d_0 and standard deviation σ:[8]

$$\frac{M(d_0,\sigma,t)}{M_s} = \int_0^\infty \left(\frac{1}{1+(\omega\tau)^2} + i\frac{(\omega\tau)^2}{1+(\omega\tau)^2} \right) \left(Coth\left[\alpha d^3 H(\omega,t)\right] - \frac{1}{\alpha d^3 H(\omega,t)} \right) g(d_0,\sigma,d) dd \quad (1)$$

where $H(\omega,t)$ is the RF driving field, which varies sinusoidally with amplitude H and angular frequency ω, $\alpha = \frac{\pi M_s \mu_0}{6k_b T}$, where M_s is the saturation magnetization of the nanoparticles (446 kA/m for magnetite), μ_0 is $4\pi \times 10^{-7} Hm^{-1}$, k_b is the Boltzmann constant, $1.38 \times 10^{-23} JK^{-1}$, and T is the temperature in Kelvin; τ is the effective relaxation time for the particle moment to reverse in an alternating magnetic field, $\tau = \tau_B \tau_N / (\tau_B + \tau_N)$, where τ_N is the Neel relaxation,

$$\tau_N = \frac{\sqrt{\pi}}{2} \tau_0 \frac{\exp[K\rho]}{K\rho^{1/2}}, \quad (2)$$

where K is the magnetocrystalline anisotropy constant, $\rho = \frac{\pi d^3}{6k_b T}$ and τ_0 is taken to be 10^{-10} s, and τ_B is the Brownian relaxation, $\tau_B = \frac{3V\eta}{k_b T}$, where V is the hydrodynamic volume of the particle, and η is the viscosity of the suspending fluid

(0.89 mPa s for water). Finally, $g(d_0, \sigma, d)$ represents the distribution of diameters in the sample, and can be well-approximated[6] using a log-normal distribution function:

$$g(d_0,\sigma,d)=\frac{1}{\sigma d\sqrt{2\pi}}\exp\frac{-(\ln(d/d_0))^2}{2\sigma^2}, \tag{3}$$

where σ is the standard deviation of the distribution, and d_0 is the median diameter.

3. RESULTS & DISCUSSION

By carefully controlling the size of our particles, we were able to demonstrate that MPI signal varies dramatically with their diameter, *d*. This is illustrated in Figure 1 where measured signal per mg iron is seen to vary over nearly three orders of magnitude, with some particles exhibiting a 30 fold sensitivity increase over commercial counterparts with comparable iron concentration.

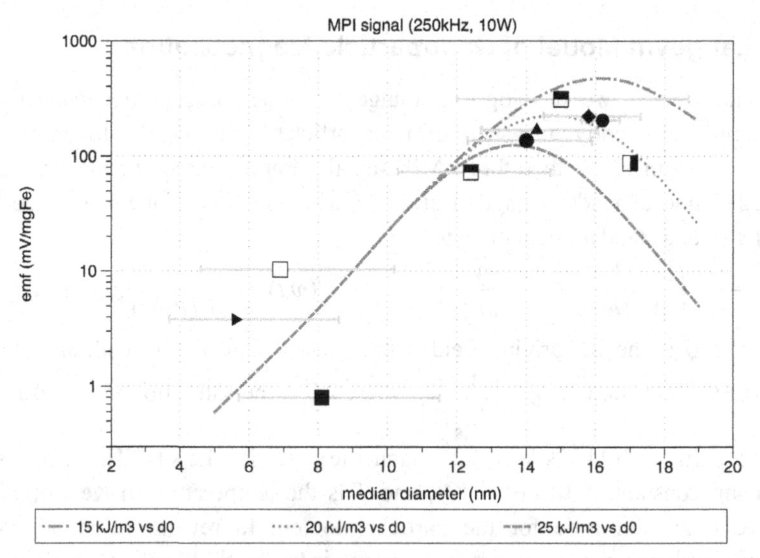

Figure 1: MPI signal testing results. Symbols represent nanoparticle samples (particle details are listed in table 1). The error bars in x are not uncertainty, but rather delineate the first standard deviation of the sample diameter distribution. The grey curves are simulated data for particles with the listed anisotropy constant (eq. 2), and a log-normal distribution with standard deviation 0.1.

Most striking is the observed peak in the harmonic signal vs diameter, indicating that there is an optimum nanoparticle size for MPI at 250 kHz. Strictly speaking, this optimal size depends on the drive frequency and the anisotropy constant *K* (eq. 2), and can be predicted for other frequencies using the Langevin model discussed in section 2.3. For 250 kHz MPI, the optimum particle diameter is

~15 nm. Detailed information about the nanoparticle samples shown in Figure 1 is provided in Table 1. Also included in Fig. 1, are three simulated curves, for Magnetite samples of increasing diameter, having anisotropy constants K of 15, 20, and 25 kJ/m^3, respectively, each with a log-normal size distribution with standard deviation, $\sigma = 0.1$.

Table 1. Details of Magnetite nanoparticle samples used in MPI signal testing.

Sample	MPI signal (mV/mgFe)	mgFe/ ml	D0 (nm)	σ
Feridex IV (Bayer)	10	2.21	6.9	0.40
mf090401	4	0.24	5.6	0.42
ak090309	<1	1.68	7.5	0.28
mf090806	72	0.68	12.4	0.18
mf090810p	136	1.56	14.0	0.12
mf090903p	168	2.72	14.3	0.17
mf090910p	310	1.10	15.0	0.22
mf090917p	221	3.64	15.8	0.09
mf090924p	204	3.12	16.3	0.07
mf091001p*	88	1.73	17.0	n/a

Maximum signal was produced by sample mf090910p in Table 1. The height and location of the peak in measured signal vs diameter (Fig 1) quantitatively match the predicted values for magnetite nanoparticles with an anisotropy constant K of~ 20 kJ/m^3. Measured values of K for magnetite typically range between 23-41 kJ/m^3,[9] while theory predicts 11 kJ/m^3.[10] The decrease in MPI signal for larger particles implies that, though the 10 $mT\mu_0^{-1}$ excitation field is sufficiently large to generate harmonics, it is not large enough to shorten the effective relaxation time τ, and instead relaxation is determined by particle size as discussed in section 2.3. In fact, shortening should only occur at higher applied fields, H_a, such that $H_a >> H_K$, where $H_K = 2K / M_s$ is the anisotropy field.[11] The signal voltage per mg iron curve has a 9% average uncertainty, due to errors in the iron concentration and MPI signal voltage measurements. Some deviation from simulated data beyond this uncertainty

* Size for sample MF091001p, which had an open loop at room temperature, was determined by TEM (FEI Tecnai G2 F20), and by the ratio of precursors relative to the other samples

is visible, but this is to be expected considering the size distribution for each sample differed from the value used for the simulated data ($\sigma = 0.1$ was chosen from within the range of measured values, and represents our assumption of what constitutes an achievable "narrow dispersion"). For the measured range of size distributions, we expect deviation of plus or minus a factor of 2 from the simulated data, based on theoretical projections using the described equations. Therefore, while our best sample (mf090910p) gives substantial improvement over commercial agents, its efficiency for MPI imaging at 250 kHz can be even further improved by narrowing its size distribution. We expect at least a factor of two improvement in efficiency by reducing σ from 0.22 to our targeted value of 0.1.

ACKNOWLEDGMENTS

This work was supported by NIH NHLBI RO1 HL073598, NIBIB R21 EB008192, and partial support for RMF from the University of Washington Center for Nanotechnology (CNT).

REFERENCES

1 Gleich B, Weizenecker J. Tomographic Imaging Using the Nonlinear Response of Magnetic Particles. *Nature* 2005; **435(7046):** 1214.

2 Park J, An K, Hwang Y, Park J, Noh HJ, Kim JY, Park J, Hwang N, Hyeon T. Ultra-Large-Scale Syntheses of Monodisperse Nanocrystals. *Nature materials* 2004; **3(12):** 891.; Yu W, Falkner J, Yavuz C, Colvin V. Synthesis of Monodisperse Iron Oxide Nanocrystals By Thermal Decomposition of Iron Carboxylate Salts. *Chemical Communications* 2004; 2306.; Puntes VF, Krishnan KM, Alivisatos AP. Colloidal Nanocrystal Shape and Size Control: The Case of Cobalt. *Science* 2001; **291(5511):** 2115.; Gonzales M, Krishnan K. Synthesis of Magnetoliposomes With Monodisperse Iron Oxide Nanocrystal Cores for Hyperthermia. *Journal of Magnetism and Magnetic Materials* 2005; **293:** 265.; Bao Y, Pakhomov A, Krishnan K. A General Approach to Synthesis of Nanoparticles With Controlled Morphologies and Magnetic Properties. *J. Appl. Phys. (USA)* 2005; **97(10):** 10.; Krishnan K, Pakhomov A, Bao Y, Blomqvist P, Chun Y, Gonzales M, Griffin K, Ji X, Roberts B. Nanomagnetism and Spin Electronics: Materials, Microstructure and Novel Properties. *Journal of Materials Science* 2006; **41:** 793.

3 Jana N, Chen Y, Peng X. Size- and Shape-Controlled Magnetic (Cr, Mn, Fe, Co, Ni) Oxide Nanocrystals Via a Simple and General Approach. *Chemistry of materials* 2004; **16(20):** 3931.

4 Soenen SJH, De Cuyper M. Assessing Cytotoxicity of (Iron Oxide-Based) Nanoparticles: An Overview of Different Methods Exemplified With Cationic Magnetoliposomes. *Contrast Media and Molecular Imaging* 2009; **4 (5):** 207.
5 Gonzales M, Mitsumori LM, Kushleika JV, Rosenfeld ME, Krishnan KM. "Synthesis and Toxicity of Monodisperse Iron Oxide Nanoparticles. *Contrast Media and Molecular Imaging* (in Press).
6 Chantrell R, Popplewell J, Charles S. Measurements of Particle Size Distribution Parameters in Ferrofluids. *IEEE Transactions on Magnetics* 1978; **Mag-14(5):** 975.
7 Ferguson R, Minard K, Krishnan K. Optimization of Nanoparticle Core Size for Magnetic Particle Imaging. *Journal of Magnetism and Magnetic Materials* 2009; **321:** 1548.
8 Chikazumi S *Physics of Magnetism.* New York: John Wiley & Sons, 1964.
9 Rosensweig. Heating Magnetic Fluid With Alternating Magnetic Field. *Journal of Magnetism and Magnetic Materials* 2002; **252:** 370.
10 Morrish AH *The Physical Principles of Magnetism.* New York: Wiley, 1965.
11 Shliomis MI. Magnetic Fluids. *Soviet Physics-Uspekhi* 1974; **17(2):** 153.

A SPECTROMETER TO MEASURE THE USABILITY OF NANOPARTICLES FOR MAGNETIC PARTICLE IMAGING

SVEN BIEDERER, TIMO F. SATTEL, TOBIAS KNOPP,
MARLITT ERBE, KERSTIN LÜDTKE-BUZUG

Institute of Medical Engineering, University of Lübeck,
Ratzeburger Allee 160, Lübeck, Schleswig-Holstein, 23538, Germany
Email: biederer@imt.uni-luebeck.de

FLORIAN M. VOGT, JÖRG BARKHAUSEN

Clinic for Radiology and Nuclearmedicine, University Hospital Schleswig Holstein,
Ratzeburger Allee 160, Lübeck, Schleswig-Holstein, 23538, Germany
Email: florian.vogt@uk-sh.de

THORSTEN M. BUZUG

Institute of Medical Engineering, University of Lübeck,
Ratzeburger Allee 160, Lübeck, Schleswig-Holstein, 23538, Germany
Email: buzug@imt.uni-luebeck.de

Magnetic Particle Imaging is an imaging modality for measuring the spatial distribution of superparamagnetic nanoparticles. Here, the imaging quality and resolution depends on the raised harmonics caused by the nanoparticles, when exposed to alternating magnetic fields. The more harmonics are measureable the better the imaging quality. In this contribution, a magnetic particle spectrometer is presented for measuring the originated harmonics. Based on these measurements, two different performance indicators are introduced to classify different nanoparticles for magnetic particle imaging.

1. INTRODUCTION

Magnetic Particle Imaging (MPI) is a new tomographic imaging technique for determining the spatial distribution of superparamagnetic iron oxide nanoparticles (SPIOs) [1]. MPI is capable of measuring 3D volumes in real-time[2,3]. The achievable image resolution and quality is strongly dependent on the iron core diameter of the SPIOs[4]. For the currently used SPIOs, only a fraction of about 3% contributes to the particle signal. By increasing this fraction, it is expected that the sensitivity of MPI can be increased up to a factor of 30. Thus, new nanoparticle synthesis processes for

MPI are of major interest[5,6]. During these processes, a tool for measuring the MPI performance of SPIOs is indispensable. Therefore, a Magnetic Particle Spectrometer (MPS) is presented for measuring the particle performance.

2. MATERIAL AND METHODS

The MPS is based on the same physical effect as exploited in MPI. It excites the SPIOs with a pure sinusoidal magnetic excitation field and simultaneously measures the particle magnetization. The frequency of the excitation field is set to 25 kHz, which is currently used in most MPI devices[1-3,7]. The sinusoidal waveform is generated with a standard digital-to-analog converter card (SMT8036, Sundance Multiprocessor Technology Ltd.). After amplifying the signal with a power amplifier (DCU2250-28, MT MedTech Engineering GmbH), it is band-pass filtered to suppress harmonics potentially contained in the signal. The solenoid transmit coil is matched by a capacity voltage divider to the impedance of the power amplifier. A feedback loop controls the current in the transmit coil. The nanoparticle magnetization is measured with a solenoid receive coil. The voltage in the receive coil is directly proportional to the time derivation of the particle magnetization. However, the transmit signal, which is several magnitudes higher than the particle signal, directly couples into the receive coil. To suppress this signal, a band-stop filter is added before the signal is amplified by a low noise amplifier. Finally, the signal is digitized at a sampling rate of 12.5 MHz by the same data acquisition card as used for generating the transmit signal. A schematic overview of the signal chain is given in Figure 1. The coil setup is sketched in Figure 2. After integration and Fourier transformation of the measured signal, the nanoparticle magnetization spectrum is obtained.

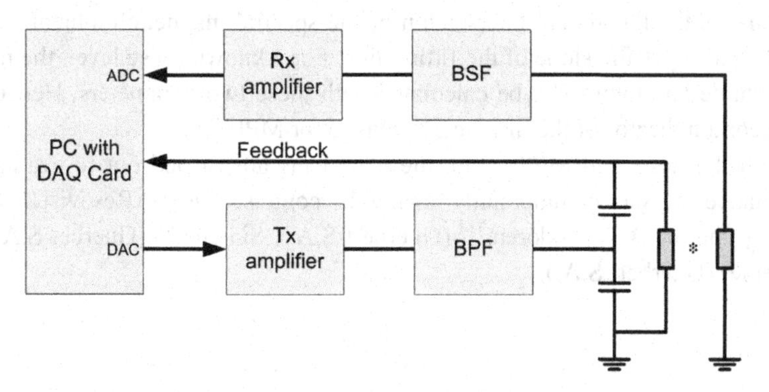

Fig. 1. Signal chain of the MPS.

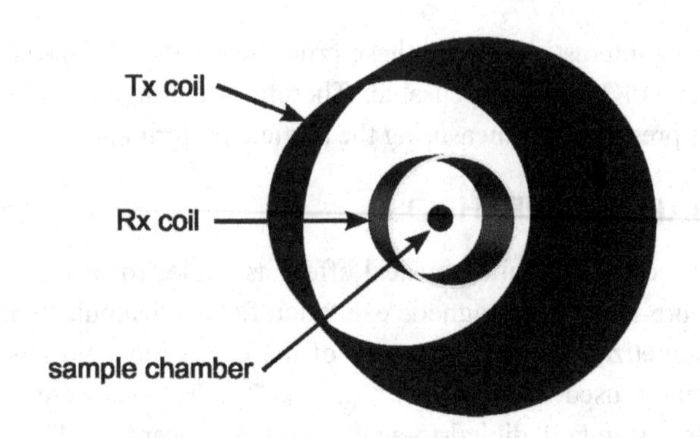

Fig. 2. Coil setup of the MPS.

In an MPI system, the sensitivity and, thus, the image quality depend on the magnitude of the received frequency components. Thus, a first measure of the SPIO performance is the total harmonic distortion (THD)

$$\mathrm{THD} = 20 \cdot \log_{10}\left(\frac{1}{m_{\mathrm{AC}}} \sqrt{\frac{1}{N-1} \sum_{n=2}^{N} \hat{m}(f_k)^2} \right), \tag{1}$$

where $\hat{m}(f_k)$ is the spectral magnetic moment of the kth harmonic, N is the number of harmonics above noise level, and m_{AC} is the magnetic moment of the applied magnetic field.

The image resolution in MPI mainly depends on the number of detectable harmonics. A linear regression can be carried out with the spectral magnetization $\hat{m}(f)$ in a semi-logarithmic scale by solving the minimization problem

$$\min_{\hat{m}_{\mathrm{o}}, \hat{m}_{\mathrm{s}}} \left\| 20 \cdot \log_{10}\left(\hat{m}_{\mathrm{o}} \cdot 10^{\hat{m}_{\mathrm{s}} \cdot f_k}\right) - 20 \cdot \log_{10}\left(\hat{m}(f_k)\right) \right\|_2, \tag{2}$$

where $\hat{m}_{\mathrm{o}}$ is the theoretical intersection of the spectral magnetic moment with the ordinate and $\hat{m}_{\mathrm{s}}$ is the slope of the fitting line. For a known noise level, the number of detectable harmonics can be calculated with these two parameters. Hence, they are a second indicator of the SPIO performance for MPI.

With the described MPS setup, measurements are carried out to evaluate the performance of the commercially available contrast agents Resovist® (Bayer Schering Pharma AG), Endorem™ (Guerbert S.A.), Sinerem® (Guerbet S.A.), and Lumirem® (Guerbert S.A.).

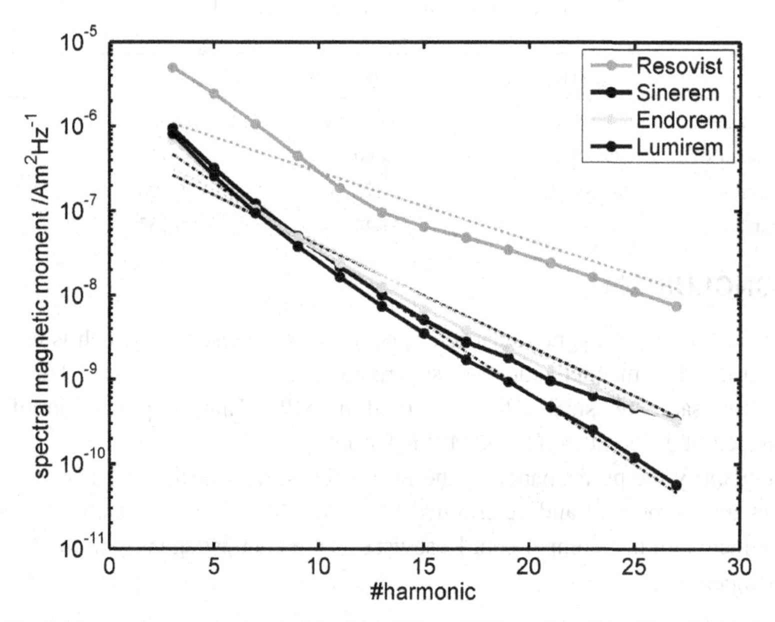

Fig. 3. Measured magnetization (solid) of the different SPIOs and the line of best fits (dashed).

3. RESULTS AND DISCUSSION

Measurements are performed with a magnetic excitation field strength amplitude of 20 mT/μ_0. The measured spectral magnetic moments are shown in Figure 3. For comparison, the magnetization of the four different contrast agents are normalized to an iron content of 1 mol (Fe)/l. Due to the symmetry of the excitation field, the even harmonics are negligible and only the odd harmonics are shown. In Figure 3, the calculated lines of best fit are illustrated as well.

In Table 1, the THD as well as $\hat{m}_0$ and $\hat{m}_s$ are given. Resovist® has the highest THD and $\hat{m}_0$, while it has the lowest slope $\hat{m}_s$. Thus, it is the SPIO with the best performance for MPI. Sinerem® and Endorem™ perform almost the same. Lumirem® has the steepest slope $\hat{m}_s$ and, therefore, the weakest performance. However, Lumirem® is an oral contrast agent, and, thus, it is provided in a concentration, which is about 100 times smaller than that of the other three SPIOs. Thus, for MPI experiments it is necessary to concentrate the nanoparticles.

Table 1. Performance values of the measured SPIOs.

	THD / dB	$\hat{m}_0$ / µAm^2	$\hat{m}_s$ / $dB_{Am^2Hz^{-1}}$
Resovist®	-76,5	1.89	-0.081
Sinerem®	-94.4	0.60	-0.119
Endorem™	-96.6	0.75	-0.126
Lumirem®	-95.3	1.46	-0.167

4. CONCLUSION

In this contribution, a magnetic particle spectrometer is presented, which is capable of measuring the magnetization of superparamagnetic nanoparticles. The MPS exploits the same physical effects as used in MPI. Thus, a prediction of the performance of different SPIOs for MPI is feasible.

To quantify the performance of the SPIOs for MPI, two different performance measures are introduced and determined for four different commercially available contrast agents. In this comparison, Resovist® is the contrast agent with the highest performance.

ACKNOWLEDGMENTS

We thank B. Gleich, J. Weizenecker, I. Schmale, J. Rahmer and J. Borgert for numerous fruitful discussions about MPS and Magnetic Particle Imaging in general.

This work was financially supported by the Innovation Foundation (ISH) of the state of Schleswig-Holstein, Germany (project id 2007-60). It is also part of the University Research Program "Imaging of Disease Processes", University of Luebeck.

REFERENCES

1 Gleich B, Weizenecker J. Tomographic imaging using the nonlinear response of magnetic particles. *Nature 2005*; **435(7046)**: 1214-1217.

2 Gleich B, Weizenecker J, Borgert J. Experimental results on fast 2D-encoded magnetic particle imaging. *Physics in Medicine and Biology 2008*; **53(6)**: N81-N84.

3 Weizenecker J, Gleich B, Rahmer J, Dahnke H, Borgert J. Three-dimensional real-time in vivo magnetic particle imaging. *Physics in Medicine and Biology 2009;* **54(5)**: L1-L10.

4 Weizenecker J, Borgert J, Gleich B. A simulation study on the resolution and sensitivity of magnetic particle imaging. *Physics in Medicine and Biology 2007*; **52**:6363-6374.
5 Lüdtke-Buzug K, Biederer S, Sattel TF, Knopp T, Buzug TM, Synthesis and Spectroscopic Analysis of Super-Paramagnetic Nanoparticles for Magnetic Particle Imaging, *Suppl Mol Imaging Biol 2009*; **11**: J054.
6 Lüdtke-Buzug K, Biederer S, Sattel TF, Knopp T, Buzug TM, Preparation and Characterization of Dextran-Covered Fe3O4 Nanoparticles for Magnetic Particle Imaging, *Proc. 4th European Congress for Medical and Biomedical Engineering, Springer IFMBE Series 2008*; **22**: 2343-2346.
7 Sattel TF, Knopp T, Biederer S, Gleich B, Weizenecker J, Borgert J, Buzug TM. Singlesided device for magnetic particle imaging. *Journal of Physics D: Applied Physics 2009*; **42(1)**: 1-5.

EVIDENCE OF AGGREGATES OF MAGNETIC NANOPARTICLES IN SUSPENSIONS WHICH DETERMINE THE MAGNETISATION BEHAVIOUR

D. EBERBECK, F. WIEKHORST, AND L. TRAHMS

Physikalisch-Technische Bundesanstalt, Berlin, Germany

Email: dietmar.eberbeck@ptb.de

Magnetization measurements on Resovist® MNP, the agent presently used for magnetic particle imaging (MPI), reveal that there are small single core MNP as well as clusters of MNP within the size range of 20-50 nm, in good agreement with electron microscopic data and light scattering results. The data of the integral measurement method of magnetorelaxometry also support the existence of (magnetic) aggregates. From the calculatated relative MPI signal strength we conclude that mainly these aggregates contribute to the MPI signal.

1. INTRODUCTION

Magnetic nanoparticles (MNP) find wide biomedical application, for example as a contrast agent for MRI[1], like Resovist®. Recently, Magnetic Particle Imaging (MPI) was introduced as a new quantitative method of imaging the spatial distribution of MNP[2]. In order to achieve a high sensitivity the magnetite particle cores should be monodispersed with core diameters around 40 nm and the cores should have a magnetic anisotropy as small as possible[2].

In the present study we demonstrate, how the particle size parameters and the magnetic anisotropy can be assessed using an integral quasistatic magnetic measurement method (magnetization measurement) and a fast dynamic method, magnetorelaxometry (MRX). The results will be compared with data obtained by Small Angle X-ray Scattering (SAXS) and Transmission Electron Microscopy (TEM). On the base of measurement magnetization curve we modeled the MPI signal strength.

2. MATERIALS AND METHODS

2.1. Sample

We investigated the MNP-suspension Resovist® (Bayer Health Care, Berlin. Germany). Resovist® comprise magnetite cores, where predominantly single cores are coated with carboxy methyl dextran.

2.2. Measurement methods

The device and the method for the measurement of the magnetic relaxation (MRX) were described in detail in[3]. In short, a sample of 140 µl volume (within a PE micro vial) is placed in the 10 mm bore of the magnetizing coil. A magnetic field of 1.5 kA/m is applied for 1 s to align the magnetic moments in the sample. After switching off the field within about 500 µs, the decay of the magnetization is measured by a low-Tc SQUID at a distance of 10 mm above the sample.

The relaxation curves of total magnetic moment of a fluid suspensions can be described by the cluster moment superposition model (CMSM)[4], where mainly the Brownian relaxation time $\tau_B \propto V_h$ determines the relaxation of the magnetization. The relaxation curve is described by the superposition of the contribution of the differently sized objects, MNP and optionally of clusters of MNPs with the hydrodynamic volume V_h. In order to get an integral information about the core size distribution and the magnetic anisotropy constant, we describe the relaxation of the magnetic moment of a suspension of immobilised MNP by the Moment Superposition Model[5], getting a distribution of effective energy barriers $E_A = K_{eff}V$.

The magnetization of the samples was measured by a commercial susceptometer MPMS (Quantum Design) as a function of applied magnetic field, *M*(*H*), at room temperature. We describe the *M*(*H*) curves of the fluid suspensions by a superposition of the Langevin functions, optionally with a bimodal distribution function

$$M(H) = \phi M_S (1-\beta_2) \int_{d_C} f_{C,1}(\mu_{C,1}, \sigma_{C,1}, d_C) L(d_C, M_S, T, H)\, \mathrm{d}d_C + \\ + \beta_2 \int_{d_C} f_{C,2}(\mu_{C,2}, \sigma_{C,2}, d_C) L(d_C, M_S, T, H)\, \mathrm{d}d_C \qquad (1)$$

where ϕ is the volume fraction of the cores (magnetite) and β_2 is the fraction of particles belonging to f_2. As mean values for the size we use in the following the diameter which is associated with the mean volume, denoted by index V, e.g. d_{CV}.

3. RESULTS AND DISCUSSION

3.1. Magnetization behaviour

First, we measured fluid suspensions of Resovist with various MNP concentrations (Fig. 1). Above about 100 mmol/l iron the relaxation curves do no longer scale with the concentration. This is also oberserved for the *M*(*H*) data.

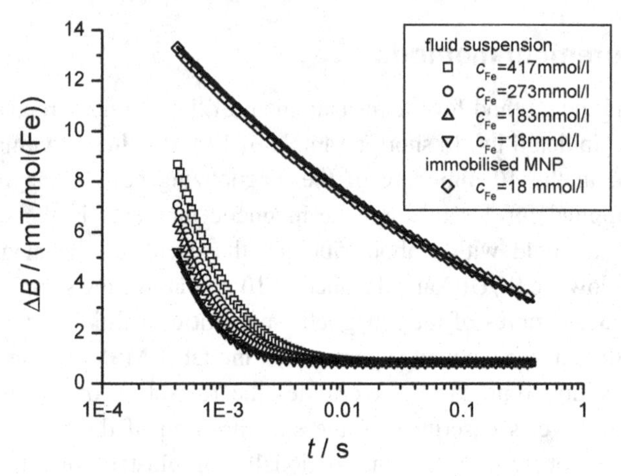

Figure 1. MRX curves for fluid suspensions of Resovist at different concentrations and for a diluted freeze dried sample (immobilised MNP). The best fit curves of the moment superposition model (1) and cluster moment superposition model, applied to the diluted samples with c_{Fe} = 18 mmol/l, are added

Analysing the *M*(*H*) data using eq. (1) with a monomodal distribution function (dotted line in figure 3a), i.e. β_2=0, leads to a broad size distribution with σ_C=0.82 (mean size is d_{CV}=3.7 nm) which did not fit to the value of 0.32 estimated from TEM pictures[6]. However, if we used the model with a bimodal distribution function according to eq. (1), the fit yielded one mean diameter of $d_{mV,1}$=(4.9±0.1) nm and a second one of $d_{mV,2}$=(23.2±0.3) nm as well as more reasonable distribution parameters (Table). The smaller deviation of the fit curve from the data (Fig. 2, bottom part) indicate that the bimodal model is better suited to explain the data than the monomodal distribution.

Next, we extracted information from measurements on freeze dried samples about the behaviour of magnetic moments within the particles, i.e. about the effective Néel relaxation. Figure 1 clearly shows that the freezing of the Brownian mobility leads to a strong slowing of the relaxation rate, i.e. to increasing relaxation times. Analyzing the MRX curve of the freeze dried sample with eq. (1) yields a mean volume corresponding to d_V=(16±2) nm, a size dispersion of 28% (Table 1) and an anisotropy constant of 5000 J/m³.

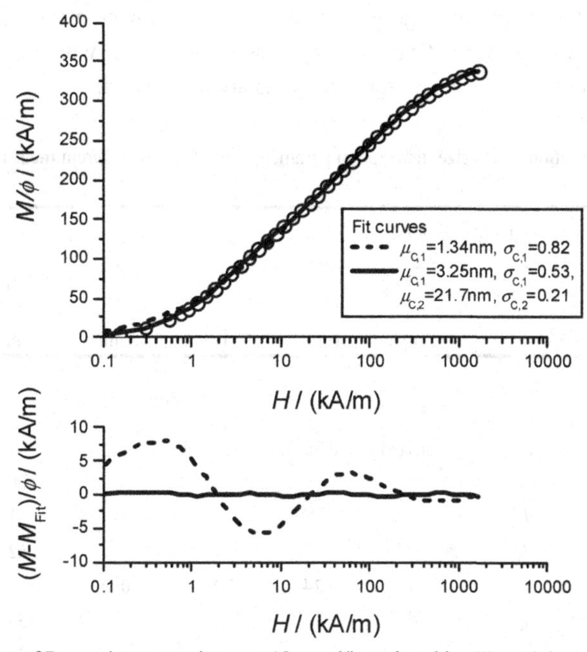

Figure 2. $M(H)$ curves of Resopvist suspension, c_{Fe}=18 mmol/l, analysed by (1) applying a monomodal size distribution (β_2=0) and a bimodal size distribution (see text).

3.2. Comparison of Size Distributions

The mean size of single particles, obtained from a TEM picture[6] and confirmed by Wang et al.[7], is about 5 nm (Table 1). SAXS being sensitive to scattering cross section inhomogeneities reveals the existence of larger units with a bimodal size distribution having its maxima at 10 nm and 20 nm, respectively. Obviously both peaks represent aggregates of the single core particles in agreement with earlier findings on similar MNP suspensions[8]. Note, that the scattering intensity of scatters scale with V^2, where V is the volume of the scatter, so that the small single MNP give only a relative small contribution to the signal. Within the $M(H)$ signal ($\propto V$), on the other hand, we found contributions of small magnetic moments associated with 5 nm single core MNP. The second fraction of 23 nm magnetic entities is obviously associated with clusters of MNPs. This value is near the value obtained from MRX data measured on immobilized MNP. Note, that the calculation of both effective diameters is based on a saturation magnetization of 358 kA/m and 330 kA/m, respectively which is an overestimate of the real magnetization of aggregates because its MNP core volume fraction is less than 1 and because the magnetic moments of the individual cores are not completely parallel oriented. Therefore, the magnetic aggregate size is rather a lower estimate for the particle cluster size. Hence, it is at present not possible to say to which kind of aggregates (Table 1) these magnetic structure elements are associated.

Table 1. Compilation of the size distribution parameters obtained by different measurement methods.

Method	Quantity	Size					Reference
		$\bar{d}_{1,V}$ (nm)	$\frac{\Delta d_1}{\bar{d}_{1,V}}$ (nm)	$\bar{d}_{2,V}$ (nm)	$\frac{\Delta d_2}{\bar{d}_{2,V}}$ (nm)	$\bar{d}_{3,V}$ (nm)	
TEM	d	5					7
TEM	d	4.7(3)	0.30(3)				this study
PCS	d_h					60	7
PCS	d_h					61	9
PCS+A4F	d_h			30		62	10
SAXS+A4F	d_s	10	0.24	20	0.16		10
MRX	d_C					53(3)	this study
MRX	d_C					54(2)	7
M(H)	d_m	4.9(1)	0.53(1)	23.2(3)	0.21(1)		this study
MRX	d_m			16(2)	0.28(2)		this study

d – single core diameter, d_h - hydrodynamic diameter, d_s – diameter of scatter elements (single core particles and clusters), d_m – effective diameter of magnetic domain, d_C - (hydrodynamic) diameter of clusters, A4F - flow field-flow fractionation.

The size of the largest aggregates observed by MRX on fluid suspensions (Brownian rotation) of 53 nm is in good agreement with the data of earlier PCS (photon correlation spectroscopy) measurements on other Resovist samples revealed mean hydrodynamic diameter of about 60 nm [4,7,9,10] which was in good agreement with the mean cluster size $d_{C,V}$ [4,9].

Finally, based on our $M(H)$ data we calculated the harmonic MPI response spectrum for a sinoidal excitation of 10 mT, normalized to the response spectrum of ideal MNP, producing a step like magnetisation curve with the same saturation value. We obtained a value of about 7%. On the other hand, for 10 nm MNP (which is a favorable estimate for the mean core size in Resovist), Gleich and Weizenecker[2] calculated a value of about 1%. In the light of our findings in this study we may attribute this discrepancy and, thus, the improved MPI-performance of Resovist to the presence of clusters.

In conclusion, we believe it is important to know the degree of aggregation in an MNP system, to better understand its magnetic behavior, and, in particular, its response to MPI.

ACKNOWLEDGMENTS

The research was supported by BMBF project Nanomagnetomedizin FKZ-13N9150. Furthermore, we thank P. Zirpel and K. Schwarz for their excellent technical support.

REFERENCES

1 Sosnovik DE, Nahrendorf M, Weissleder R. Magnetic nanoparticles for MR imaging: agents, techniques and cardiovascular applications. *Basic Res. Cardiol.* 2008, **103**: 122-30.
2 Gleich B, Weizenecker J. Tomographic imaging using the nonlinear response of magnetic particles. *Nature* 2005; **435**: 1214-1217.
3 Matz H, Drung D, Hartwig S, Groß H, Kötitz R, Müller W, Vass A, Weitschies W, Trahms L. A SQUID measurement system for immunoassay, *Appl. Supercond.* 1999; **6**: 577-583.
4 Eberbeck D, Bergemann C, Wiekhorst F, Glöckl G. Quantificationof aggregates of magnetic nanoparticles in different suspension media by magnetorelaxometry. *Magnetohydrodynamics* 2005 **41**: 305-316.
5 Eberbeck D, Hartwig S, Steinhoff U, Trahms L. Description of the magnetisation decay in ferrofluids with a narrow particle size distribution, *Magnetohydrodynamics* 2003; **39**: 77-83.
6 Ramírez Rios L. private information.
7 Wang Y, Ng YW, Chen Y, Shuter B, Yi J, Ding J, Wang SC, Feng SS. Formulation of Superparamagnetic Iron Oxides by Nanoparticles of Biodegradable Polymers for Magnetic Resonance Imaging. *Adv. Func. Mater.* 2008; **18**: 308-318.
8 Eberbeck D, Lange A, Hentschel M. Identification of aggregates of magnetic nanoparticles in ferrofluids at low concentrations. *J. Appl Cryst.* 2003; **36**: 1069-1074.

9 Eberbeck D, Wiekhorst F, Steinhoff U, Trahms L. Aggregation behaviour of magnetic nanoparticle suspensions investigated by magnetorelaxomery, *J. Phys.: Condens. matter* 2006; **18**: S2829-S2846.

10 Thünemann AF, Rolf S, Knappe P, Weidner S. In situ analysis of a bimodal size distribution of superparamagnetic nanoparticles. *Anal. Chem.* 2009; **81**: 296–301.

INVESTIGATION OF THE MAGNETIC PARTICLE IMAGING SIGNAL'S DEPENDENCY ON FERROFLUID CONCENTRATION

J.-P. GEHRCKE[1]
jgehrcke@physik.uni-wuerzburg.de

M.A. RÜCKERT[1,2]
mnruecke@physik.uni-wuerzburg.de

T. KAMPF[1]
tskampf@physik.uni-wuerzburg.de

W.H. KULLMANN[2]
Walter.Kullmann@fhws.de

P.M. JAKOB[1,3]
peja@physik.uni-wuerzburg.de

V.C. BEHR[1]
behr@physik.uni-wuerzburg.de

1: Department of Experimental Physics 5, University of Würzburg, Am Hubland, D - 97074 Würzburg, Germany

2: University of Applied Sciences Würzburg-Schweinfurt, Ignaz-Schön-Straße 11, D - 97421 Schweinfurt, Germany

3: Research Center Magnetic Resonance Bavaria (MRB) e.V., Am Hubland, D - 97074 Würzburg, Germany

Evaluation of the Magnetic Particle Imaging (MPI) signal in terms of LANGEVIN's single particle model of paramagnetism (SPM) is well-established. The SPM does not consider interparticle interactions and therefore is only valid for very low ferrofluid concentrations c, yielding a linear relation between single harmonics' amplitudes A and c. Motivated by MPI applications that potentially bear local particle densities significantly exceeding the SPM's scope of validity, the impact of increasing ferrofluid concentration on the MPI signal was investigated experimentally. The results exhibit a significant nonlinear relation between c and A and therefore show a strong deviation from the SPM, even for relatively small concentrations. Considering this fact can be crucial for image reconstruction in MPI.

1. INTRODUCTION

Magnetic Particle Imaging (MPI) is a new method to acquire the spatial concentration distribution $c(\boldsymbol{r})$ of superparamagnetic particles in biological systems at high spatial and temporal resolution[3].

Superparamagnetic particles are homogeneously magnetized (single-domain) ferromagnetic particles with diameters on the order of 10 nm. For medical applications, they are stabilized by a biocompatible coating (e.g. Dextran) and come as colloidal suspensions, so-called ferrofluids. The particle core material commonly is an iron oxide (such particles are called SPIOs), e.g. Magnetite (Fe_3O_4).

In MPI, the detection of SPIOs is based on a nonlinear effect: a fluid containing particles at concentration c is exposed to a harmonically oscillating magnetic field H. Due to the nonlinearity of the ferrofluid's magnetization curve $M(H, c)$, the response field is distorted. Its FOURIER spectrum shows higher harmonics of the fundamental frequency, which prove the existence of SPIOs. The magnetic moments in biological systems are several orders of magnitude lower than the SPIO ones. Hence, regarding excitation field strengths used in MPI (which are on the order of 10 mT), such biological systems respond linearly, ideally leading to no false-positive MPI background signal in medical applications.

$M(H, c)$ is the transfer function between input (irradiated field) and output (fluid magnetization). Therefore, it is the key quantity to calculate the MPI signal for a known configuration. For tomography, $c(\boldsymbol{r})$ has to be reconstructed from the MPI signal. Thus, the contact with reality of the theory describing the concentration dependency of the magnetization curve is essential for image reconstruction.

Until now, LANGEVIN's single particle model of paramagnetism is considered to understand the MPI signal generation and used for linear image reconstruction[5]. Particle interactions are neglected, which is valid only in the limit $c \to 0$.

In this work the impact of particle concentration on the spectroscopical MPI signal is investigated. It is shown that concentration effects introduce significant deviations from the single particle model, which is important to consider when particles e.g. agglomerate in cell vesicles, as is the case for SPIO labeled cells.

2. SINGLE PARTICLE MODEL

In this part the theoretical ferrofluid magnetization curve is discussed in terms of LANGEVIN's single particle model (SPM), which is well-established in MPI literature[5].

Assuming spherically shaped particles, the magnetic dipole moment m of a particle in dependence of its magnetic-core diameter x is given by

$$m(x) = \frac{\pi}{6} M_s x^3, \tag{1}$$

where M_s is the bulk saturation magnetization of the core material.

Polydispersity of particle diameters is neglected in this discussion. This does not change the scaling behavior of the magnetization with respect to particle concentration. For a ferrofluid containing monodisperse particles of diameter x at normed density $\rho(c) \in [0,1]^a$, the SPM yields the magnetization curve

$$M_{SPM}(H, \rho) = \rho M_s \, \mathcal{L}\left(\frac{\mu_0 m(x) H}{k_B T}\right). \tag{2}$$

T is the temperature, k_B is the BOLTZMANN constant. The LANGEVIN function

$$\mathcal{L}(a) = \coth(a) - \frac{1}{a} \tag{3}$$

is the classical limit of the BRIOULLIN function[b]. It describes a single paramagnetic particle's relative magnetization in an external field. Hence, the model does not include interparticle interactions. Within the SPM, the relative ferrofluid magnetization is independent of particle concentration, while the absolute magnetization is linear in ρ, as given by equation (2).

Describing highly concentrated magnetic fluids with the SPM dramatically underestimates the initial susceptibility and results in considerably decreased magnetization values for field strengths below saturation[4]. Thus, concentration effects most noticeably appear in the regime of weak fields, which is the regime of MPI drive fields. Here, the SPM predicts a too small curvature (second derivative) of $M(H, \rho)$, which is a gauge for nonlinearity of the magnetization curve and - with that - a gauge for the creation of higher harmonics in MPI.

As a result of this discussion, for measuring the amplitude A of single harmonics in the MPI signal with changing ferrofluid concentration c, a deviation from the SPM, manifesting itself in a nonlinear relation between the two quantities c and A, is expected. For increasing concentration, the real signal amplitudes must be higher than the ones predicted by the SPM, due to particle coupling effects.

---

[a] $\rho = 1$ (maximum density) is corresponding to the bulk core material.

[b] While the BRIOULLIN function depends on the total angular momentum quantum number J, the LANGEVIN function describes the classical limit $J \rightarrow \infty$, which is valid for systems consisting of a huge number of atoms with parallel spin-alignment, as is the case for superparamagnetic particles.

3. EXPERIMENT

The harmonics' amplitude A was analyzed for one ferrofluid at five different concentrations c, using a self-built MPI spectrometer.

The apparatus' harmonic drive circuit is based on a signal generator, two integrated audio-amplifier chips in parallel (LM3886T, National Semiconductor) and a solenoid as transmission coil (field homogeneity $\geq 99\,\%$; 340 windings; length 7 cm, inner diameter 3 cm, central field efficiency $6\,\mathrm{mT/A}$). During all experiments, the transmission coil's current was held constant (0.95 A RMS at 15.65 kHz). For signal detection, a coil made of litz wire (field homogeneity $\geq 96\,\%$; 800 windings; length 4 cm, inner diameter 5.5 mm) is used. An 11-pole Type I CHEBYSHEV high-pass filter effectively damps detected harmonics up to the cutoff frequency at 99.4 kHz. Filter characteristic and excitation frequency optimize the setup for detecting the 7th harmonic. Low-noise amplified (AD604, Analog Devices) time signal detection was done with a digital storage oscilloscope (TDS1001, Tektronix).

To obtain FOURIER spectra with high signal to noise ratio (SNR), all recorded time signals were averaged 128 times before evaluation. During measurement, the appropriate ferrofluid sample was centered within the receive coil, which itself was centered within the excitation coil. Systematic errors were minimized by evaluating the difference between the signal with and without a sample within the receive coil.

The samples used in the experiments were customized ferrofluids[1], consisting of Dextran coated Magnetite cores (mean diameter: 8.5 nm) with water as solvent. Their iron concentration $c\,[\mathrm{mol/l}]$ is known from production and measurement (ultraviolet-visible spectrophotometry). The error in c, which is estimated to $\pm 0.02\,\mathrm{mol/l}$, is the dominating error in the experiments.

4. RESULTS

The experimental result for the 7th harmonic of the MPI signal is presented in Fig 1. Additionally, the linear relation given by the first two data points is shown.

Systematic deviations of the data points from the linearity shown imply that the measured signal amplitudes are nonlinear dependent on c. Since the SPM is only correct in the limit $c \to 0$, the straight line extrapolated from the first two points overestimates the slope we would get from the SPM. Hence, the real deviation of the measured values from the SPM is larger than the difference visualized here.

Additionally, in results not shown, a strong nonlinear c-A-dependency was also verified for experimentally observable harmonics higher than the 7th.

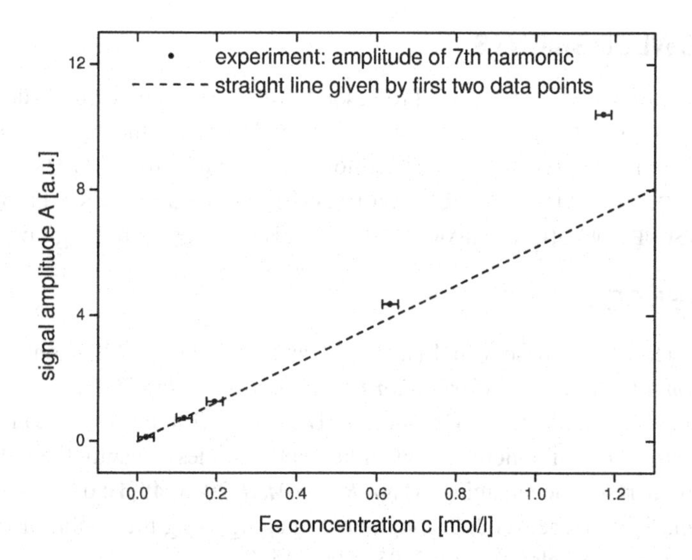

Fig. 1. Measured 7th harmonic amplitude A in arbitrary units (a.u.) of the MPI signal in dependence on iron concentration c. The straight line, which is the linearity given by the first two data points, has an overestimated slope in comparison with the slope of the linearity the SPM would predict. Due to high SNR and minimized systematic errors, the error in A is negligible compared to the error in c.

5. DISCUSSION AND CONCLUSION

It was shown that LANGEVIN's single particle model of paramagnetism is insufficient to describe the MPI signal of concentrated ferrofluids. It strongly underestimates the amplitudes of higher harmonics for increasing concentration. In biological applications of MPI local particle densities significantly exceeding SPM's scope of validity won't be uncommon. A prime example - leading to iron concentrations of $0.2 - 5$ mol/l - is the agglomeration of SPIOs in cells[2].

Regarding quantitative tomography, a problem for image reconstruction is identified: the spatial concentration distribution is the searched-for quantity and it is related to the MPI signal in a nonlinear way, while current image reconstruction schemes base on the SPM using linear methods[5].

In the future, other ferrofluid magnetization models, which are valid for wide concentration ranges, have to be considered to predict the MPI signal correctly. It has to be discussed, to what extent image reconstruction methods need to be adjusted to the nonlinear relation between MPI signal and ferrofluid concentration.

ACKNOWLEDGMENTS

We are grateful to the group of Professor SCHENK (University of Würzburg), in particular to REINER BERINGER and STEFFEN BLÖMER, for preparation of the analyzed ferrofluid samples. Furthermore, we thank the GERMAN FEDERAL MINISTRY OF EDUCATION AND RESEARCH (BMBF grant number FKZ 1745X08) and the DEUTSCHE FORSCHUNGSGEMEINSCHAFT (SFB 688) for supporting this work.

REFERENCES

1 Beringer R. Synthese von Eisenoxid-Nanopartikeln als MR-Kontrastmittel. *Diploma thesis, Julius-Maximilian-Universität Würzburg* 2007.

2 Billotey C, Wilhelm C, Devaud M, Bacri JC, Bittoun J, Gazeau F. Cell internalization of anionic maghemite nanoparticles: quantitative effect on magnetic resonance imaging. *Magn Reson Med.* 2003; **49(4)**: 646–54.

3 Gleich B, Weizenecker J. Tomographic imaging using the nonlinear response of magnetic particles. *Nature* 2005; **435**: 214–7.

4 Pshenichnikov AF. Equilibrium magnetization of concentrated ferrocolloids. *J. Magn. Magn. Mater.* 1994; **145**: 319–326.

5 Rahmer J, Weizenecker J, Gleich B, Borgert J. Signal encoding in magnetic particle imaging: properties of the system function. *BMC Medical Imaging* 2009; **9:4**.

MAGNETIZATION HARMONICS AS A REMOTE METHOD FOR MONITORING ENDOCYTOSIS OF NANOPARTICLES

ADAM M. RAUWERDINK

Thayer School of Engineering, Dartmouth College, 8000 Cummings Hall
Hanover, NH 03755, USA
Email: adam.rauwerdink@dartmouth.edu

ANDREW J. GIUSTINI

Thayer School of Engineering and Dartmouth Medical School
Hanover, NH 03755, USA

P.J. HOOPES

Department of Surgery, Dartmouth Medical School, Dartmouth-Hitchcock Medical Center
Lebanon, NH, 03756 USA

JOHN B. WEAVER

Department of Radiology, Dartmouth Medical School, Dartmouth-Hitchcock Medical Center
Lebanon, NH, 03756 USA
Email: john.b.weaver@hitchcock.org

Magnetic nanoparticles have shown much promise in the clinical and pharmaceutical fields. Their non-linear magnetization has been exploited to produce in vivo spatial images of particle distribution, but the particle environment can also affect this magnetization. Here we show that endocytosis of the particles causes pronounced changes to the magnetization's harmonic spectrum. Various concentration-independent metrics can be used to monitor these effects and gain insight into the mechanisms responsible. Incorporation of this technology into a magnetic particle imaging system should allow for monitoring of molecular level events in vivo.

1. INTRODUCTION

Magnetic nanoparticles (MNP) offer much potential for medical imaging, therapy, targeted drug delivery, monitoring binding kinetics, and a myriad of other pharmaceutical and clinical applications[1,2]. Many of these applications are impacted by cellular interactions with the MNPs whether through surface binding or uptake. The impact of MNP size and shape on cellular response has been studied with TEM and fluoroscopy techniques[3,4]. Following endocytosis of the MNPs into the cells, clusters of MNPs are seen within vesicles[4]. This clustering or aggregation of the MNPs causes significant changes to their dynamic magnetization, as has been demonstrated with magnetic relaxometry and AC susceptibility[5,6]. The dynamic magnetization of MNPs has been exploited for a number of other applications. McNaughton et al used the nonlinear magnetization of MNPs to monitor changes in viscosity or binding dynamics[7]. Binding of the MNPs to a larger substrate significantly influences the magnetization of the MNPs allowing for binding kinetics to be monitored[8]. These effects have been monitored *in vivo* using spatially resolved relaxometry but with limited resolution[9].

Magnetic particle imaging (MPI) offers a means of high resolution, high sensitivity mapping of the spatial location of MNPs *in vivo*[10,11]. Much of the work in the field of MPI to date has used MNP concentration as the primary source of image contrast. We have shown previously that concentration-independent MNP measurements can be acquired by using a ratio of the 5th and 3rd harmonic amplitudes. A theory-driven relationship between the effects of temperature and magnetic field amplitude on this ratio has been presented as a means of quantitatively mapping MNP temperature[12,13]. Dynamic effects like viscosity have also been shown to impact this ratio[14]. The magnetic moment of a MNP can align itself with an applied field via two methods, Neel and Brownian relaxation. Both of these relaxation methods are governed by time constants that impact the MNP's relaxation. The dynamic magnetization of MNPs has been approximated using the Debye theory[14,15] and more robust equations can be borrowed from the field of magnetohydrodynamics[16,17].

Multifunctional nanoparticles capable of incorporating guidance, imaging, and therapy components have been produced using a number of approaches[18,19]. Here we show how MPI should be capable of utilizing the motion of the MNPs themselves to monitor biological processes. Incorporation of such technology into MPI systems should significantly broaden the scope of its applications. Using a cancer cell line, we monitor endocytosis of MNPs *in vitro* using harmonic phase and a ratio of harmonic magnitudes. We compare endocytosis's impact on these various metrics to the effects of viscosity and aggregation.

2. METHODS AND MATERIALS

Iron oxide MNPs (MicroMod GmbH, Germany) with a biocompatible dextran coating were used in all experiments. The hydrodynamic size distribution of the

MNPs was measured with a Malvern ZetaSizer Nano ZS. The mean hydrodynamic diameter was found to be 122 nm with a polydispersity index of 0.125. The magnetic core of these particles consists of multiple crystals in the 15-20 nm range. The lectin Concanavalin-A (Sigma Aldrich, L7647), which crosslinks dextran, was used to cause aggregation of the MNPs. Glycerol was added according the formulas of Cheng to produce solutions of different viscosities[20].

MTG-B murine breast adenocarcinoma cells were grown in Eagle's Minimum Essential Medium. Cells were removed from the growth medium by scraping as these cells were found to uptake MNPs more efficiently than cells that had been trypsinized. Cells were resuspended in media using an approximate concentration of 1 million cells/mL and MNPs were added.

Nanoparticle magnetization measurements were performed using a MNP spectrometer described previously[21]. The harmonic signals were analyzed using a Stanford Research SR830 Lock-In Amplifier. Measurements for this study focused on the magnitude and phase of the 3rd and 5th harmonics.

3. RESULTS AND DISCUSSION

Our experimental study of endocytosis's impact on MNPs' harmonic spectrum analyzed concentration-dependent measures, 3rd and 5th harmonic amplitude, and concentration-independent measures, the ratio of the 5th over 3rd harmonic amplitudes and angles of the 3rd and 5th harmonics. All data was acquired with drive field amplitude of 26 mT/μ_0 using frequencies of 270 and 790 Hz. The drive amplitude is comparable to those currently used in MPI while the frequencies are substantially lower. The signal changes due to viscosity and aggregation presented here rely on changes in the MNPs' Brownian motion. For this reason small core particles which relax predominantly through the Neel mechanism should be avoided. We previously showed that the effect of viscosity on the 5th/3rd ratio can be changed by varying the frequency, which could allow for contrast selection[14].

We used MTG-B cells that have shown pronounced uptake of dextran-coated MNPs in previous magnetic fluid hyperthermia work. Cells were prepared as described above, and the 1mL solution was placed in a 2mL microcentrifuge tube which fit securely in our spectrometer's receive coil. MNPs (0.125 mg Fe) were added to this solution at time 0. The amplitude and phase of the 3rd and 5th harmonics were recorded every 1.5 minutes using a drive field frequency of 270 Hz, see Figure 1. After approximately 15 hours, the amplitudes of the 3rd and 5th harmonics had dropped to 16% and 40%, respectively, of their values at time 0. The concentration-independent metrics all changed by over 100 standard deviations in that same time period. The standard deviations of repeat measurements were 0.16°

and 0.44° for the 3rd and 5th angles, respectively, and 5.32E-4 for the ratio. At the end of the experiment, visual inspection of the cell suspension revealed a cell pellet with a region of white cells, which had not taken up MNPs, covered by darker MNP laden cells. The supernatant liquid, though lighter than at time 0, still appeared to contain MNPs in solution.

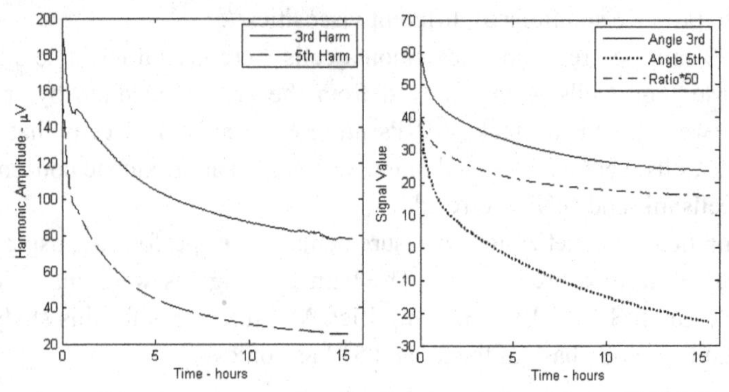

Fig. 1. Harmonic spectrum changes versus time for dextran-coated particles and MTG-B cells using an applied field of 270 Hz and 26 mT/μ_0. The ratio is unitless and is multiplied by 50 to match the scale of the harmonic angles.

To improve cellular uptake of the MNPs, a similar MNP and cell solution was incubated in a rotating stage at 37°C. At the end of this 24 hour incubation, visual inspection of the vial showed a supernatant liquid very close in color to the cell media and a completely dark cell pellet. Further experiments with different particle concentrations showed a mixture model like result corresponding to different quantities of cell associated and cell unassociated particles. This vial of endocysed MNPs was measured in the spectrometer, and the signal compared to that of a control sample of MNPs in cell media but without cells, see Figure 2. In an attempt to ascertain what physical changes to the MNPs were responsible for the observed changes in our MNP measurements, we aggregated the control with Concanavalin-A. We also dispersed the MNPs in various glycerol/water mixtures of known viscosities. At both 270 and 790 Hz the effect of aggregation closely resembled the effect of endocytosis of the MNPs for all three of our concentration-independent metrics. Though a sample of increased viscosity could cause a change in one metric comparable to aggregation or endocytosis, the other two metrics were far different. Further, the viscosity which resulted in a 3rd harmonic angle comparable to aggregation at 270 Hz was far different from the viscosity needed at 790 Hz. Addition of Concanavalin-A to the endocysed MNPs' vial resulted in minimal change in the signals, which would suggest a lack of free MNPs in the solution.

To confirm that the MNPs were truly being taken into the cells and forming aggregates within vesicles, a sample of the cell/MNP solution was fixed with glutaraldehyde and TEM images taken, see Figure 2c. The gray body of a cell can be seen throughout most of the image. On the left side of the image, MNPs are seen associated with the cell wall, while in the gray cell mass they are seen as clusters within vesicles. Extensive TEM imaging of these particles and cells for related magnetic fluid hyperthermia work has consistently confirmed the endocytosis and aggregation of the particles in vesicles.

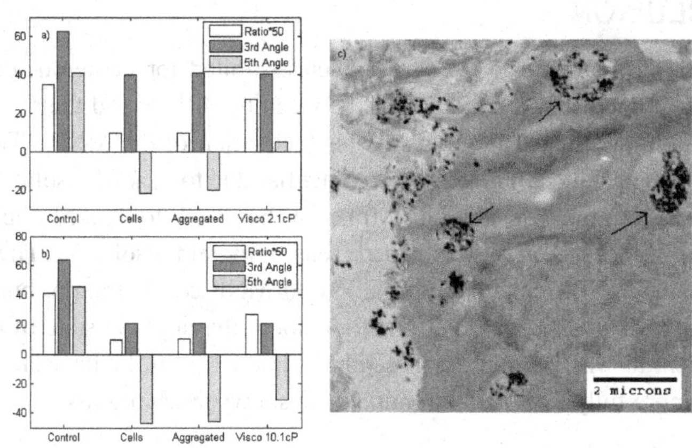

Fig. 2. a,b) Comparison of the effects of MNP endocytosis with the effects of viscosity and aggregation. a) 790 Hz - 26mT, b) 270 Hz - 26mT. c) TEM image confirming endocytosis of the MNPs by the cells.

Though the cellular endocytosis results of Figure 2 closely resemble the effects of aggregation, the various influences on the MNPs' dynamic magnetization need to be examined more thoroughly across numerous amplitudes and frequencies. Interestingly the method of aggregation for Concanavalin and endocytosis are likely different though they gave similar results. Concanavalin forms a chemical cross-link between particles while endocytosis likely involves a packing of particles. The impact of a singular influence such as binding[22], viscosity[14], or aggregation can be shown, but *in vivo* several of these effects are likely to be present at one time. Data from harmonics beyond the 5th, or from even harmonics in the presence of static fields, though not included here are likely to add additional information about the physical state of the MNPs. Numerous other concentration-independent metrics that incorporate information from multiple harmonics can also be explored. The harmonic spectrum can be analyzed against known changes in frequency and AC/DC amplitude giving extensive data about the MNPs. The full extent to which this data can be interpreted remains to be seen.

The use of MPI for monitoring changes in a MNP's state will likely require unique image acquisition sequences. MRI generally relies on fixed magnetic coils, but through the creative use of pulse sequences new applications are still being envisioned and implemented. In a similar fashion, changes to the "pulse sequence" of an MPI system should allow for various biological processes to be used as contrast in the images. Incorporation of the techniques presented here, as well as others yet to be explored, should make MPI a more robust imaging modality.

4. CONCLUSION

The magnetic properties of MNPs have been exploited for numerous clinical and pharmaceutical applications. Interactions between the MNPs and their environment have been monitored using the dynamic magnetization of the MNPs. The existing magnetic techniques have limited *in vivo* potential due to lack of resolution or strict limitations on sample preparation. MPI can be used to record the magnetic properties of MNPs remotely with superb sensitivity and resolution. The harmonic spectrum of the MNPs contains information on MNP concentration, but as shown here it can also contain valuable information about the physical state of the MNPs. The full extent to which information can be extracted from the harmonic spectrum needs to be more fully explored, but initial data shows much promise.

REFERENCES

1 Pankhurst QA, Thanh NKT, Jones SK, Dobson J. Progress in applications of magnetic nanoparticles in biomedicine. *J Phys D: Appl Phys* 2009; **42**: 224001.

2 Kim DH, Rozhkova EA, Ulasov IV, Bader SD, Rajh T, Lesniak MS, Novosad V. Biofunctionalized magnetic-vortex microdiscs for targeted cancer-cell destruction. *Nature Mater* 2009; DOI:10.1038/NMAT2591

3 Jiang W, Kim BYS, Rutka JT, Chan WCW. Nanoparticle-mediated cellular response is size-dependent. *Nature Nanotechnology* 2008; **3**: 145-150.

4 Chithrani BD, Ghazani AA, Chan WCW. Determining the size and shape dependence of gold nanoparticle uptake into mammalian cells. *Nano Letters* 2006; **6**: 662-668.

5 Eberback D, Wiekhorst F, Steinhoff U, Trahms L. Aggregation behaviour of magnetic nanoparticle suspensions investigated by magnetorelaxometry. *J Phys: Condens Matter* 2006; **18**: S2829-S2846.

6 Petersson K, Ilver D, Johansson C, Krozer A. Brownian motion of aggregating nanoparticles studied by photon correlation spectroscopy and measurements of dynamic magnetic properties. *Anal Chim Acta* 2006; **573-574**: 138-146.

7 McNaughton BH, Agayan RR, Wang JX, Kopelman R. Physiochemical microparticle sensors based on nonlinear magnetic oscillations. *Sensor Actuat B* 2007; **121**: 330-340.

8 Eberbeck D, Bergemann C, Wiekhorst F, Steinhoff U, Trahms L. Quantification of specific bindings of biomolecules by magnetorelaxometry. *J Nanobiotechnology* 2008; **6**.

9 Jurgons R, Seliger C, Hilpert A, Trahms L, Odenbach S, Alexiou C. Drug loaded magnetic nanoparticles for cancer therapy. *J Phys: Condens Matter* 2006; **18**: S2893-S2902.

10 Gleich B, Weizenecker J. Tomographic imaging using the nonlinear response of magnetic particles. *Nature* 2005; **435**: 1214-9.

11 Weizenecker J, Gleich B, Rahmer J, Dahnke H, Borgert J. Three-dimensional real-time in vivo magnetic particle imaging. *Phys Med Biol* 2009; **54**: L1–L10.

12 Rauwerdink AM, Hansen EW, Weaver JB. Nanoparticle temperature estimation in combined ac and dc magnetic fields. *Phys Med Biol* 2009; **54**: L51-L55.

13 Weaver JB, Rauwerdink AM, Hansen EW. Magnetic nanoparticle temperature estimation. *Med Phys* 2009; **36**: 1822-1829.

14 Rauwerdink AM, Weaver JB. Viscous effects on nanoparticle magnetization harmonics. *J Magn Magn Mater* 2009; **322**: 609-613.

15 Rosensweig RE. Heating magnetic fluid with alternating magnetic fields. *J Magn Magn Mater* 2002; **252**: 370-374.

16 Felderhof BU, Jones RB. Nonlinear response of a dipolar system with rotational diffusion to an oscillating field. *J Phys: Condens Matter* 2003; **15**: S1363-S1378.

17 Raikher YL, Shliomis MI. The effective field method in the orientational kinetics of magnetic fluids. *Adv Chem Phys* 1994; **87**: 595-751.

18 Santra S, Kaittanis C, Grimm J, Perez JM. Drug/Dye loaded multifunctional iron oxide nanoparticles for combined targeted cancer therapy and dual optical/magnetic resonance imaging. *Small* 2009; **5**: 1862-1868.

19 Nasongkla N, Bey E, Ren J, Ai H, Khemtong C, Guthi JS, Chin SF, Sherry AD, Boothman DA, Gao J. Multifunctional polymeric micelles as cancer-targeted MRI-ultrasensitive drug delivery systems. *Nano Letters* 2006; **6**: 2427-2430.

20 Cheng NS. Formula for viscosity of glycerol-water mixture. *Ind Eng Chem Res* 2008; **47**: 3285-3288.

21 Weaver JB, Rauwerdink AM, Sullivan CR, Baker I. Frequency distribution of the nanoparticle magnetization in the presence of a static as well as a harmonic magnetic field. *Med Phys* 2008; **35**: 1988-1994.

22 Rauwerdink AM, Weaver JB. Measurement of molecular binding using the Brownian motion of magnetic nanoparticle probes. *Appl Phys Lett* 2010; **96**: 033702.

MAGNETIC PARTICLE SPECTROMETRY FOR THE EVALUATION OF FIELD-DEPENDENT HARMONICS GENERATION

THILO WAWRZIK, JAN HAHN, FRANK LUDWIG, MEINHARD SCHILLING

Institut für Elektrische Messtechnik und Grundlagen der Elektrotechnik, TU Braunschweig, Hans-Sommer-Str. 66
Braunschweig, 38106, Germany
Email: t.wawrzik@tu-bs.de

A modified setup of a Magnetic Particle Spectrometer is described. It allows the spectrum to be evaluated at different static field levels. The additional degree of freedom enables a parameter-based verification of the magnetic particle model derived for the sample.

1. INTRODUCTION

Magnetic Particle Imaging (MPI) is a new imaging method capable of measuring the spatial distribution of magnetic nanoparticles [1]. The encoding scheme for two- or three-dimensional MPI heavily depends on the structure of the harmonic spectrum varying with a static offset field. In a MPI system the offset field is provided by a gradient field consisting of a field-free point (FFP) at its center.

The Magnetic Particle Spectrometer (MPS) helps to understand the dynamics of the tracer material and its applicability for MPI [2]. The extended MPS setup described here also enables the investigation of the MPI encoding scheme properties.

In combination with other magnetic methods, such as AC susceptibility (ACS) and magnetorelaxometry (MRX) MPS qualifies as a standard method for magnetic nanoparticle characterization [3].

2. METHODS

Figure 1 shows a schematic view of the spectrometer setup consisting of four coils. The excitation signal generated by a D/A converter card (NI PCI-6733) is amplified with an audio power amplifier driving a single elongated solenoid. On the center line of the excitation coil a pair of detection coils is located. These coils are wired in anti-serial configuration forming a gradiometer setup.

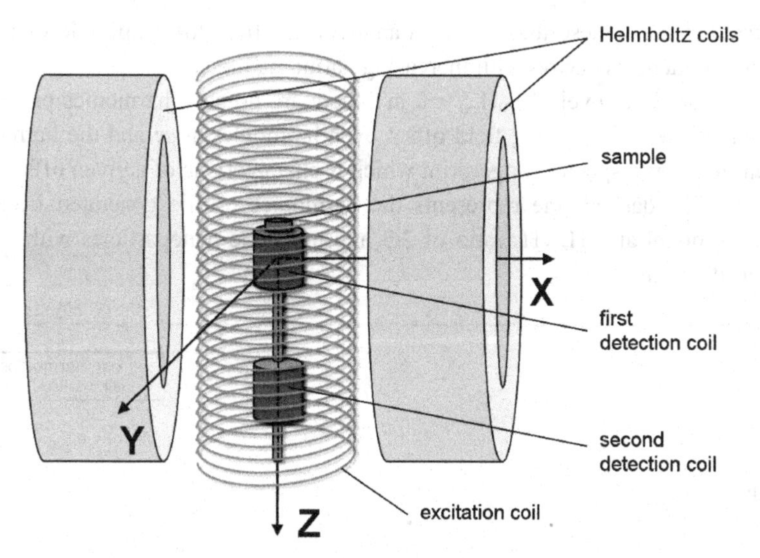

Fig. 1. Schematic view of the MPS system.

The gradiometer cancels the excitation frequency from the detection signal and effectively picks up the stray-field generated by the magnetic sample placed in the upper coil of the gradiometer (first detection coil). The resulting signal is digitized with a 24bit D/A converter card (NI PCI-4462) at a sampling rate of 204.8 kS/s. In addition, two larger coils in Helmholtz-type configuration are orientated orthogonally to the excitation and detection coils. They are capable of generating a static offset field of up to 15 mT.

With the described setup one can now measure the generation of higher harmonics in dependence on the excitation signal amplitude H_0 and the field strength H_{ext} of the static offset field.

Measurements were performed on an aqueous suspension of MagPrep 25 silica magnetite nanoparticles (from Merck KGaA) with a mean core diameter of 25 nm covered with a silica shell.

3. RESULTS AND DISCUSSION

The number of higher harmonics which can be measured and used for spatial encoding depends on the signal-to-noise ratio (SNR) of the system, as well as on the provided magnetic nanoparticle sample. For generation of higher harmonics the magnetic sample has to be driven into saturation, where the slope of the magnetization curve scales with the particle core diameter. For particles with a magnetization curve described by the Langevin function, the amplitude of higher harmonic frequencies decays with increasing harmonic index.

At a static field level of $\mu_0 H_{ext} = 0$ mT there are no even harmonics present in the spectrum. With increasing field offset even harmonics arise and the harmonics spectrum features a spectral fingerprint which is characteristic of a given offset field (figure 2). The dashed line represents the harmonics profile generated from the simulation model at a H_{ext}/H_0 ratio of 2/3 and magnetic nanoparticles with a core diameter of 25 nm.

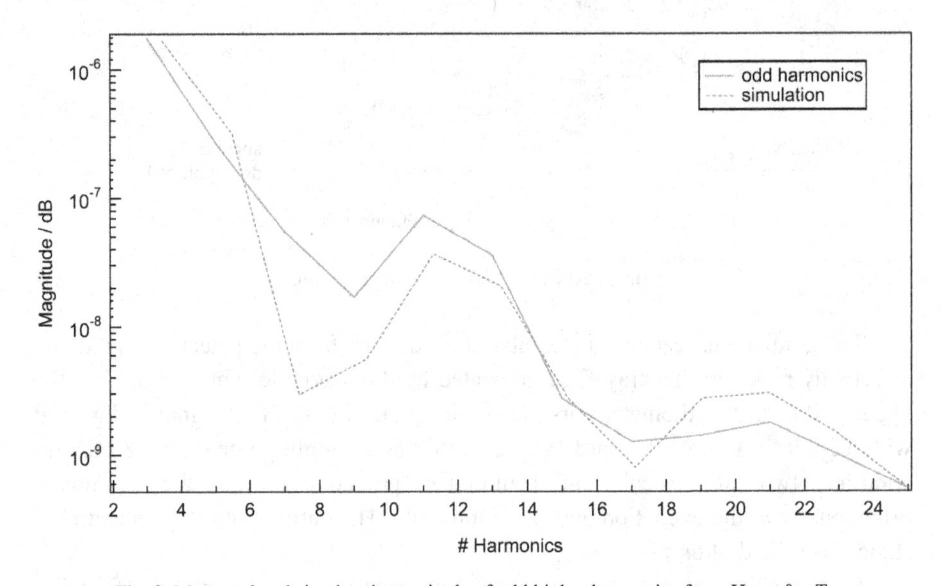

Fig. 2. Measured and simulated magnitude of odd higher harmonics for $\mu_0 H_{ext} > 0$ mT.

Figure 3 shows the dependence on the magnitude of odd harmonic frequencies on an applied offset field. It is apparent that higher harmonics decay faster corresponding to a narrow region around the FFP movement in imaging. The decay of the amplitude to higher harmonics is noticeable from the plot as well.

Due to the orthogonal orientation of the static field to the direction of the excitation field, the abscissa in figure 3 has to be rescaled to match a uni-axial system or single-directional simulation. For this reason, the absolute scale of static field axis can differ when comparing the results from MPS with other setups, such as a 1-dimensional MPI system or simulations.

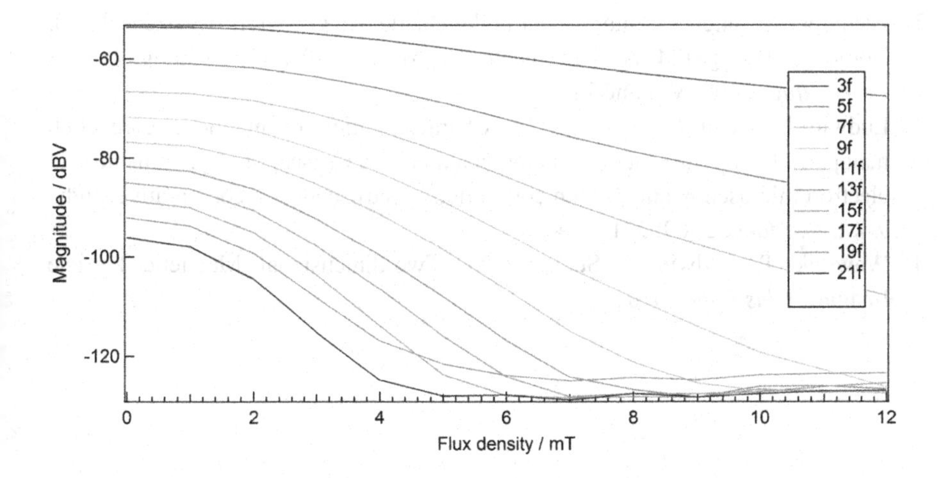

Fig. 3. Measured magnitudes of odd harmonics in dependence on the offset field level.

In principle, measuring a series of spectra at different offset levels allows the determination of the system matrix for 1-dimensional spatial encoding of an ideal MPI system [4].

4. CONCLUSION

The described system can be used to evaluate the generation of higher harmonics of the excitation frequency. In advance to previous MPS configurations the system allows the parametric measurement of the harmonic spectrum in dependence on excitation field amplitude and static offset field.

With the experimental backup it is possible to derive and verify a method-independent model for magnetic nanoparticles, describing the dynamic behavior of the tracers in ACS, MRX and MPS/MPI.

ACKNOWLEDGMENTS

Financial support of the DFG via SFB 578 is acknowledged.

REFERENCES

1 Gleich B, Weizenecker J. Tomographic imaging using the nonlinear response of magnetic particles. *Nature* 2005; 435/7046: 1214.

2 Biederer S, Sattel T, Knopp T, Lüdtke-Buzug K, Gleich B, Weizenecker J, Borgert J, Buzug TM. A Spectrometer for Magnetic Particle Imaging. *IFMBE Proceedings* 2008; Volume 22.
3 Ludwig F, Heim E, Schilling M. Characterization of magnetic core shell nanoparticles by fluxgate magnetorelaxometry, ac susceptibility, transmission electron microscopy and photon correlation spectroscopy – a comparative study. *J. Magn. Mater.* 2009; 321: 1644.
4 Wawrzik T, Ludwig F, Schilling M. Two-dimensional Magnetic Particle Imaging. *This Book* 2010.

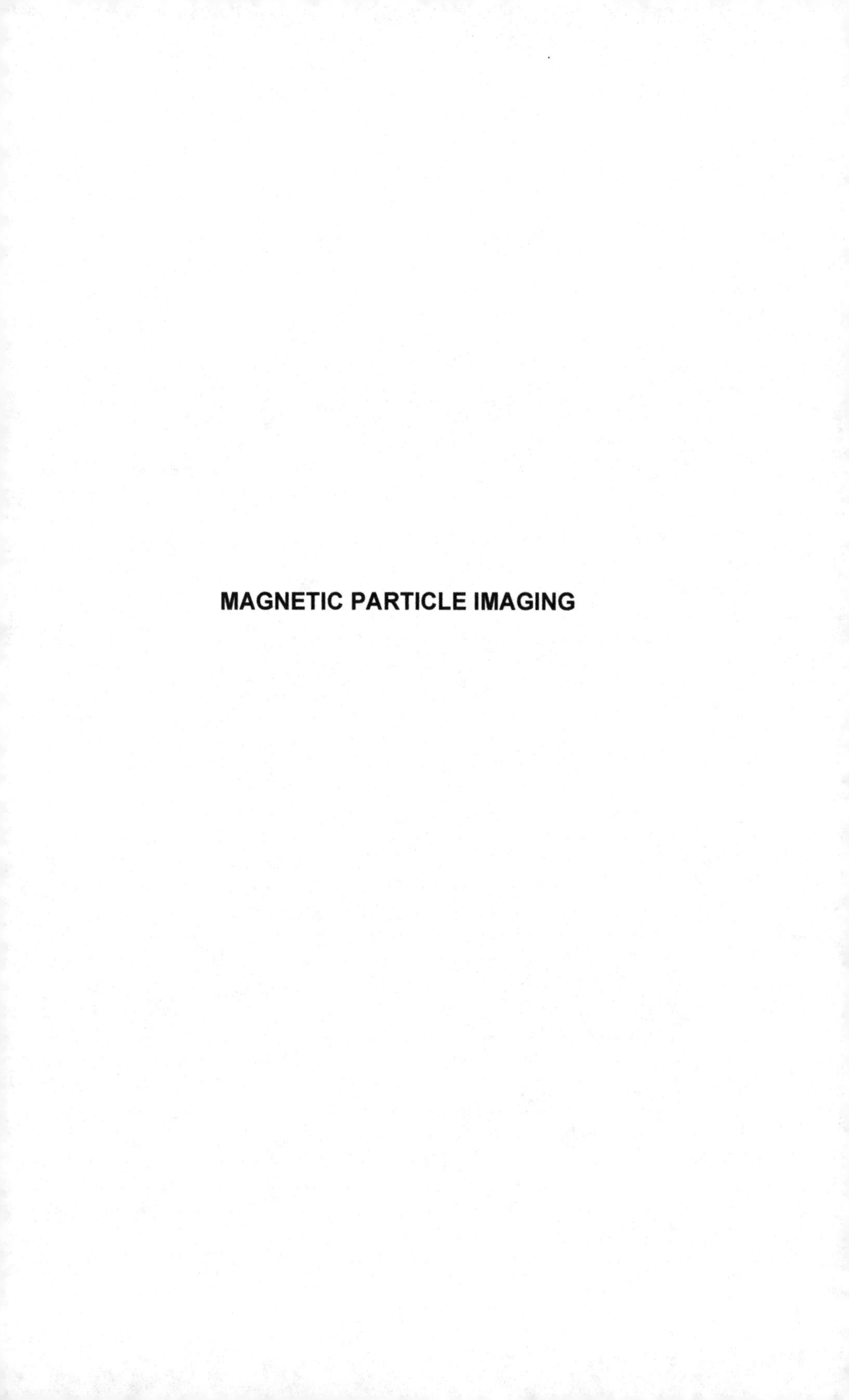

MAGNETIC PARTICLE IMAGING

NARROWBAND MAGNETIC PARTICLE IMAGING IN A MOUSE

PATRICK GOODWILL†

UC SF / UC Berkeley Joint Graduate Group in Bioengineering,
University of California, Berkeley CA 94720 USA
Email: goodwill@berkeley.edu

STEVEN CONOLLY

Department of Bioengineering
Berkeley, CA 94720 USA
Email: sconolly@berkeley.edu

The Magnetic Particle Imaging (MPI) method directly images the magnetization of Super-Paramagnetic Iron Oxide (SPIO) nanoparticles, which are contrast agents commonly used in MRI. MPI, as originally envisioned, requires a high-bandwidth receiver coil and preamplifier, which are difficult to optimally noise match. This paper demonstrates how we have scaled Narrowband MPI, which dramatically reduces bandwidth requirements and increases the signal-to-noise ratio for a fixed specific absorption rate, to a system that fits a mouse.

1. INTRODUCTION

Magnetic Particle Imaging (MPI) is a new[1] imaging modality that promises detection of nanomolar concentrations of super-paramagnetic iron oxide (SPIO) nanoparticles without depth limitations. The MPI method directly detects the bulk magnetization from a SPIO nanoparticle whose saturation magnetization approaches $0.6T\mu_0^{-1}$. The MPI method has extraordinary promise for sensitivity and contrast because this bulk SPIO magnetization is 10 million times more intense than the nuclear paramagnetism of water detected with a 7 Tesla MRI scanner.

2. MAGNETIC PARTICLE IMAGING OVERVIEW

MPI detects the unique signature of ferromagnetic nanoparticles in a confluence of static and dynamic magnetic fields. The static magnetic field is a very strong gradient (4000 mT/m) with a *field-free-point* (FFP) at the midpoint between the

† Work partially supported by the California Institute for Regenerative Medicine.

magnets. The gradient field effectively saturates all nanoparticles outside of the FFP.

In recent literature, Weizenecker *et. al.* have recently demonstrated a wide-bandwidth MPI system capable of imaging a beating mouse heart in real-time[10]. MPI is not restricted to small animals, and Sattel *et. al.* have recently demonstrated MPI using a single-sided device that holds great promise for human use[6]. Much progress has been made on theoretically understanding the received signal as we search to better ways to reconstruct the signals received by MPI [3,4,11].

3. NARROWBAND MPI THEORY

3.1. Intermodulation

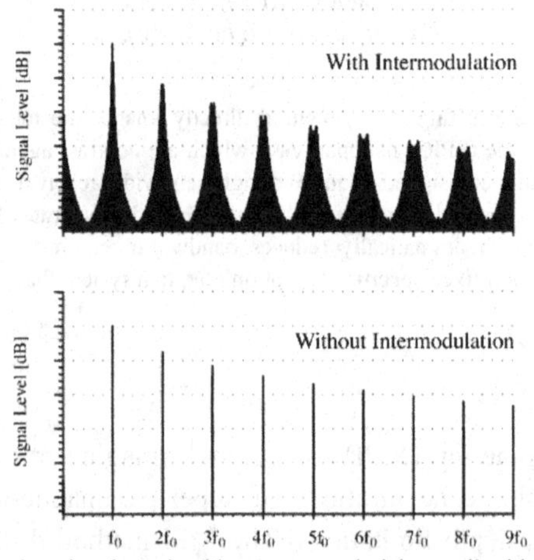

Figure 1: Simulation showing signal received by an untuned pickup coil with intermodulation (top) and without intermodulation (bottom). The fundamental (f_0) is not useful because it is contaminated by direct feedthrough from the excitation field. Intermodulation generates useful intermodulation tones around the main harmonics. The amplitude and phase of the IM tones vary as a function of position.

Intermodulation in MPI is discussed in more detail by Goodwill *et. al.*[2] At DC field strengths used in MPI of $B_{\max} < 1$ Tesla, tissue is largely unaffected by the magnetic field, but a SPIO particle undergoes a nonlinear change in magnetization described by the Langevin theory of paramagnetism[8].

$$M = M_0 L\left[\frac{mH}{k_B T}\right] = M_0\left(\coth\left(\frac{mH}{k_B T}\right) - \frac{k_B T}{mH}\right)$$

where L is the Langevin function, *m* is the magnetic moment of the particle, *H* is the applied field, and T is the absolute temperature. This relation only holds strictly true at DC.

In the original MPI protocol, a single sinusoidal magnetic field is applied to the magnetic nanoparticle. Here we analyze the magnetization response to two simultaneously applied sinusoidal magnetic fields with a large frequency separation:

$$H(t) = H_0 \sin(2\pi f_0 t) + H_1 \cos(2\pi f_1 t)$$

where we assume $f_0 >> f_1$.

The nonlinear Langevin function acts as a non-linear mixer when subjected to these two fields simultaneously, producing a rich output spectrum that reveals the quantity of magnetic nanoparticles at the FFP. Specifically, the SPIO nanoparticle's time varying magnetization will contain a rich spectrum with tones at the sum and difference products of the two input frequencies:

$$M(t) = \sum_{m=1}^{M} \sum_{n=-N}^{N} A_{m,n} \exp(i2p(mf_0 + nf_1)t)$$

where *M* and *N* occur because only a finite number of harmonics are detectable. Note that m=1 is not detected in this paper as it is overwhelmed by fundamental feed-through from the source directly to the detector.

Intermodulation enables us to choose f_0, H_0, f_1 and H_1 independently. SAR is dominated by f_0 and H_0 since f_0>>f_1, and SAR grows as H^2f^2 . Imaging speed and detection bandwidth are limited by f_1 since imaging data will show up as sidebands surrounding $m\supseteq f_0$. Thus, to prevent aliasing between the sidebands, we must restrict the scanning speed so that the sidebands do not overlap. There is a limit to increasing f_1 to increase imaging speed because the received signal bandwidth must be less than the bandwidth of the receiver coil. Last, SNR and the size of the Point-Spread-Function (PSF) are strongly linked to the magnitude of H_{total}=H_0+H_1. Increasing H_{total} increases the total signal received at the expense of widening the PSF. Increasing H_1 increases the received signal while affecting SAR negligibly. This allows trading increased signal for reduced resolution.

3.2. MPI System Construction

We constructed a narrowband MPI imaging system (Fig. 2) using NdFeB permanent magnets. The permanent magnet gradient is built using two ring magnets

(OD=15.24 cm, ID=7.62 cm, THK=1.9 cm) mounted on G10. The magnetic field down the bore has a gradient field strength measured at dB/dz=6.5 T/m. Coronal gradients are simulated to be smaller at dB/dx=dB/dy=3.25 T/m.

The interfacing electronics (Fig. are designed to prevent intermodulation in the RF and LF amplifier output stages and in the preamplifier through the use of high-pass, low pass, and notch filters. The battery-powered preamplifier uses low-noise op-amps (Texas Instruments OPA211) with noise power e_n= 1.1 $nV/(Hz)^{-1/2}$, i_n= 1.7 $pA/(Hz)^{-1/2}$ matched to a high-Q coil[7]. The receiver is a home-built phase coherent control console and detector[9]. The coherent detector directly samples at 65 MSPS (Analog Devices AD6644) and digitally down converts the RF signal to baseband (Analog Devices AD6620). The down-sampled signal has a bandwidth of 31.25 kSPS centered at $2f_0$=300 kHz. Samples are translated through the bore using a 3D stage controlled by the console. The digitized signal is quadrature demodulated at multiples of the intermodulation frequency ($\pm f_1, \pm 2f_1, \ldots, \pm Nf_1$) and brick-wall filtered at 20 Hz.

RF is generated by a signal-generator (Tektronix Inc AFG3102) phase locked to the coherent detector. The RF amplifier (Tomco Technologies BT00400-AlphaA-CW) drives a matched, water cooled resonant transmit coil to generate a $B_0 = 10$ mTpp sinusoidal magnetic field at $f_0 = 250$ kHz.

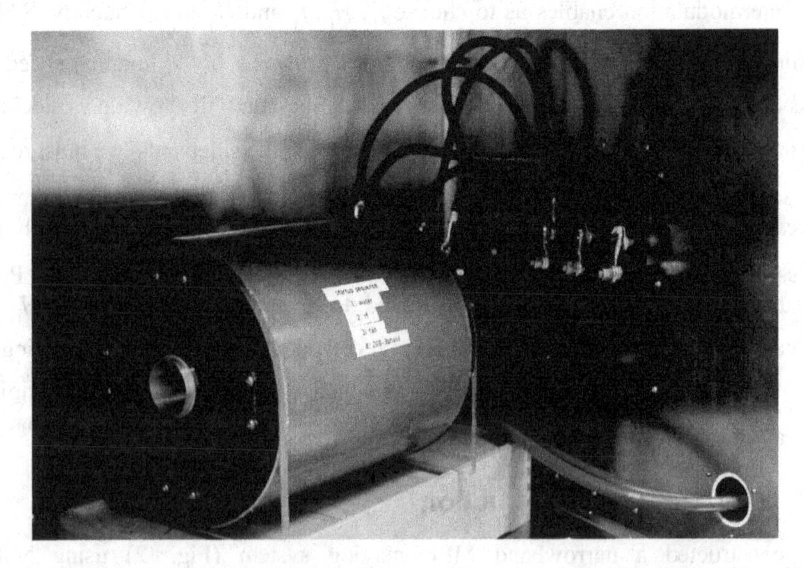

Figure 2: Photo of the MPI mouse imaging system. The system is water cooled with a 30 psi pressurized water system.

Water cooled intermodulation coils, driven by MRI gradient amplifiers (Copley Controls model 234) can move the FFP up to 3cm in any direction. Phantoms are constructed of milled acrylic and filled with undiluted 50 nm SPIO nanoparticles (Chemicell GmbH fluidMAG-D) or injected into preserved mouse (Carolina Biological Supply).

4. RESULTS AND DISCUSSION

4.1. Imaging

The PSF from a single point of 50 nm SPIO nanoparticles shows the complex interplay between the magnetic particle and the field-free point. In Fig. 3 we see the measured two-dimensional PSF for the first eight sidebands when acquired using the intermodulation method. The measured PSF is of higher SNR in the lower sidebands ($2f_0$, $2f_0 \pm f_1$), but contains more high frequency spectral content in the upper sidebands ($2f_0 \pm 2f_1$, $2f_0 \pm 3f_1$, ...).

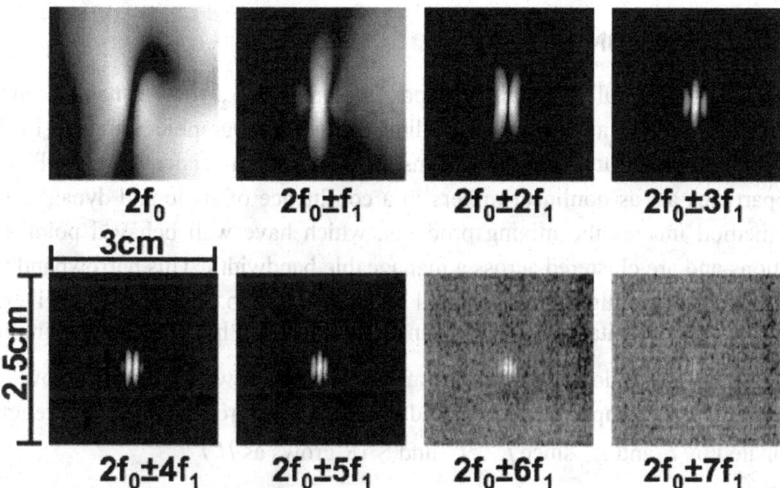

Figure 3: (TOP) Measured point spread functions from a point source containing 25 μgrams Fe with B_0=10 mTpp at 150 kHz, and B_1=10 mTpp at 128 Hz. FOV: 2.5x3cm.

To demonstrate 3D imaging and our ability to acquire signal in an animal, we have acquired a full three-dimensional image in a mouse (Fig. 4). As expected, there is no endogenous signal from the animal. The method is quantitative, and we have tested that the signal increases linearly with the quantity present.

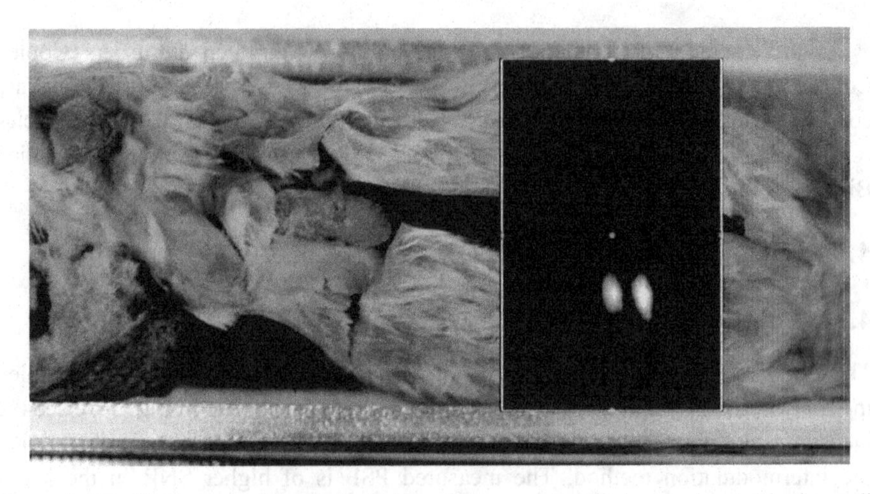

Figure 4: Full 3D Maximum Intensity Projection of preserved mouse phantom injected in the small intestine with 100 μgrams Fe. FOV: 3x3x2 cm, 7 minute acquisition time. The MIP is rendered in OsiriX[5].

5. CONCLUSION

We have successfully simulated and implemented a new imaging method, narrowband MPI, capable of three-dimensional tomographic imaging of SPIO nanoparticles without depth limitations in a mouse. In Narrowband MPI, SPIO nanoparticles act as nonlinear mixers in a confluence of static and dynamic fields. Our method images the mixing products, which have well behaved point spread functions and are clustered across a manageable bandwidth. This narrowband signal is detected using a high-Q receive coil noise matched to a low-noise receiver. The high frequency excitation field f_0 can be chosen so that the receive frequency enables body noise dominance, a desirable result. Narrowband MPI improves SNR for a fixed SAR compared to wideband MPI. SAR and received signal strength are dominated by f_0 and H_0 since $f_0 >> f_1$, and SAR grows as H^2f^2.

ACKNOWLEDGMENTS

The authors would like to thank the California Institute for Regenerative Medicine (CIRM) for a graduate fellowship (Training Grant Number T1-00007), University of California Berkeley Bioengineering for a graduate fellowship, and the National Institutes of Health for a training grant. The contents of this publication are solely the responsibility of the authors and do not necessarily represent the official views of CIRM or any other agency of the State of California.

REFERENCES

1 Gleich B, and Weizenecker J, "Tomographic imaging using the nonlinear response of magnetic particles," *Nature*, vol. 435, no. 7046, pp. 1214–7, Jun 2005.

2 Goodwill P, Scott S, Stang P, and Conolly S. "Narrowband Magnetic Particle Imaging," *IEEE Trans. Med. Imag.* vol 28., No. 8, pp 1231-1237, Aug 2009.

3 Knopp T, Biederer S, Sattel T, Weizenecker J, Gleich B, Borgert J, and Buzug TM, "Trajectory analysis for magnetic particle imaging," *Phys. Med. Biol.*, vol. 54, no. 2, pp. 385–397, Dec 2008.

4 Rahmer J, Weizenecker J, Gleich B, and Borgert J. "Signal encoding in magnetic particle imaging: properties of the system function," *BMC Med. Img.* vol. 9 no. 2, pp. 4, 2009

5 Rosset A, Spadola L, and Ratib O, "OsiriX: An Open-Source Software for Navigating in Multidimensional DICOM Images," *J Digit Imaging*, vol. 17, no. 3, pp. 205–216, Sep 2004.

6 Sattel TF, Knopp T, Biederer S, Gleich B, Weizenecker J, Borgert J, and Buzug TM. "Single-sided device for magnetic particle imaging," *J. Phys. D: Appl. Phys.,* vol. 42, no. 2, 2008.

7 Scott G, Conolly C, and Macovski A, "Low Field Preamp Matching Design for High Q Receiver Coils," *In: Proceedings of the 4th Annual Meeting of ISMRM, New York, NY*, p. 396, Jan 1996.

8 Spaldin NA, Magnetic Materials: Fundamentals and Device Applications, Jan 2003.

9 Stang P, Conolly S, Pauly J, and Scott G, "MEDUSA: A Scalable MR Console for Parallel Imaging," *In: Proceedings of the 16th Annual Meeting of ISMRM, Berlin, Germany*, p. 925, 2007.

10 Weizenecker J, Gleich B, Rahmer J, Dahnke H, and Borgert J. "Three-dimensional real-time in vivomagnetic particle imaging." *Phys. Med. Biol.*, vol. 54, no. 5, pp. L1-L10, 2009.

11 Weizenecker J, Borgert J, and Gleich B, "A simulation study on the resolution and sensitivity of magnetic particle imaging," *Phys Med Biol*, vol. 52, no. 21, pp. 6363–74, Nov 2007.

TWO-DIMENSIONAL MAGNETIC PARTICLE IMAGING

THILO WAWRZIK, FRANK LUDWIG, MEINHARD SCHILLING

Institut für Elektrische Messtechnik und Grundlagen der Elektrotechnik, TU Braunschweig, Hans-Sommer-Str. 66
Braunschweig, 38106, Germany
Email: t.wawrzik@tu-bs.de

A setup for two-dimensional magnetic particle imaging (MPI) is described. The system uses two orthogonal drive fields creating a Lissajous trajectory in the imaging area. A single pair of detection coils picks up the resulting signal and allows the reconstruction of a 2-dimensional image from the signal spectrum.

1. INTRODUCTION

A simple MPI experiment can be performed by moving the sample mechanically through the coil assembly. It has been shown that for faster image acquisition the field free point (FFP) can be moved through the sample area by a drive field [1]. Our first practical realization of such a system was able to acquire line scans of magnetic samples in a quasi-static fashion [2]. The method has been enhanced by 1-dimensional spatial encoding which allows the image reconstruction from the harmonic spectrum. Here we are taking the next step towards dynamic 2-dimensional imaging. A setup similar to the original setup [1] is described using two orthogonal drive fields but one detection coil only.

2. METHODS

2.1. Physical Setup

The physical setup of the two-dimensional MPI scanner, as shown in figure 1, consists of four pairs of coils. The gradient field is generated by coils in Maxwell-type configuration. A gradient of about 3.5 T/m is achievable. The drive field coils in z-direction, parallel to the field gradient, and the orthogonal drive field coils in x-direction are constructed as Helmholtz-type pairs [1, 2].

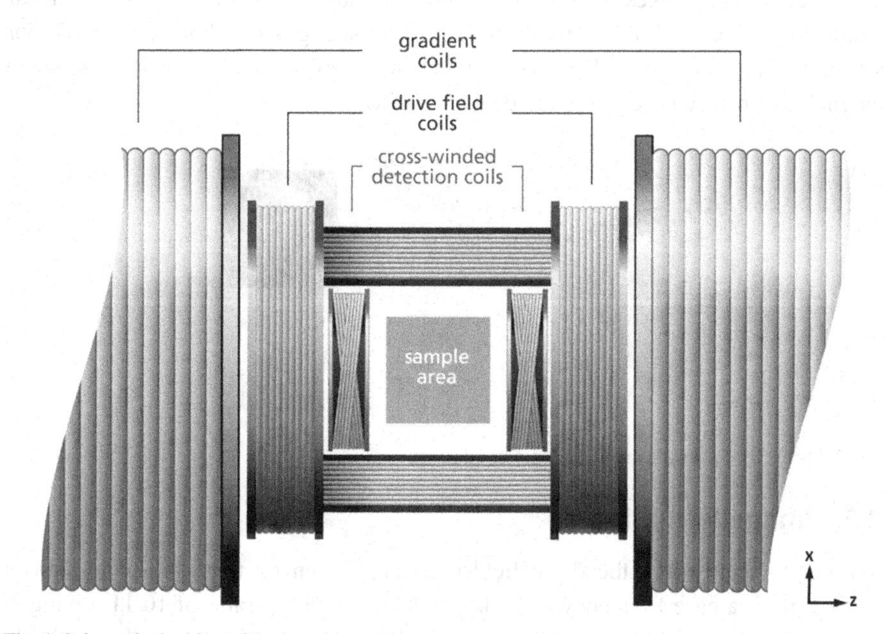

Fig. 1. Schematic drawing of the imaging system

The drive field signal is generated by a custom-built audio power amplifier with a current feedback loop to minimize total harmonic distortion (THD). No additional filtering is applied in the transmit chain. The phase of the resulting current is shifted against the excitation signal generated by the D/A converter. Therefore, the voltage drop across a shunt resistor in series with the drive field coils is used to verify and stabilize the phase as well as the frequency and amplitude of the drive field.

The Helmholtz-type detection coils are positioned in parallel to the z-coils. Since for two-dimensional imaging two field components have to be registered, a special cross winding technique is used to form the detection coils. With this configuration a small signal component from x-direction can be measured in addition to the aligned z-direction. The detection coils are placed close to the sample to pick up as much signal as possible. The detection signal is directly fed into a differential amplifier with prefixed phase-shift circuit subtracting the drive field signal electronically and suppressing the drive frequencies from the signal.

The sample used for the imaging experiments is based on a plastic cuboid with dimensions of 10x10x7 mm³ (figure 2a). A hole (diameter 1 mm) in the solid is stuffed with a small stripe of Vitrovac, an isotropic amorphous metal with soft magnetic properties. Since the foil is kept perpendicular to the imaging plane, its cross section resembles a point-like sample. Vitrovac consists of a non-linear magnetization curve and requires a low field strength of about 25-50 μT for saturation [3]. It is well suited for an MPI experiment because its steep magnetization curve is close to an ideal (step-like) one.

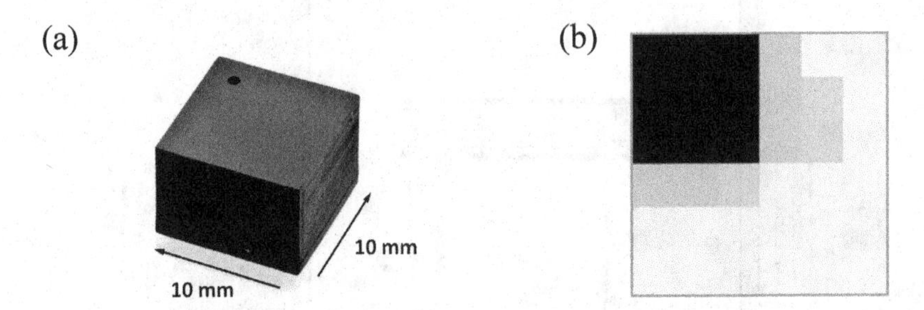

Fig. 2. Photo (a) of a sample and (b) reconstructed image

2.2. Image formation

For image acquisition, the drive field coils are driven by two sinusoidal signals derived from a base frequency of 20 kHz with a frequency ratio of 10/11, giving f_1 = 2 kHz and f_2 = 1.81 kHz, respectively. With this configuration the resulting Lissajous pattern has a repetition time of t_r = 5.5 ms (181.81 Hz). For each image the acquired spectrum is averaged over 250 periods, entailing a total acquisition time of about 1.3 seconds. Because image quality is currently limited by the THD of the power amplifier and the signal-to-noise ratio (SNR) of the detection path, up to 20 image data sets are stacked to form the final image.

The frequency spectrum of the detection signal contains both drive field frequencies and their harmonics as well as mixing components originating from the nonlinear magnetization curve of the magnetic sample (figure 3). The harmonics of the drive frequency carry spatial information about the respective drive field direction whereas the mixing components enclose both spatial directions. However, in this setup only multiples of the drive frequencies are used for reconstruction.

The encoding scheme for MPI is based on the characteristic spectral pattern of each spatial point [4]. For reconstruction, the reference response of the magnetic sample in the image plane has to be determined. This can be done by means of performing reference scans on a point-like sample.

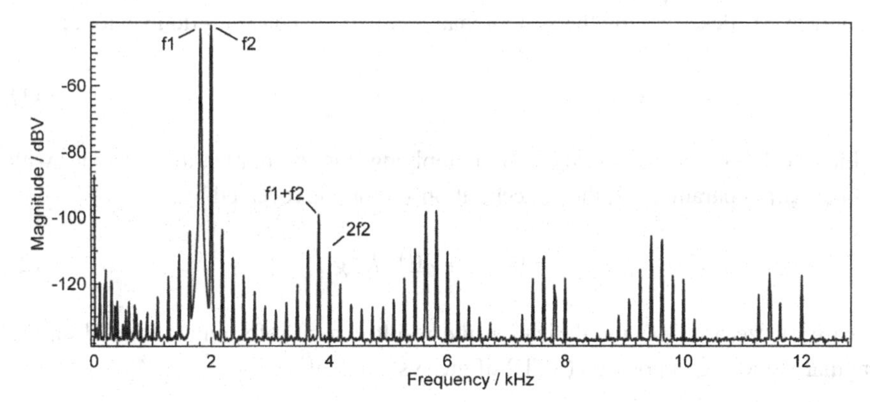

Fig. 3. Spectrum of a measured detection signal containing both drive frequencies

The system matrix for constructing a 1-dimensional image contains the spectral signature (harmonics of the drive frequency) for each point on a line (figure 4). To extend 1-dimensional encoding to the second dimension, an additional drive frequency is introduced. As this second drive field is orientated orthogonally to the first one, it allows spatial encoding in the second dimension. If frequency components for both drive frequencies are registered simultaneously, the system matrix can also be extended to represent 2-dimensional images. The reconstruction algorithm takes all spatial dimensions at once, collapsing the spatial indices into one sequential index.

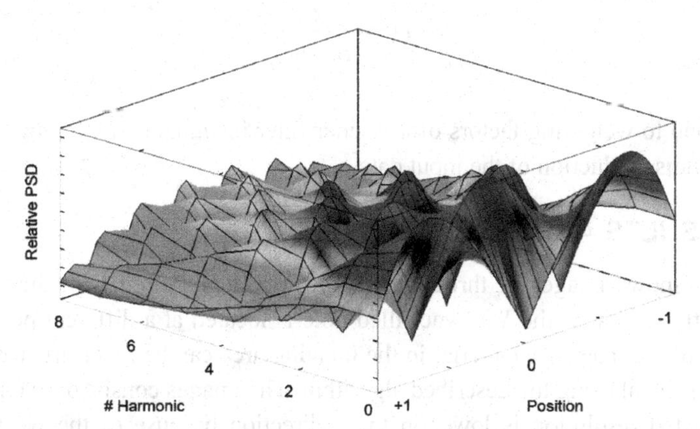

Fig. 4. Graphical representation of the simulated 1-dimensional system matrix (power spectral density (PSD) over harmonic number and position)

The experiments are performed using a Tikhonov regularization method [1, 5]. Here the image g is described by the system matrix K and the concentration vector c:

$$Kc = g \tag{1}$$

Taking a least square approach and applying the regularization scheme with regularization parameter λ, the concentration vector c is revealed by

$$c = \left(K^T K + \lambda \mathrm{E}\right)^{-1} K^T g \,. \tag{2}$$

In case of "zero order" regularization the result can be reformulated based on the singular value decomposition (SVD) of the system matrix K

$$SVD(K) = U\Sigma V^* \,, \tag{3}$$

consisting of two unitary matrices U and V (or the conjugate transpose V^*) and the diagonal matrix Σ containing the singular values σ_i. We arrive at a simpler expression to reconstruct the concentration vector c:

$$c = VDU^* g \tag{4}$$

The elements D_{ii} of the diagonal matrix D given by

$$D_{ii} = \frac{\sigma_i}{\sigma_i^{\,2} + \lambda^2} \tag{5}$$

correspond to weighting factors of a Wiener filter in signal conditioning, promising the best noise reduction of the input data.

3. RESULTS AND DISCUSSION

Figure 5 shows images of three magnetic samples measured with the system. In each of these images the Vitrovac-filled hole is located at a different position. The position of the magnetic material in the imaging area can be reconstructed from the detection signal using the described algorithm. The images consist of 6x6 pixels, but the expected resolution is lower in the x-direction because of the weaker signal picked up by the detection coils and the lower gradient strength in this direction. It is also apparent that the contrast of the image depends on the position of the sample.

The contrast by visual inspection is better in the right image compared to the left one.

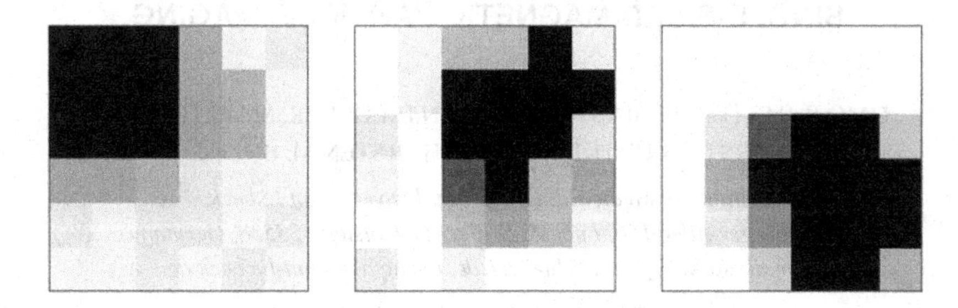

Fig. 5. Three images (10x10 mm^2) of Vitrovac samples acquired with the system

4. CONCLUSION

The first images of Vitrovac samples acquired with the described MPI system show that spatially resolved 2-dimensional imaging is feasible. However, improvements to the hardware and optimization of the reconstruction algorithms have to be completed in order to take higher resolved images.

ACKNOWLEDGMENTS

Financial support of the DFG via SFB 578 is acknowledged.

REFERENCES

1 Gleich B, Weizenecker J. Tomographic imaging using the nonlinear response of magnetic particles. *Nature* 2005; 435/7046: 1214.
2 Wawrzik T, Ludwig F, Schilling M. Assembly for One-dimensional Magnetic Particle Imaging. *IFMBE Proceedings* 2009; Volume 25.
3 Hinnrichs C, Pels C, Schilling M. Noise linearity of a fluxgate magnetometer in racetrack geometry. *J. Appl. Phys.* 1987; 9: 7085.
4 Rahmer J, Weizenecker J, Gleich B, Borgert J. Signal encoding in magnetic particle imaging: properties of the system function. *BMC Medical Imaging* 2009; 9: 4.
5 Golub GH, Van Loan CF. Matrix Computations 3rd Edition. Baltimore: John Hopkins University Press, 1996.

RESOLUTION DISTRIBUTION IN SINGLE-SIDED MAGNETIC PARTICLE IMAGING

TIMO F. SATTEL, TOBIAS KNOPP, SVEN BIEDERER, MARLITT ERBE, KERSTIN LÜDTKE-BUZUG, THORSTEN M. BUZUG

Institute of Medical Engineering, University of Lübeck, Ratzeburger Allee 160, Lübeck, Schleswig-Holstein, 23538, Germany

Email: satttel@imt.uni-luebeck.de, buzug@imt.uni-luebeck.de

In most coil geometries used for magnetic particle imaging (MPI), the specimen has to be positioned in-between the coil sets for investigation. This poses a size limitation, which is overcome when using a single-sided coil configuration. First measurements documenting the feasibility of this concept have been published. In this contribution, properties of the magnetic field generated by a symmetrical and a single-sided MPI scanner are compared. The spatially dependent resolution distribution of single-sided MPI is investigated and related to the simulated magnetic field properties.

1. INTRODUCTION

Magnetic particle imaging (MPI) is an imaging method capable of determining the spatial distribution of super-paramagnetic iron oxide nanoparticles (SPIOs).[1] The first coil configuration used for MPI is a symmetric assembly, where the object of interest has to fit in-between the coils (Fig. 1). So far, only small scanner devices have been realized, where small animals such as mice can be imaged. To overcome this limitation, one can apply a single-sided coil configuration (Fig. 2), where all transmit and receive coils are situated on one side of the specimen. As a proof of concept, a basic experimental setup has been implemented for 1D imaging.[2]

In both setups, the physical principle utilized for imaging is the same. To obtain information about the spatial nanoparticle distribution, a field-free point (FFP) is generated and steered through the volume of interest on a defined trajectory. This trajectory approximately defines the field of view (FOV). The applied alternating magnetic fields cause the nanoparticle magnetization to change in the direct vicinity of the FFP, while other nanoparticles are barely affected. In this way, signals are induced in receive coils, which allow for image reconstruction of the spatial particle distribution.

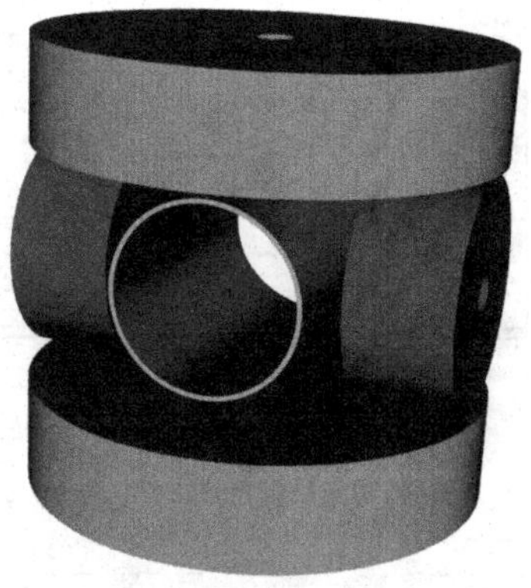

Fig. 1. Symmetrical coil setup for 3D-imaging.1 The FOV is situated in the center of the coil assembly.

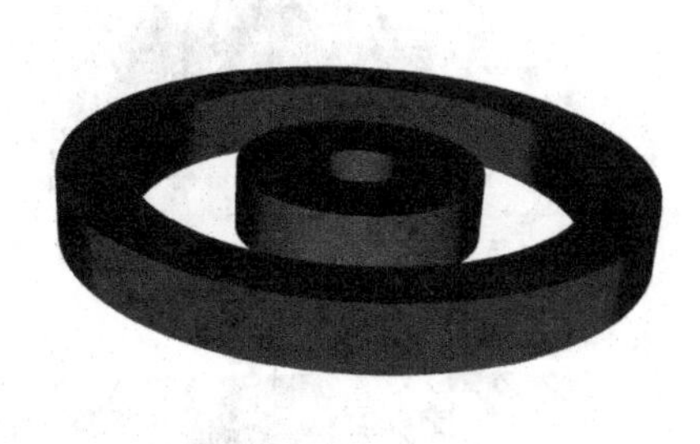

Fig. 2. Single-sided coil setup for 1D-imaging.[2] The FOV is situated in front of the coil assembly.

Weizenecker et al. simulated and discussed the achievable resolution of MPI in general, but did not investigate inhomogeneous resolution distributions in MPI.[3]

The introduced setups differ not only in coil geometry and thus in generated magnetic field geometry, but also in potential imaging quality. The reason is a pronounced inhomogeneity of the gradient distribution of the selection field generated by the single-sided setup. In this contribution, the gradient distribution of both coil setups is investigated for 1D-imaging in a simulation study. Finally, the image quality of single-sided measurements is investigated by means of full width half maximum (FWHM) and related to theory.

2. THEORY

The achievable image resolution in MPI depends on different parameters. According to Rahmer et al., the spatial resolution Δx in x-direction is given by

$$\Delta x = \frac{k_B T}{\mu_0 m G_x} c \text{, with } c \approx 4.16, \tag{1}$$

assuming a sufficiently high signal-to-noise ratio and a sufficiently dense FFP-trajectory.[4] The parameters hence are the particle magnetic moment m, the absolute temperature T, and the selection field gradient strength G_x in x-direction. The particle moment m in turn comprises of the saturation magnetization M_S (0.6 T/μ_0 for magnetite) and the particle core diameter d:

$$m = \frac{\pi}{6} M_S d^3. \tag{2}$$

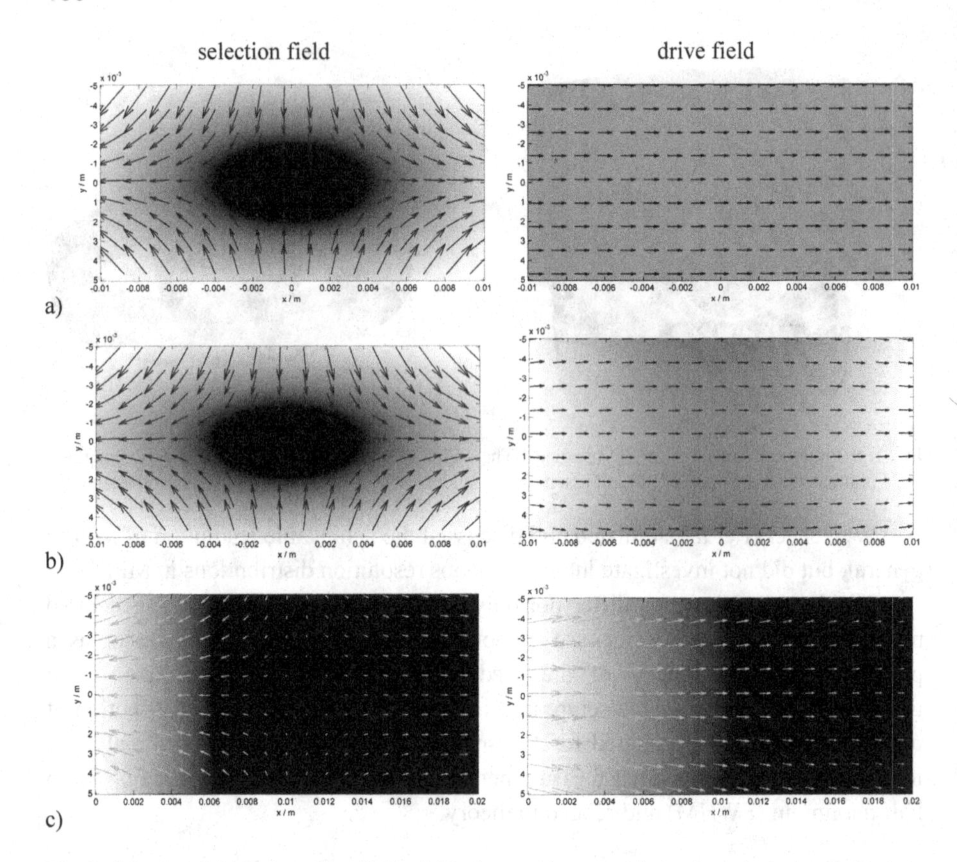

Fig. 3. Selection field and gradient field. a) ideal case, b) symmetrical setup, c) single-sided setup. Arrows indicate the strength and direction of the magnetic flux density B. The absolute value |B| is coded in gray values in the background (dark: low value, bright: high value) individually for each plot.

For improved image resolution, it is the aim to provide both, nanoparticles with high magnetic moments, and a high selection field gradient. Optimizing magnetic nanoparticles for MPI is an actual field of research.[5,6] To understand and to compare the gradient distribution of the magnetic field, the following paragraphs first introduce ideal magnetic field geometries, the magnetic field geometries generated by the symmetrical setup, and the ones generated by the single-sided setup. For simplicity, the 1D-imaging case is considered here. That means that only one drive field is applied and the FFP moves on a line.

In simulation, one can apply a homogeneous magnetic field gradient distribution. That means that G is constant in the entire area. This field provides an FFP with linearly increasing field strength in all directions. To move the FFP, a

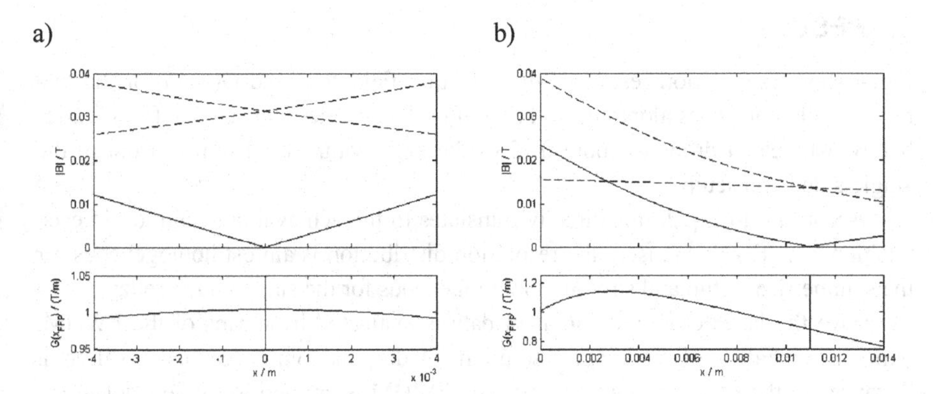

Fig. 4. Generated magnetic flux density |B(x)| of the static selection field and normalized $G(x_{FFP})$. a) symmetrical setup, b) single-sided setup. |B(x)| is plotted for each coil separately as dashed line and its sum as solid line.

homogeneous drive field can be applied (Fig. 3a) with the same magnetic field vector at each position.

Using the symmetric setup, one aims to generate homogeneous magnetic fields. With this intent, the coil pairs are applied in Maxwell configuration and Helmholtz configuration respectively. The magnetic fields generated by the Maxwell coil pair cancel out each other in the center of the setup. To move the FFP, the drive field is generated by superimposing a current on these coils such that they operate in Helmholtz configuration (Fig. 3b). Due to the coil geometry itself, complete field homogeneity cannot be achieved. The field geometry is derogated, which is more pronounced when leaving the center of the setup.

To generate a selection field using a single-sided setup, static currents are applied in opposite directions to two concentrically mounted coils. The resulting magnetic field and its spatial gradient are strongly inhomogeneous. The FFP can simply be moved by superimposing an alternating current on at least one of both coils. Here, the inner coil is used for this drive field generation (Fig. 3c).

When dealing with inhomogeneous fields in MPI, it is required not only to consider the geometry of the selection and the drive field separately but rather their combination. During one excitation period, the FFP moves to positions $x_{FFP}(t)$ in space. To investigate the achievable resolution at each position x_{FFP}, it is required to measure or simulate the field gradient $G(x_{FFP})$, which is the gradient of the resulting field at this very position and time.

3. RESULTS

Fig. 4 shows simulation results of the selection field $B(x)$ and $G(x_{FFP})$ for the two named coil geometries along the coil axes. For the symmetrical setup, $G(x_{FFP})$ varies barely, whereas it drops to about 0.75 of the mean value at 14 mm in front of the single-sided coil setup.

According to Eq. 2, this directly translates to the achievable resolution in each position x_{FFP}. For this reason, the resolution distribution is almost homogeneous for the symmetrical setup and strongly inhomogeneous for the single-sided setup.
To prove the latter case, measurement data is evaluated by means of the FWHM, which is a measure of the image resolution[2]. A dot phantom is scanned at different distances to the scanner front (Fig. 5). The FWHM is applied to the left dot in the image series (Fig. 6). As expected from the simulation results in Fig. 4 and Eq. 2, the resolution is best directly in front of the scanner device and decreases with larger distances.

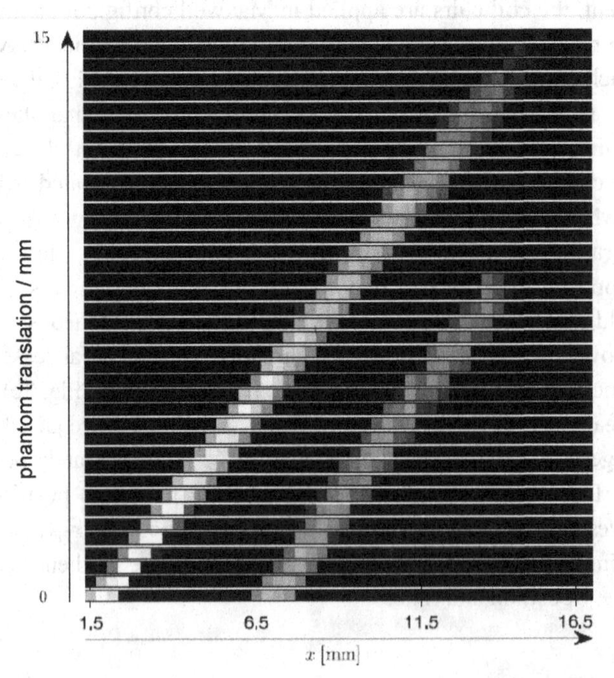

Fig. 5. Reconstructed measurement results. 2-dot phantom shifted to different positions and imaged with the single-sided setup.

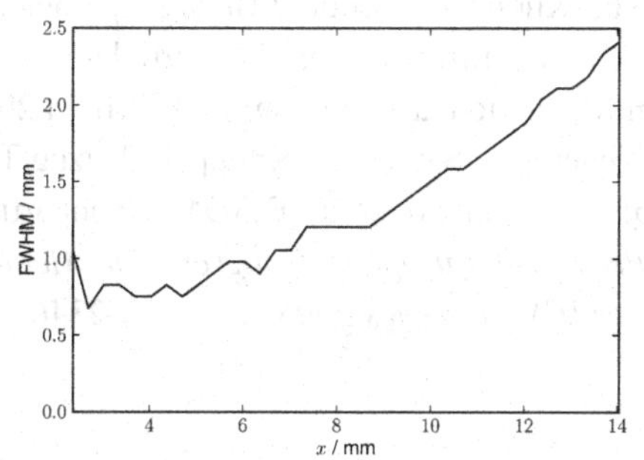

Fig. 6. FWHM depending on the position, evaluated at the left dot of the reconstructed 1D-images in Fig. 5.

4. DISCUSSION

As stated in Rahmer et al. and proven in the previous chapter, the achievable resolution in MPI is constrained by field gradient strength.[3] We investigated the spatial dependency of the magnetic field gradient when steering the FFP to different positions. For symmetrical setups, an almost position-independent image resolution can be achieved within a certain FOV. One aspect of magnetic field geometry optimization for MPI in general is to provide a homogeneous resolution all over the FOV. However, using single-sided coil setups, this is a challenging task. Using the basic coil setup, this can hardly be fulfilled. Here, only the inner coil was used to apply the drive field. Image resolution homogeneity might be improved by generating the drive field using both coils and adjusting the amplitude and relative phase of the applied currents. To obtain most information from the measured data with nominal inhomogeneous resolution, it is necessary to apply position-dependent regularization during the reconstruction process.

REFERENCES

1 Gleich B, Weizenecker J. Tomographic imaging using the nonlinear response of magnetic particles. *Nature* 2005; **435(7046)**: 1214-1217.

2 Sattel T, Knopp T, Biederer S, Gleich B, Weizenecker J, Borgert J, Buzug TM. Single-sided device for magnetic particle imaging. *Journal of Physics D: Applied Physics 2009*; **42(1)**: 1-5.

3 Weizenecker J, Borgert J and Gleich B. A simulation study on the resolution and sensitivity of magnetic particle imaging, *Phys. Med. Biol 2007*; **52**: 6363-6374

4 Rahmer J, Weizenecker J, Gleich B and Borgert J. Signal encoding in magnetic particle imaging *BMC Med. Imaging.* 2009 **9** 4.

5 Biederer S, Sattel TF, Knopp T, Lüdtke-Buzug K, Gleich B, Weizenecker J, Borgert J, Buzug TM, The Influence of the Particle-Size Distribution on the Image Resolution in Magnetic Particle Imaging, ESMRM 2009
6 Lüdtke-Buzug K, Biederer S, Sattel TF, Knopp T, Buzug TM, Preparation and Characterization of Dextran-Covered Fe3O4 Nanoparticles for Magnetic Particle Imaging, *Proc. 4th European Congress for Medical and Biomedical Engineering, Springer IFMBE Series 2008*; **22**: 2343-2346.

THE EFFECT OF RELAXATION ON MAGNETIC PARTICLE IMAGING

YONG WU, ZHEN YAO, GARETH KAFKA, DAVID FARRELL, MARK GRISWOLD, ROBERT BROWN

MG is in the *Department of Radiology;* all others are in the *Department of Physics*
Case Western Reserve University, 10900 Euclid Avenue,
Cleveland, OH, 44106, USA

In Magnetic Particle Imaging, resolution and SNR are highly dependent on, and grow with, the particles' size. In this paper, we study the fact that the magnetization relaxation time, also depends sensitively on particle diameter. Analytical derivations and simulations of the effects of response time are carried out and a trade-off between sensitivity and resolution is discussed.

1. INTRODUCTION

Magnetic particle imaging (MPI) is a new tomographic method [1] based on the nonlinear response of superparamagnetic iron oxide (SPIO) nanoparticles. It has promise for fast imaging with certain advantages in resolution, sensitivity, contrast, and cost. A static but spatially inhomogeneous field (selection field) and homogeneous oscillating field (drive field) are applied for spatial encoding. The selection field has a very strong gradient in order to saturate the nanoparticle domains outside the field-free-point (FFP). The oscillating drive fields can move the FFP around the whole field of view by using different driving frequencies in different directions. Only the FFP region yields a detectable signal. The average magnetization has been assumed to respond immediately to changes in the applied field [1-8]. However, delays due to magnetization relaxation lead to limitations on the response time and it is the purpose of the present paper to augment previous simulations [2, 3] by taking into account relaxation time effects.

2. THEORY

2.1. The MPI Signal from SPIO Nanoparticles

The voltage signal induced in a receive coil with uniform and normalized sensitivity can be written as

$$V(t) = -\mu_0 \int_{FOV} s(\vec{r},t)d\vec{r}\,, \tag{1}$$

where $s(\vec{r},t) = -\,d\vec{M}(\vec{r},t)/dt$ with $\vec{M}(\vec{r},t)$, the magnetization. The higher harmonics $S_n (n \geq 2)$ are obtained by the Fourier transform of $s(\vec{r},t)$.

The magnetized particle equilibrium (temperature T) distribution is given by the Langevin equation [9] $M_L(\xi) = M_0(\coth(\xi) - 1/\xi)$ where M_0 is the saturation magnetization and $\xi = \mu_0 mH / k_B T$ with particle magnetic moment m and external field H.

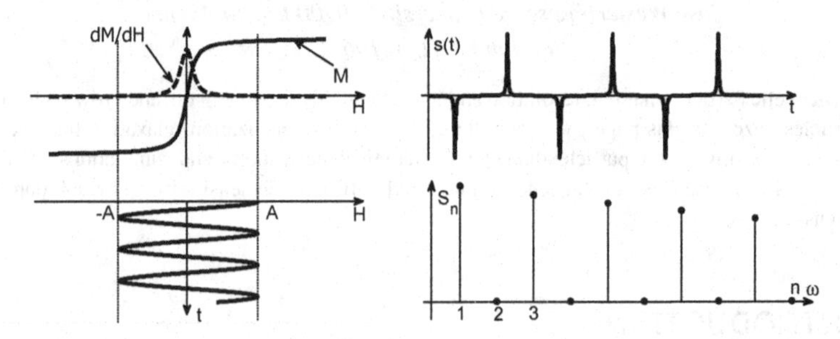

Fig. 1. Illustration of MPI signal. M(H) is the Langevin magnetization, s(t) = dM(H(t))/dt, S_n is the Fourier transform of s(t). ω is the drive-field frequency.

With a harmonic external field, the typical shape of $M_L(\xi)$, the signal $s(\vec{r},t)$, and the corresponding S_n are plotted in Fig. 1. Sufficiently large amplitudes for the higher-order harmonics, such as the example shown in the figure, facilitate our ability to find the inverse Fourier transform of (1).

2.2. Relaxation Time of SPIO Ferrofluids

In much of the early MPI modeling the time dependence of the magnetization response to the changes in the external magnetic fields has been ignored. Therefore, the time dependence of this response is the principal focus of this paper. Generally speaking, there are two major relaxation mechanisms in magnetic fluids when no interaction between the particles is considered [10]. The first one assumes the particles are magnetically hard, which means the direction of the magnetic moment is fixed compared to the particles' crystal structure. In this case, the viscous rotation, or Brownian relaxation, of the whole particle determines the relaxation time $\tau_B = 3V\eta / k_B T$ where V is the volume of the particle and η is the dynamic viscosity of the liquid. The other kind of relaxation stems from the change of the magnetic moment inside the particles. It takes place if the thermal energy is large enough to climb an energy barrier between two different states. The additional state arises from the anisotropic nature of the particle crystal structure. This response is called magnetically weak with Neel relaxation time, $\tau_N = \tau_0 \exp(KV / k_B T)$. Here, K is an anisotropy constant and τ_0 is a time constant on the order of 10^{-9}s for usual SPIO ferrofluids. The effective relaxation time τ is the combination of the Neel and Brownian relaxation times, $\tau^{-1} = \tau_B^{-1} + \tau_N^{-1}$.

Comparing these, we can see that the Neel relaxation time is much more sensitive to the volume of the particles than the Brownian relaxation time. The Neel relaxation time is very large and on the order of hundreds of seconds when the diameter of the particles is about 30nm, or larger, at room temperature. If the nanoparticles of principal interest in MPI have a diameter in the neighborhood of 20 nm, then the Brownian response dominates and it is assumed that $\tau \simeq \tau_B$. That is, the critical diameter for transition from Neel to Brownian relaxation is about 13 nm [10]. The field dependent dynamics equation for Brownian-dominated relaxation has the Bloch form

$$d\vec{M} / dt = \vec{S} \times \vec{M} / I - (\vec{M} - \vec{M}_L(\xi)) / \tau_B \tag{2}$$

where $\vec{S}$ (I) is the angular momentum (inertia) volume density. The precession term in (2) can be ignored for the range of particle sizes considered.

2.3. 1D Ideal Particles

The derivative of the Langevin magnetization to the magnetic field shown in Fig. 1 is nearly a delta function, which is the "ideal" case. For 1D ideal particles without relaxation, J. Rahmer et al. [8] show that the mathematical form of the signal S_n under a harmonic driving field is

$$S_n = -4M_0 iU_{n-1}(Gx / A)\sqrt{1-(Gx / A)^2} / T_H . \tag{3}$$

Here, T_H is the period of the driving field, U_{n-1} is the second-kind Chebyshev polynomial, G is the gradient of the selection field and A is the amplitude of the driving field.

Solving (2) for the case where the relaxation time is smaller than the duration time of the measurement (usually of the order of ms), we find the steady state shown in Fig. 2. Generalizing the analysis of 1D ideal particles, we have derived (in the Appendix) the mathematical form of S_n

$$S_n = -\frac{(-1+\exp(2\,i\,n\,\arccos(Gx/A)))M_0\omega}{\pi(1+i\,n\,\tau_B\,\omega)}. \tag{4}$$

As a comparison, the first few harmonics at $x = 0$ are plotted in Fig. 3. In a comparison with the uniform amplitudes of the harmonics without relaxation, the signal vanishes rather faster when relaxation is taken into account. The decrease of signal will reduce the SNR and thus blur the image and lower the resolution. For the more realistic Langevin equilibrium magnetization, the numerical results are simulated with, and without, relaxation; see Fig. 3.

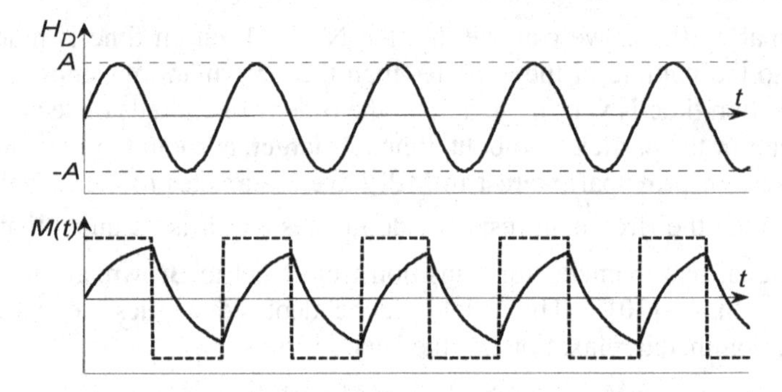

Fig. 2. Steady state of ideal particles. The upper figure is the harmonic field where x = 0, the dashed line in the lower figure is the magnetization curve of ideal particles. The solid line is the simulated magnetization curve of ideal particles, but now including relaxation. The relaxation time is chosen to be 2.5 times the period of the harmonic field, for comparison with the other simulations of this paper.

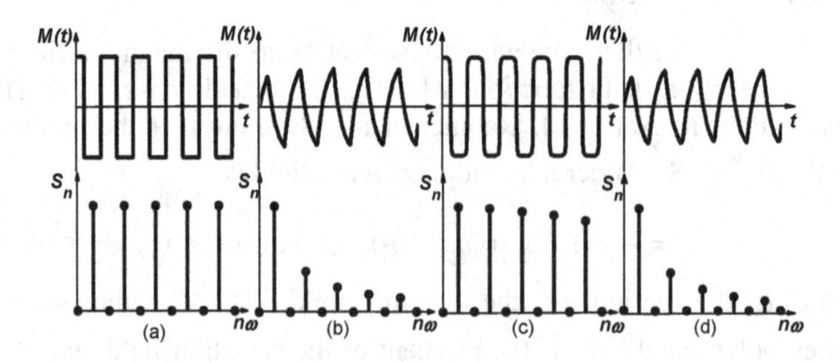

Fig. 3. Magnetization response M(t) and signal strength S_n for (a) ideal particles without relaxation, (b) ideal particles with relaxation, (c) realistic particles without relaxation, and (d) realistic particles with relaxation. (a) and (b) are calculated using (7) and (8), (c) and (d) are numerical solutions. The relaxation times for (b) and (d) are all set to be 10^{-5} s. The signal S_n is normalized by S_1.

3. SIMULATION

A slice with 3D dimensions of 1mm × 32mm × 16mm is used as the phantom. The 2D are divided into a 64 × 32 matrix so each pixel is 1mm × 0.5mm × 0.5mm. A sufficiently large Maxwell coil pair is assumed along the y-axis, which provides two selection fields with gradients of 1.25 mT/mm μ_0^{-1} in the y-direction and 2.5 mT/mm μ_0^{-1} in the z-direction, respectively. The two corresponding drive fields have the same amplitude of 20 mT μ_0^{-1} and different frequencies of 25.51 kHz and 25.25 kHz separately, as in [2]. The total duration of the scan is 3.88 ms and the sample frequency is 2.5 MHz. Two receiving coils with uniform sensitivities are oriented with y-direction and z-direction axes, respectively, and lead to a sum-of-squares signal. In the original simulation [2], the sensitivity, and hence the resolution, was seen to be significantly improved by considering larger diameters in the 30-50 nm range. We turn now to the change due to relaxation.

4. RESULTS AND DISCUSSION

With the increase in the total relaxation time, which is dominated by τ_B, the SNR and spatial resolution drop dramatically. And the relaxation time varies from 10^{-6} s to 10^{-4} s, as the diameter of the particles is changed from 10 to 50 nm. The 50-nm particles, which by simulation have the best spatial resolution with no relaxation, actually give a significantly poorer quality image when relaxation modeling is included. Fig. 4 shows the pattern used in [1], which could also stand for Physics, for different relaxation times corresponding to different diameters, as indicated in the caption. It is seen that larger particles lead to relaxation blurring; smaller particles lead to poorer resolution with some optimal size between. The underlying physical principle is when the FFP is moved to a previously saturated point, the particles at the original or final FFP do not respond quickly enough to the change at the frequency of the driving field f_0 if $1/\tau_B$ is much smaller than f_0. The signal from the final point will be reduced by the factor of $1/\tau_B$ and the signal surviving from the original point will blur the image. From our simulation results, we find that images from large particles provide high spatial resolution but are badly blurred by the relaxation time. While a growing number of interesting experimental results and theoretical studies already have been found for MPI [1-8], we conclude that relaxation should be taken into account in modeling, especially for a reliable interpretation of which particle size is dominating the imaging signal. Note added in proof: see [11] and a corresponding contribution to this workshop.

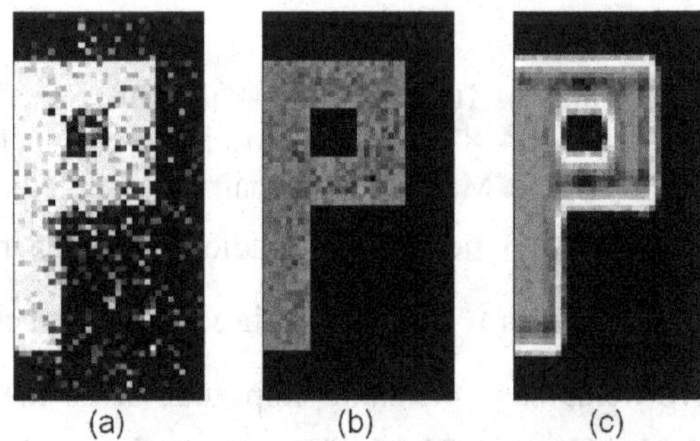

Fig. 4. MPI results of (a) 50 nm particles with relaxation time of 10^{-4} s, (b) 25 nm particles with relaxation time, $1.25 \cdot 10^{-5}$ s, and (c) 10 nm particles with relaxation time, $0.8 \cdot 10^{-6}$ s.

Appendix: Relaxation Theory of 1D Ideal Particles

As shown in Fig. 2, the magnetization reaches a steady state after several periods, and its analytic form is our immediate goal. As illustrated in Fig. 5, we assume the magnetization just before the period t_{n-1} and t_n is $M^-(t_{n-1})$, while the magnetization at the end of this period is $M^-(t_n)$. With saturation magnetization M_0 for ideal particles, we find

$$M(t)=\begin{cases} M_0\,\mathrm{sgn}(H(t))+\left[M^-(t_{n-1})-M_0\,\mathrm{sgn}(H(t))\right]e^{-(t-t_{n-1})/\tau_B} & t_{n-1}\le t<t_{n-1}+t' \\ M_0\,\mathrm{sgn}(H(t))+\left[M(t_{n-1}+t')-M_0\,\mathrm{sgn}(H(t))\right]e^{-(t-t_{n-1}-t')/\tau_B} & t_{n-1}+t'\le t<t_n \end{cases}$$

where $M(t_{n-1}+t')$ is the magnetization after the external field changes its sign. Since the steady state condition is $M^-(t_{n-1}) = M^-(t_n) = M'$, we obtain

$$M(t_{n-1}+t') = M_0 + (M'-M_0)e^{-t'/\tau_B}$$

$$M^-(t_n) = -M_0 + \left[M(t_{n-1}+t') + M_0\right]e^{-(t_n-t_{n-1}-t')/\tau_B}$$

and $M' = M_0(2e^{-(T_H-t')/\tau_B} - e^{-T_H/\tau_B} - 1)/(1-e^{-T_H/\tau_B})$. Here, T_H is the period of the driving field. For $t_{n-1} \le t < t_{n-1}+t'$, the corresponding signal is

$$s(t) = 2M_0\delta(H)\frac{\partial H}{\partial t} + \left[M'-M_0\,\mathrm{sgn}(H(t))\right]\left(-\frac{1}{\tau_B}\right)e^{-(t-t_{n-1})/\tau_B} - 2M_0\delta(H)\frac{\partial H}{\partial t}e^{-(t-t_{n-1})/\tau_B}$$

and, for $t_{n-1}+t' \le t < t_n$, it is

$$s(t) = 2M_0\delta(H)\frac{\partial H}{\partial t} + \left[M(t_{n-1}+t')-M_0\,\mathrm{sgn}(H(t))\right]\left(-\frac{1}{\tau_B}\right)e^{-(t-t_{n-1})/\tau_B} - 2M_0\delta(H)\frac{\partial H}{\partial t}e^{-(t-t_{n-1}-t')/\tau_B}$$

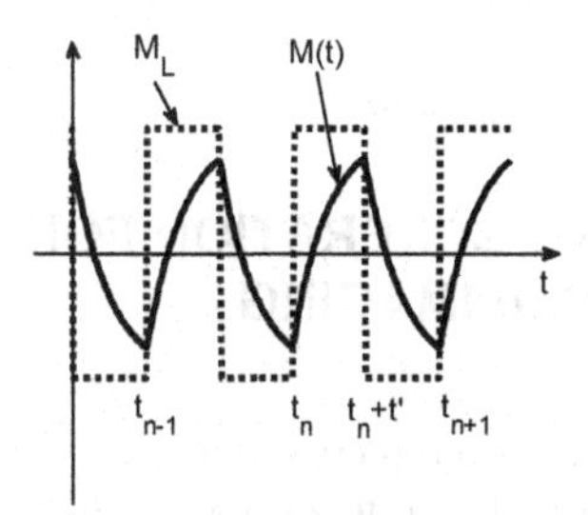

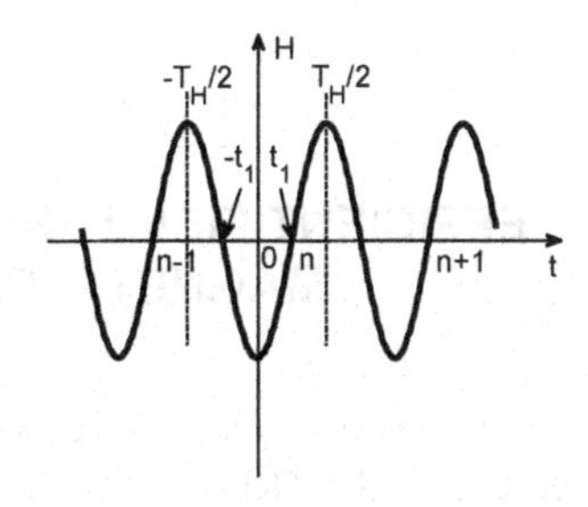

Fig. 5. The steady-state magnetization and its seminal field. The time span between t_n and t_{n+1} is the period of the steady state; $t_n + t'$ is the time when the magnetic field changes sign during this period. The origin of the time axis is chosen to be the lowest point of the external field during the period t_{n-1} and t_n, so the two zero points of the field during the integration region $-T_H/2$ and $T_H/2$ will be symmetric.

If we reset the time origin and switch the integration region in the transform, as shown in Fig. 5, in order to ensure the symmetry of the integration region, the four terms with $\delta(H)\,\partial H / \partial t$ inside will cancel each other. The integration of the remaining two terms gives us the explicit and simple result (4).

REFERENCES

1 Gleich B, Weizenecker J. Tomographic imaging using the nonlinear response of magnetic particles. *Nature* 2005; **435**:1214–1217.
2 Weizenecker J et al. A simulation study on the resolution and sensitivity of magnetic particle imaging. *Phys Med Biol* 2007; **52**:6363–6374.
3 Knopp T et al. Trajectory analysis for magnetic particle imaging. Phys Med Bio 2009; 54:385–379.
4 Weizenecker J, Gleich B, Borgert J. Magnetic particle imaging using a field free line. *J Phys D* 2008; **41**:105009.
5 Gleich B et al. Experimental results on fast 2D-encoded magnetic particle imaging. *Phys Med Biol* 2008; **53**:N81–N84.
6 Goodwill PG et al. Narrowband Magnetic Particle Imaging. *IEEE Transactions On Medical Imaging* 2009; **28**:1231–1237
7 Weizenecker J et al. Three-dimensional real-time in vivo magnetic particle imaging. *Phys Med Biol* 2009; **54**:L1–L10
8 Rahmer J et al. Signal encoding in magnetic particle imaging: properties of the system function. *BMC Medical Imaging* 2009; **9**:4
9 Rosensweig RE. Ferrohydrodynamics. *Cambridge Univ. Press* 1985.
10 Odenbach S. Magnetoviscous Effects in Ferrofluids, *Springer* 2002.
11 Ferguson R et al. Optimization of nanoparticle core size for magnetic particle imaging. *J Magnetism and Mag. Mat.* 2009; **321**:1548-1551.

EFFICIENT FIELD-FREE LINE GENERATION FOR MAGNETIC PARTICLE IMAGING

TOBIAS KNOPP, SVEN BIEDERER, TIMO F. SATTEL,
KERSTIN LÜDTKE-BUZUG, MARLITT ERBE, THORSTEN M. BUZUG

Institute of Medical Engineering, University of Lübeck,
Lübeck, 23538, Lübeck
Email: {knopp,buzug}@imt.uni-luebeck.de

Signal encoding in magnetic particle imaging is accomplished by moving a field-free point (FFP) through the region of interest. Due to saturation effects, only the particles in a certain region around the FFP contribute to the measurement signals induced in receive coils. The sensitivity of MPI depends on the gradient strength of the FFP field. Recently, a new signal encoding scheme was proposed, which has the potential to significantly increase the sensitivity of the method by taking advantage of a field-free line (FFL). However, the proposed coil assembly used to generate the FFL was unfeasible in practice due to high electrical power losses. In this work, we show that the efficiency of the setup can be considerably improved by reducing the number of coils.

1. INTRODUCTION

The quantitative imaging method magnetic particle imaging (MPI) is capable of determining the spatial distribution of superparamagnetic nanoparticles (SPIO) at high temporal and spatial resolution.[1] The method takes advantage of a magnetic gradient field featuring a field-free point (FFP). The gradient field is superimposed by a dynamic drive field, which is responsible for moving the FFP in space. As the particle magnetization reaches saturation even for low field strength, only a small number of particles in the close vicinity of the FFP contributes to the measurement signal.

Recently, it has been shown that the sensitivity of MPI could be considerably increased using a simultaneous acquisition scheme in the form of a field-free line (FFL).[2] In Fig. 1, both the FFP and the FFL field are shown for comparison. For imaging the distribution of the nanoparticles, the FFL is rapidly moved back and forth while rotating slowly.[2] This acquisition scheme essentially samples the particle distribution in Radon space,[3] which allows for reconstruction by efficient algorithms, like for instance the filtered back projection.[4] In order to realize the

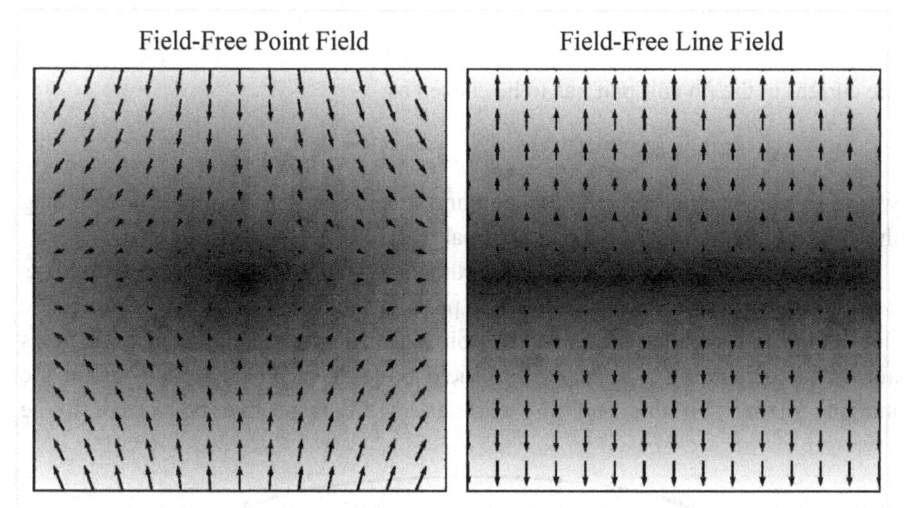

Fig. 1: Comparison of the FFP field (left) and the FFL field (right). Shown is a slice through the origin. Black indicates zero field strength whereas white indicates high field strength.

FFL encoding scheme, the coil assembly used to generate the magnetic field must be capable of rotating and translating the FFL.

Although it was shown in Ref. 2 that FFL imaging is significantly more sensitive than FFP imaging, Weizenecker *et al.* questioned the practicability of the method.[2] Their skepticism originated from the fact that the used coil assembly had a considerably higher electrical power loss than an FFP scanner of comparable size and gradient strength. In this work, it is shown, that practical implementations of the FFL become feasible by reducing the number of coils.

2. COIL ASSEMBLY

The initially proposed coil assembly capable of rotating a magnetic FFL consists of 32 small coils, which are positioned at equidistant angles on a circle.[2] A sketch of the setup is shown in Fig. 2. The clear space of the scanner is determined by the circle diameter d_{circle}. To generate an FFL, the currents are chosen in such a way that two opposing coils have the same current flowing in converse direction. Thus, both coils form a Maxwell coil pair such that the complete setup consists of $L = 16$ Maxwell coil pairs. The currents consist of a static and a dynamic part. The latter depends on the desired FFL direction and is varied to perform an FFL rotation. To establish an FFL along direction

$$\mathbf{d}_{\mathrm{FFL}}^{\alpha} = (\cos(\alpha),\ \sin(\alpha),\ 0)^{\mathrm{T}}, \tag{1}$$

the current in the lth coil pair has to be chosen as

$$I_l(\alpha) = A\left(\tfrac{3}{2} - \cos(2\varphi_l - 2\alpha)\right), \tag{2}$$

where φ_l is the angle of the lth coil pair and A is the current amplitude determining the gradient strength of the field orthogonal to the FFL.

For translating the FFL, two large orthogonal Helmholtz coil pairs are used, as is illustrated in Fig. 2. Each of the coil pairs generates a homogeneous magnetic field along the symmetry axis of the coil pair. The superposition of both fields allows for generating a homogeneous field pointing in any direction within the imaging plane.[2] To this end, the currents in the respective coils have to be

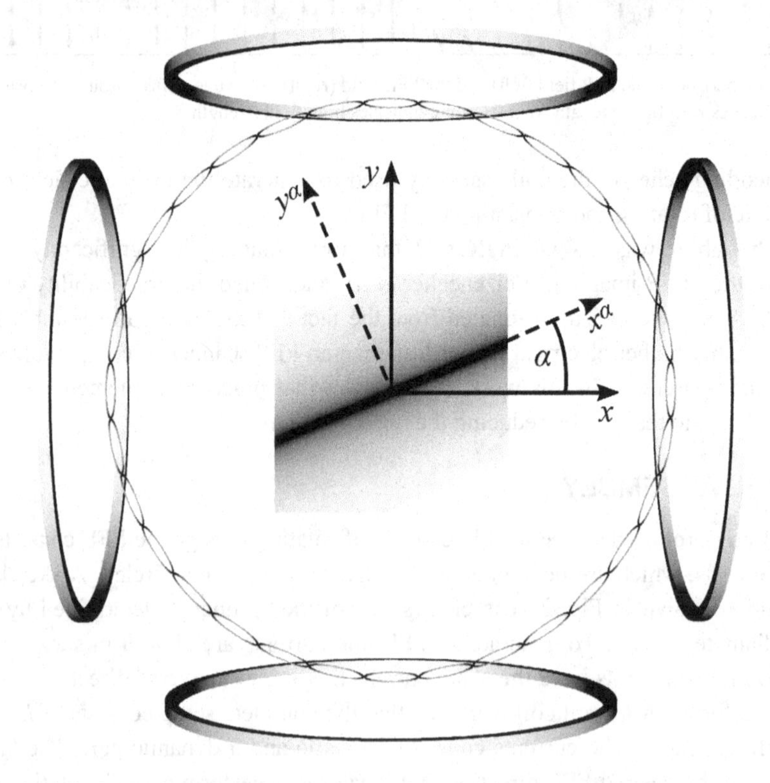

Fig. 2: Coil setup for generation and translation of a magnetic FFL. 32 small coils are positioned at equidistant angles on a circle enclosing the clear space of the setup. Each pair of opposing coils is arranged in Maxwell configuration with current flowing in converse direction. Using appropriate currents (2), these coils generate a rotating FFL. Two large Helmholtz coil pairs are responsible for FFL translation.

Table 1. Relative power loss of the FFL coil setup compared to that of the FFP setup for different Maxwell coil pair numbers L.

L	3	4	8	16
$P_{\mathrm{FFL}}^{L} / P_{\mathrm{FFL}}$	3.1	6.5	70.7	1026.8

appropriately chosen. To translate the FFL, the direction of the translation field is adjusted to point in the direction orthogonal to the FFL. Then, by applying a sinusoidal current, the FFL moves back and forth.

Using 32 small coils for generation and rotation of the FFL leads to high currents and in turn high electrical power losses. Therefore, in this work, it is proposed to reduce the number of coils used to generate the FFL. Obviously, this leads to lower electrical power consumption. However, the question remains, whether the field quality degrades by using a fewer number of coils. In this work, this question is investigated in a simulation study.

3. SIMULATION

The electrical power loss of FFL coil assemblies for different coil pair numbers L = 3, 4, 8, 16 is determined using magnetic field simulations.[5] For simplicity, the translation field is neglected in this work. The coils have a diameter such that they can be placed on a circle of diameter d_{circle} without intersection, i.e.

$$d_L = d_{\mathrm{circle}} \tan \frac{\pi}{2L}. \tag{3}$$

The circle diameter is chosen as $d_{\mathrm{circle}} = 0.5$ m. The current parameter A is adapted such that the gradient strength orthogonal to the FFL is 1.0 $\mathrm{Tm}^{-1}\mu_0^{-1}$.

The electrical power loss of the setup is compared to that of an FFP scanner of equal size and gradient strength. In Tab. 1 the relative electrical power loss is listed for different L. As can be seen, the electrical power loss considerably increases with the number of coils. For L = 3, the electrical power loss of the FFL setup is only three times higher than that of an FFP scanner.

Next, the quality of the generated field is assessed for different coil pair numbers L. In Fig. 3, the generated field along the FFL is shown. The angle α is chosen such that the worst field quality for a certain L is obtained. We have found

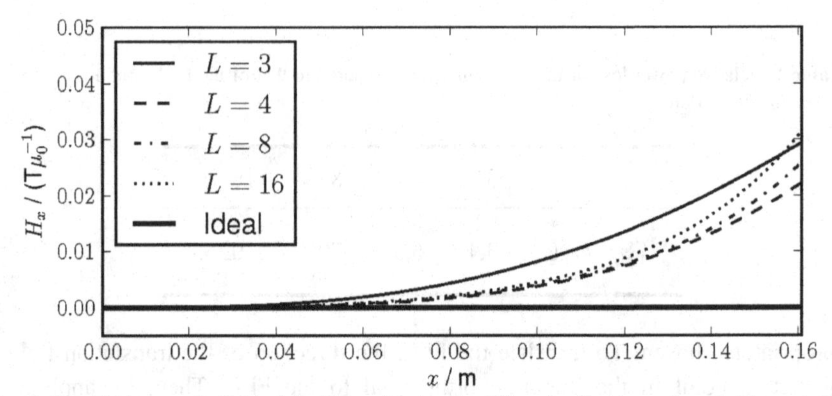

Fig. 3: Simulated magnetic field of the FFL coil setup for different coil pair numbers L. Shown is the field along the FFL.

that this is the case when the FFL is located in-between the symmetry axes of two subsequent coils, i.e.

$$\alpha_L = \frac{\pi}{2L}. \tag{4}$$

As can be seen in Fig. 2, the field along the FFL is significantly better when using less than 16 Maxwell coil pairs. Overall, the best field is obtained for $L = 4$.

4. CONCLUSION

In the present work, the efficiency of the FFL coil geometry initially proposed by Weizenecker et al. was investigated for different numbers of Maxwell coil pairs. In conclusion, the efficiency of the FFL coil geometry is considerably improved when using fewer than $L = 16$ coil pairs, which were proposed in Ref. 2. Regarding the minimum electrical power loss, $L = 3$ Maxwell coil pairs were found to be optimal. However, regarding the field quality, $L = 4$ Maxwell coil pairs generated the FFL with the lowest deviation to an ideal FFL.

ACKNOWLEDGMENTS

We thank B. Gleich, J. Weizenecker, J. Borgert and J. Rahmer for numerous fruitful discussions about field-free line imaging and magnetic particle imaging in general.

REFERENCES

1 Gleich B, Weizenecker J. Tomographic imaging using the nonlinear response of magnetic particles. *Nature* 2005; **435(7046)**: 1214–1217.

2 Weizenecker J, Gleich B, Borgert J. Magnetic particle imaging using a field free line . *Journal of Physics D: Applied Physics 2008*; **41(10)**: 1–3.
3 Radon J. Über die Bestimmung von Funktionen durch Ihre Integralwerte längs gewisser Mannigfaltigkeiten. *Berichte der Sächsischen Akadamie der Wissenschaft 1917*; **69**: 262–277.
4 Bracewell RN. Strip integration in radio astronomy. *Aust. J. Phys 1956*; **9**: 198–217.
5 Jackson JD. *Classical Electrodynamics*, New York: Wiley, 1999.

3D REAL-TIME MAGNETIC PARTICLE IMAGING: ENCODING AND RECONSTRUCTION ASPECTS

JÜRGEN RAHMER, BERNHARD GLEICH, JÖRN BORGERT

Philips Technologie GmbH, Forschungslaboratorien
Röntgenstraße 24-26, 22315 Hamburg, Germany
Email: juergen.rahmer@philips.com

JÜRGEN WEIZENECKER

Fakultät für Elektro- und Informationstechnik,
University of Applied Sciences, 76133 Karlsruhe, Germany

3D real-time magnetic particle imaging (MPI) requires rapid encoding and parallel acquisition of a large amount of information. This paper describes the signal response generated in recently published real-time *in vivo* MPI measurements, the signal processing steps, and solution of the inverse reconstruction problem. It is shown that the acquired MPI signal contains enough information for rapid encoding of 3D volumes.

1. INTRODUCTION

Any imaging technique has to collect sufficient information for reliable image reconstruction. In MPI, different approaches can be taken to generate and acquire this information[1]. One approach is to acquire information mainly in the spatial domain by measuring the MPI response of an object at many spatial positions covering the field of view. Knowing the response of a delta probe, an image can be obtained from a single frequency component by deconvolution of the delta kernel from the object measurement. In practice, several frequency components will be combined to improve SNR and resolution[1,2]. While this approach can lead to excellent image SNR and resolution, it is rather slow due to the need to measure at many spatial positions, which have to be reached either by moving the object or by applying offset fields.

Another approach is to collect object information only in frequency space. In this case, the range of the field-free point (FFP) motion has to be large enough to generate signal in the total volume of interest. A large number of signal-containing frequency components has to be generated and acquired. This approach is realized in our current scanner. Signal generation is achieved by applying three orthogonal drive fields at slightly different frequencies, from which the nanoparticles generate a wealth of harmonics and mix products. Most of these frequency components encode different spatial information. Combined with broad-band detection to enable fully parallel acquisition of this information, this approach allows very rapid imaging. It is comparable to frequency encoding in MRI, where a single readout allows full 1D encoding. The MPI approach, however, encodes in 3D.

2. SETUP AND IMAGING SEQUENCE

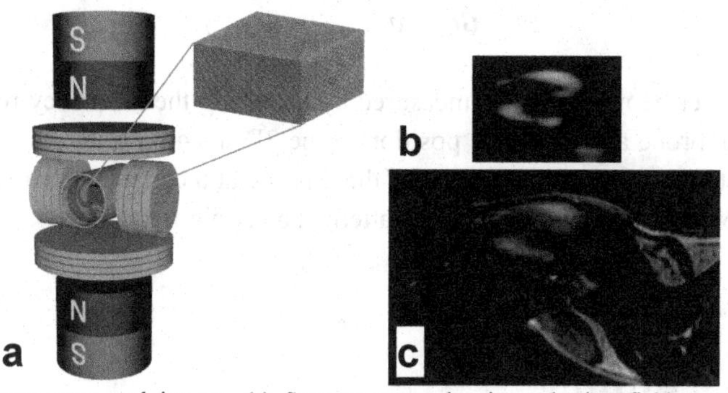

Fig. 1. Scanner setup and images. (a) Scanner setup showing selection field permanent magnets (red/green), drive field coils (green) and receive coils (blue). The blue box is an enlarged view of the region covered by the trajectory of the FFP. (b) Sagittal slice of a 3D volume extracted from a video sequence of a mouse brain. (c) Overlay of MPI data (orange) on reference MRI measurement.

Fig. 1a shows the scanner setup used in real-time *in vivo* measurements[3]. Fig. 1b,c shows images of a mouse brain measurement acquired after tail vein injection of Resovist at a dosage of 56 μmol(Fe)/kg. Three sets of drive field coils are driven at frequencies f_{0x} = 25.25 kHz, f_{0y} = 26.04 kHz, and f_{0z} = 24.51 kHz to move the FFP in a dense 3D Lissajous-type trajectory (cf. Fig. 1a). The employed frequency ratios lead to a repetition time of the applied field sequence of 21.5 ms, corresponding to an imaging rate of 46.4 volumes per second. With a selection field gradient of 5.5 T/m/μ_0 in the vertical direction and half of this value in the orthogonal directions as well as drive field amplitudes of 18 mT/μ_0, the FFP motion covers a region of 13.1 × 6.5 × 13.1 mm^3. Since signal is also generated at a certain distance to the FFP[5], data was reconstructed to a larger grid with extension 20.4 × 12 × 16.8 mm^3 and isotropic voxel size (0.6 mm)^3.

3. SIGNAL SPECTRUM AND SPECTRAL SELECTION

Signal from three sets of receive coils was sampled at 20 MS/s and Fourier transformed. Due to limited sensitivity, signal only occurs in the frequency range up to 1 MHz, so that higher frequencies are discarded. Spectral resolution is 46.4 Hz, corresponding to the repetition time of the sequence.

The spectrum contains signal only at frequencies which are direct multiples of the drive frequencies or mix terms thereof. To select these relevant frequencies, the possible signal content at each frequency can be determined. This information is contained in the system function matrix $\boldsymbol{G}$, which describes, how a spatial particle distribution vector $\boldsymbol{c}$ is mapped to a frequency response vector $\boldsymbol{v}$ in the measurement process:

$$\boldsymbol{Gc} = \boldsymbol{v} \tag{1}$$

$\boldsymbol{G}$ can either be modelled[4] or measured by acquiring the frequency response of a small δ-like probe at each voxel position in the 3D imaging grid. A column of $\boldsymbol{G}$ corresponds to the frequency response of the δ probe at a certain spatial position. A row corresponds to the spatial response pattern at a certain frequency.

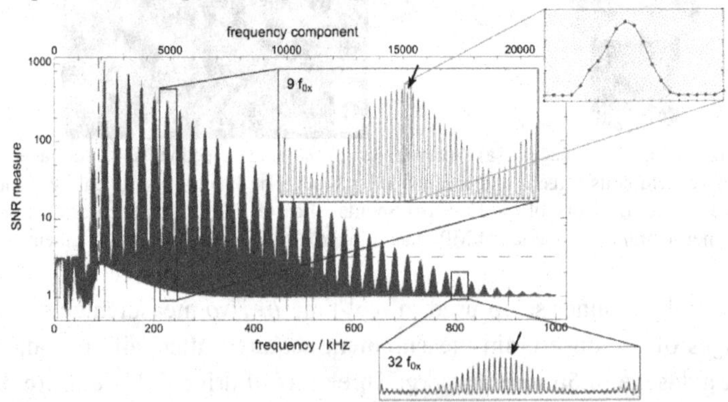

Fig. 2. SNR measure plotted versus frequency showing the information content at a certain frequency. Regions around the 9th and 32nd harmonic of the drive frequency are enlarged to reveal the sub-structure.

Signal-containing frequency components of the system function exhibit a spatial variation that can be quantified by calculating a variance measure. If this measure is determined for calibration scans with and without δ probe, their ratio gives an indication of the SNR encountered at a specific frequency. Fig. 2 shows a logarithmic plot of this SNR measure for the x channel of a system function acquired from a δ probe containing 200 nl of pure Resovist. Averaging time per scan position was 0.5 s. The broad peaks are centered at multiples of the x drive frequency f_{0x}. Peaks at 9 f_{0x} and 32 f_{0x} have been enlarged to reveal their substructure, which consists of smaller peaks with a spacing of about 740 Hz. This indicates that the corresponding frequencies relate to mix terms, e.g. with frequency $10 f_{0x} - f_{0z}$. The SNR measure can be used to select frequencies for reconstruction by applying a threshold, e.g. $\sqrt{10}$ as indicated by the dashed horizontal line in Fig. 2. Furthermore, due to a high noise level at low frequencies and close to the excitation band around 25 kHz, the lowest 1,900 frequencies are discarded, indicated by the dashed vertical line. For the x channel, this selection procedure yields 3,833 frequencies from a total of 1 MHz / 46.42 Hz = 21,542. A similar number can be selected from the y and z channel, so that about 10,000 frequencies are used for reconstructing 19,040 voxels. However, in a real-time *in vivo* measurement, the number of signal-containing frequencies in the object measurement vector $\boldsymbol{v}$ may be much smaller, since it depends on available SNR and object shape.

4. INFORMATION CONTENT OF SELECTED FREQUENCIES

Different frequency components encode different spatial information. This is indicated in Fig. 3a, where slices from the 3D patterns found at frequencies around $9 f_{0x}$ and $32 f_{0x}$ are shown, respectively. Obviously, the higher frequencies around 32 f_{0x} relate to finer spatial patterns. It can be shown that these patterns are related to tensor products of Chebyshev functions of the 2nd kind[5]. These functions form a basis set that satisfies an orthogonality relation. To reveal the relation between the spatial patterns encoded at different frequencies, their orthogonality has been calculated as the inner product of the normalized system function columns. The magnitude of the product of the first 600 selected frequencies is plotted as gray values in Fig. 3b. If all components were linearly independent, only the diagonal would be non zero. Obviously, there are linearly dependent components and thus some redundancy in the spatial information encoded at different frequencies, but the vast majority of scalar products is close to zero. On the one hand, redundancy requires acquisition of more frequency components than voxels, if full voxel resolution is to be encoded. On the other hand, it has the benefit that information from missing frequencies is not lost, but is still encoded at other frequencies. Therefore, one can expect that removal of the first 1,900 frequencies for excitation band suppression does not lead to a significant loss of image information.

From these considerations it follows, that after selection of frequencies, the inversion of Eqn. 1 is an underdetermined problem. This information mismatch can be handled using regularization. Since the current physical MPI resolution is lower than the voxel resolution anyway[3], regularization basically interpolates a low-resolution image to a high-resolution grid.

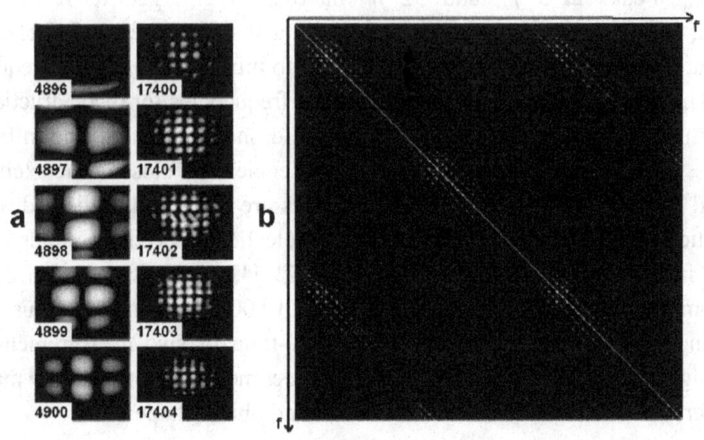

Fig. 3. System function components and orthogonality plot. (a) *xz* slices from 3D spatial pattern of frequency component with indicated number. The two columns correspond to components in the single peaks indicated by arrows in the SNR subspectra in Fig. 2. (b) Orthogonality plot between the first 600 selected frequencies. Aside from the main diagonal, only few non-zero components appear, showing good orthogonality of the basis function set.

5. RECONSTRUCTION

After selecting relevant signal components in the system function $\boldsymbol{G}$ and the object measurement vector $\boldsymbol{v}$, Eqn. 1 can be solved as the regularized least squares problem using the reduced quantities $\widetilde{\boldsymbol{G}}$ and $\widetilde{\boldsymbol{v}}$:

$$\text{minimize} \qquad \left\|\boldsymbol{W}\,(\widetilde{\boldsymbol{G}}\boldsymbol{c} - \widetilde{\boldsymbol{v}})\right\|^2 + \lambda\|\boldsymbol{c}\|^2 \qquad (2)$$

The regularization parameter λ allows balancing image SNR versus resolution. The matrix $\boldsymbol{W}$ has been introduced to allow weighting of frequency components, e.g. to increase resolution by putting more weight on components with fine spatial structure. To solve equation (2), a row-based iterative algorithm is applied[6] that allows the inclusion of a non-negativity constraint for the particle concentration image, i.e. $c_i > 0$. The MPI image shown in Fig. 1b was reconstructed using a weighting matrix $\boldsymbol{W}$ that applied the inverse of the SNR measure plotted in Fig. 2 to the respective frequency components.

6. CONCLUSION

Broadband detection with high sensitivity allows the parallel acquisition of sufficient information for 3D real-time magnetic particle imaging. One specific data processing approach used for reconstruction of *in vivo* data has been described here. However, systematic investigation of the effects of frequency component selection and weighting as well as their interplay with regularization and non-negativity constraints applied in reconstruction is necessary in the future and promises improved image quality in real-time MPI.

ACKNOWLEDGEMENT

This work was supported by the Germany Federal Ministry of Education and Research (BMBF) under the grant number FKZ 13N9079.

REFERENCES

1 Gleich B, Weizenecker J. Tomographic imaging using the nonlinear response of magnetic particles. *Nature.* 2005;**435**:1214-7.
2 Goodwill PW, Scott GC, Stang PP, Conolly SM. Narrowband magnetic particle imaging. *IEEE Trans Med Imaging.* 2009;**28**:1231-7.
3 Weizenecker J, Gleich B, Rahmer J, Dahnke H, Borgert J. Three-dimensional real-time in vivo magnetic particle imaging. *Phys Med Biol.* 2009;**54**:L1-L10.
4 Knopp T, Sattel TF, Biederer S, Rahmer J, Weizenecker J, *et al.* Model-based reconstruction for MPI. *IEEE Trans Med Imaging.* 2010;**29**:12-8.
5 Rahmer J, Weizenecker J, Gleich B, Borgert J. Signal encoding in MPI: properties of the system function. *BMC Med Imaging.* 2009;**9**:4.
6 Dax A. On row relaxation methods for large constrained least squares problems. *SIAM J. Sci. Comput.* 1993:**14**;570-584.

IMAGING TECHNOLOGY AND SAFETY ASPECTS

CONCEPT FOR A DIGITAL AMPLIFIER WITH HIGH QUALITY SINUSOIDAL OUTPUT VOLTAGE FOR MPI DRIVE FIELD COILS

CHRISTOPH LOEF[†] , PETER LUERKENS

Philips Research Laboratories Aachen
Weißhausstraße 2, 52066 Aachen, Germany
Email: christoph.loef(at)philips.com , peter.luerkens(at)philips.com

OLIVER WOYWODE

Philips Healthcare, GTC Development, Philips Medical Systems DMC GmbH
Röntgenstraße 24, 22335 Hamburg, Germany
oliver.woywode(at)philips.com

The purpose of this paper is to study the performance of a digital amplifier to supply the drive field coils of a magnetic particle image scanner with a high quality sinusoidal voltage. Available linear class A or AB amplifiers appear suitable for this application, but suffer from very high losses. Alternatively a digitally switched amplifier is proposed, which exhibits much lower losses. The characteristics of the analogue amplifier are compared to a PWM-controlled single-stage digital switching amplifier and to a solution with a multi-level inverter based topology. The characteristics of this concept are described in detail.

1. INTRODUCTION

Magnetic particle imaging (MPI) is a new method to acquire images of the interior of living bodies. It takes advantage of the magnetic non-linearity of nano-particles, incorporated in the subject. A variable external magnetic field (drive field) drives these particles in and out of saturation at defined spots in the examination volume. The change of the particles magnetization due to the external magnetic field is recorded by extremely sensitive receivers, typically on a harmonic frequency of the drive field. This requires a very high spectral purity of the drive field in order not to mask the response of the particles. The drive field is produced by exciting a coil, which can be treated electrically as an inductance with low parasitic resistance.

[†] This work is supported by grant 13N9079 of the German Federal Ministry of Education and Research.

2. ANALOGUE AMPLIFIERS

In a straight forward approach the supply unit is realized by means of a linear amplifier. In Fig. 1 a typical schematic of a linear class AB amplifier is given.

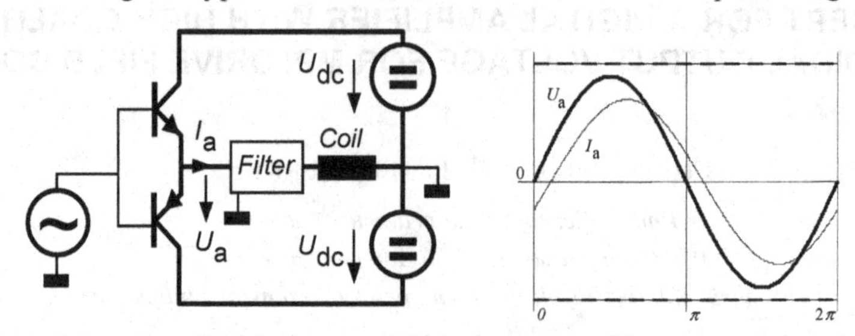

Fig. 1 : Schematic outline of a linear amplifier and typical amplifier output voltage and –current.

The amplifier consists of two transistors in a bridge configuration, which can be either bipolar or MOSFET-type transistors. The bridge output is connected via a filter to the drive field coil to reduce remaining harmonics. The transistors are controlled linearly, i.e. in a way, that the voltage drop across the transistors accounts exactly for the difference between desired output voltage and the supply voltage. Assuming sinusoidal waveform voltage and current, the maximum efficiency of an AB-type linear amplifier yields $\eta=\pi/4 \sim 78\%$, when the load power factor equals 1. As the load in this particular case is by nature a reactive load, this definition does not reflect the system characteristics in a realistic way, as there is typically very little real output power. Instead, the main output power component is reactive power.

Therefore it is more meaningful to define the required input power for a given output current. This quantity is constant for an ideal AB-class amplifier and yields $P_{in}=U_{dc} \cdot \hat{I}_{out} \cdot 2/\pi$ for sinusoidal output current. In case of almost pure reactive power, this is converted entirely into losses in the amplifier.

In a narrow-band system a filter or a match-box can be used to eliminate the reactive currents for a particular frequency, leaving only the active current component, which is required to compensate for losses in the drive coil and the filter. If the desired output frequency varies from the filter center frequency, again a relevant reactive current flow occurs which causes an increase of input power and thus, higher losses in the analogue amplifier. The amount of reactive current attenuation depends on the desired bandwidth and steepness of the filter. Practically, an attenuation of 10:1 cannot be exceeded with reasonable effort. This means, that even with an optimum filter or match-box, losses of up to 15% of the reactive power at the drive coil or 130% of the reactive power at the amplifier output have to be considered.

Due to the high demand of reactive power and the associated losses, especially under extended operating frequency range requirements, a linear amplifier is not a feasible option.

3. SWITCHED AMPLIFIERS

In contrast, switched mode amplifiers do not suffer from this effect and are able to cope with the high reactive power demand at low losses. Contrary to the analogue amplifier, digital amplifiers normally exhibit only two switching states: either the switching device is turned on or off. The output voltage is switched either to $+U_{dc}$ or to $-U_{dc}$. In either case, losses do not occur at the switching device. Though being lossless by principle, in reality current conduction losses occur at the power components, and, even more relevant, switching losses occur during change of switching states.

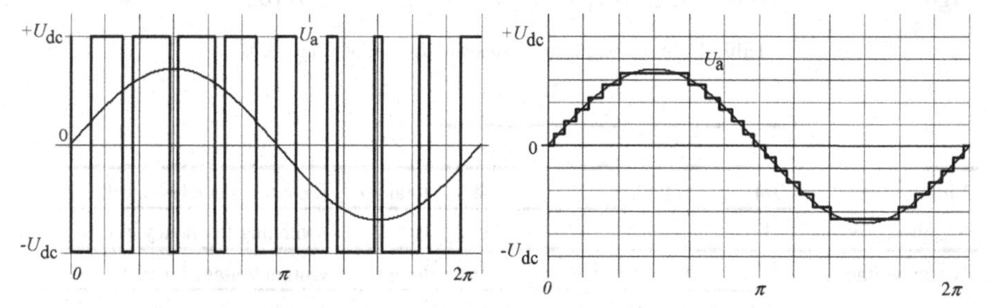

Fig. 2 Reference and output waveform of switched amplifiers, left : PWM-controlled, right : stepwise approximation, using 6 discrete voltage steps in each polarity.

3.1. Pulse-Width-Modulated Amplifier

A very common method to realize a digital amplifier is by the use of Pulse-Width-Modulation (PWM). The amplifier output is continuously switched between the two states ($\pm U_{dc}$). The duration of each state defines the average output voltage during one cycle of the switching frequency. The switching frequency of the digital amplifier has to be much higher than the desired output frequency and a sub-harmonic modulation scheme in combination with a low-pass filter is used to produce the desired base-band waveform. Preferably the switching frequency is an integer multiple of the output frequency in order to avoid beat frequencies. E.g., if output frequencies of 25kHz are desired the switching frequencies should be at least one decade higher to achieve a good output voltage quality. This will result in high switching frequencies and thus, high switching losses in the digital amplifier, as the full current is subject to the high switching frequency (Fig. 2, left).

3.2. Multilevel-Inverter Based Amplifier

High-power converters frequently use multilevel-technologies to handle the problem of high quality waveforms and limitations of switching frequency. Though normally being applied in the low frequency domain at hundreds of kilowatts up to megawatts, and switching frequency of several hundred Hertz, application of this technology can be adopted to this problem. In multilevel technology the waveform is composed by a number of discrete voltage levels. This way the sinusoidal output voltage is quantized with a certain step size. Obviously, the output quality depends on the size, and thus on the number of discrete steps. As more discrete voltage steps can be addressed, the more precisely the sinusoidal voltage reference can be approximated. A stepwise approximated sinusoidal voltage is shown in Fig. 2 (right) using 6 discrete voltage steps for each polarity, plus zero.

Table 1 : Switching frequencies and discrete voltage steps.

	Stages					
	1	2	3	4		
Linear voltage	1/4	1/4	1/4	1/4	total : 9	Output voltage level, ref. U_{dc}
Stepping	1	1	1	1	Fs	switching frequency, ref. f_1
Binary voltage	1/2	1/4	1/8	1/16	total : 17	Output voltage level, ref. U_{dc}
Stepping	1	2	4	8	fs	switching frequency, ref. f_1
Ternary voltage	2/3	2/9	2/27	2/81	total : 81	Output voltage level, ref. U_{dc}
stepping	1	3	9	27	fs	switching frequency, ref. f_1
1:5-Voltage	4/5	4/25	4/125	4/625	total:625	Output voltage level, ref. U_{dc}
stepping	1	5	25	125	fs	switching frequency, ref. f_1
3/5-level hybrid	2/5	2/5	2/25	2/25	total: 25	Output voltage level, ref. U_{dc}
stepping	1	1	5	5	fs	switching frequency, ref. f_1

While in high power systems the different levels are usually obtained by just adding equal-weighted stages, leading to a rather limited number of discrete steps and high redundancy, this is not the optimum for a power signal amplifier. Here differently weighted stages are preferred, which lead to a much higher number of different levels with a limited number of stages. It is best explained by constituting a numbering system with a given radix. In Tab. 1 the number of output voltage levels and the required switching frequencies are listed for different radici and configurations, including the high power case with equally distributed stages. As stated above, switched amplifiers can only address two voltage levels ($\pm U_{dc}$) by nature. So-called full-bridge circuits can also produce 0 as a third level, which allows creating ternary systems. The hybrid 3/5-level system is obtained by combination of two full-bridge circuits (3-level) of equal level. Two of these combinations can be combined into a hybrid two-stage 3/5-level system.

It must be noted, that despite the advantage of high resolution, high number of steps will always result into high switching frequency, which may not be feasible beyond 150 kHz and high power with currently available transistors. Indeed a good compromise appears to be the 3/5 level hybrid approach. This achieves almost the same resolution (25) as a three-stage ternary system (27), but at switching frequency factor of only 5, compared to 9 in the three-stage ternary system.

4. AMPLIFIER ARCHITECTURE

Fig. 3 and 4 show two possible implementations of hybrid 3/5-level two-stage systems. Topology ***I*** uses galvanically isolated intermediate DC-voltages. The inverter outputs are connected in series. Thus, the output voltage of the stacked inverters is determined by the sum of all inverter output voltages. The summarised output voltage is connected to the drive coil by means of a HF-filter, which reduces the remaining frequency components above eg. 50 kHz. In this topology all inverter switches carry identical load current. Two of the intermediate voltages have 2/5 of the desired output voltage, the other two 2/25 of the desired output voltage. From this, 25 different output voltage levels can be addressed using appropriate combinations of switching states at the inverters. The different voltage sources have to be kept exactly at their predefined set-points. Otherwise the step-sizes do not match each other and extra non-linear distortion will occur. Another disadvantage is the higher component count and cost.

Topology ***II*** overcomes these problems. In this topology a common DC-voltage source for all inverter modules is used. The output terminals of the inverters are connected by individual output transformers with turn ratios of 2/5 and 2/25. This means that the step sizes always fulfil a predefined ratio, given by the transformers.

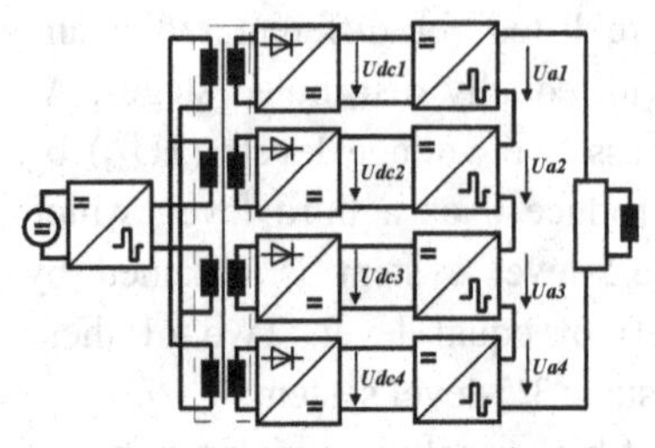

Fig. 3 Stacked inverter topology *I*.

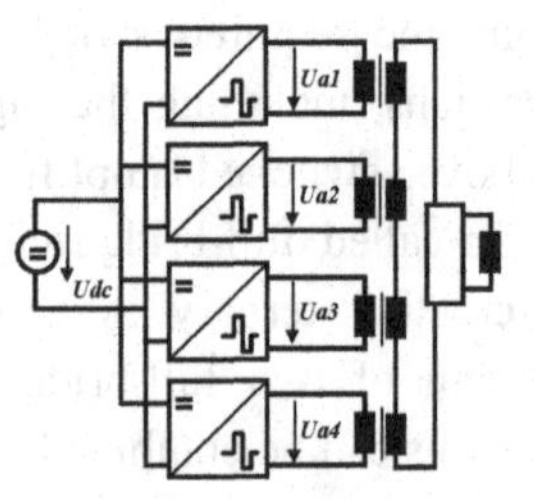

Fig. 4 Stacked inverter topology *II*.

5. RESULTS AND CONCLUSION

Fig. 5 shows the harmonic content of the two digital amplifiers referring to the fundamental sinusoidal waveform, scaled in dBc. The harmonic content of a multi-level inverter based solution is substantially lower than the harmonic content of a PWM-controlled digital amplifier. As the frequency range for magnetic particle imaging acquisition starts at the second harmonic of the drive field signal, disturbances start to become critical at 50 kHz, when the fundamental frequency of the drive field signal is 25 kHz.

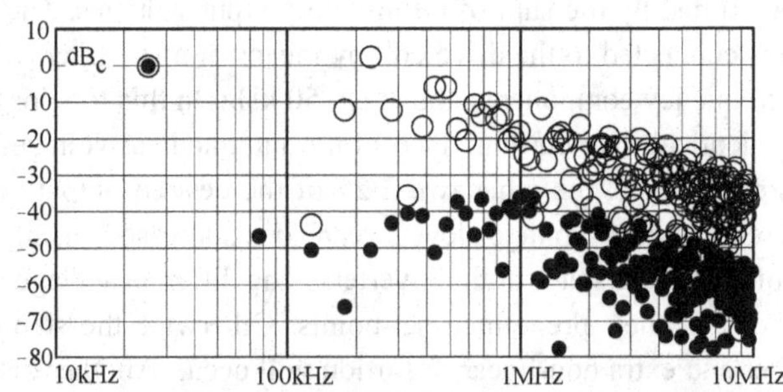

Fig. 5 Harmonic content of a PWM-controlled digital amplifier (circle, switching frequency 225 kHz) and a multi-level inverter based approach (dot, hybrid 3/5 with 25 levels).

The results suggest, that the drive coil supply for a magnetic particle imaging scanner can be efficiently realized by a multi-level inverter based digital amplifier. This concept does not suffer from the intrinsic losses of linear analogue amplifiers. Power requirements are reduced by at least one order of magnitude. Harmonic distortion can be reduced in particular in the critical range from 50 kHz to 1 MHz by a sufficient number of discrete voltage levels. Switching frequency is kept moderately low.

A NOVEL COMPENSATED COIL SYSTEM WITH HIGH HOMOGENEITY AND LOW STRAYFIELDS

R. HIERGEIST, J. LÜDKE, R. KETZLER, M. ALBRECHT

AG 2.51, Magnetic Measurements, PTB Braunschweig, Bundesallee 100
38116 Braunschweig, Germany
Email: robert.hiergeist@ptb.de

G. ROSS

Magnet-Physik Dr. Steingroever GmbH, Emil-Hoffmann-Str. 3
50996 Köln, Germany

A novel coil system as a replacement for Helmholtz coil systems will be presented. It consists of three pairs of coils with one pair having opposite polarity. In comparison to Helmholtz-coils the novel coil system has the following advantages: (a) The magnetic field amplitude on the coil axis (z-axis) outside the coil system declines with $H \sim z^{-5}$ significantly faster than in a Helmholtz coil ($H \sim z^{-3}$). (b) It provides an homogeneity up to the sixth order of the magnetic field along the coil axis. Hence a larger homogeneous volume in comparison to a Helmholtz coil system with equipollent dimensions could be achieved. The novel coil system can be applied for the stray field insensitive measurement of magnetic moments and for the generation of magnetic fields especially inside of magnetic shielding chambers whose walls should not be magnetized in any circumstance. An excellent agreement between calculated field profiles and field measurements of prototypes has been found. The homogeneity of the field profile of a prototype could be further improved by connecting a resistor in parallel to three of the six coils. This way precision measurements by nuclear magnetic resonance could be accomplished.

The most common technique to measure the magnetic dipole moment of permanent magnet samples is to integrate the induced voltage in a coil when the sample is moved. For this it is necessary to use a coil where the sensitivity in the volume of the sample is homogeneous enough. To obtain a sufficient homogeneous sensitivity for the detection coil bulky Helmholtz coils are usually used. But these Helmholtz coils – besides their dimensions – have a second significant drawback: They are not only sensitive for the sample inside but as well for other moving magnetic moments far away from the center of the coil. In order to limit influence of these magnetic disturbances a novel compensated coil was designed at the PTB[1] consisting of three pairs of coils with one pair having opposite polarity. The design of this compensated coil is shown in Fig.1.

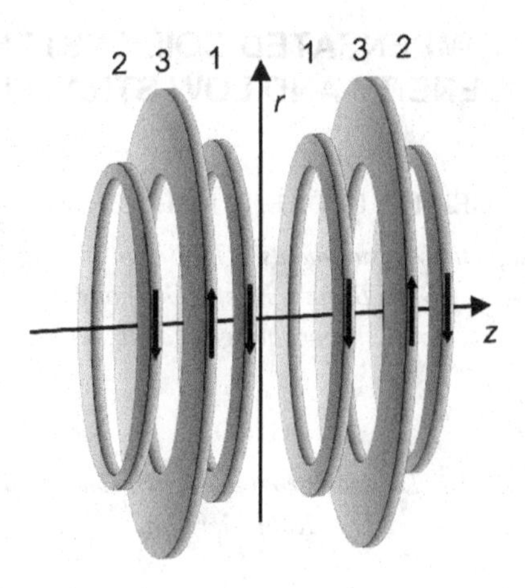

Fig. 1. Design of the compensated coil set. Winding numbers (n_1, n_2, and n_3) for the coils 1, 2, and 3 are all identical. The current directions flowing in the individual coils are indicated by arrays.

As well this concept of a compensated coil is feasible for the generation of homogeneous magnetic fields with only small stray fields outside the coil. Because of the good homogeneity obtained when field is generated with this coil design and the rapid decay of the field amplitude on the symmetry axis outside the coil, the compensated coil is excellently applicable in situations where magnetic fields have to be generated close to or in magnetic shieldings which should be prevented from being magnetized. Therefore it has recently been applied as a polarization coil for fluxgate-magnetorelaxometry of magnetic nanoparticles[3,4].

In this paper we will present experimental results of the field distribution of prototypes of compensated coils which were assembled by Magnet-Physik Dr. Steingroever, Cologne, according to fabrication data calculated by PTB-Braunschweig. These fabrication data are based on calculations where – in contrast to the calculations of Ref. 1, which were done for a model of infinitesimal thin coil filaments – realistic coil and wire dimensions were used.

In Fig. 2 the picture of an early prototype of the compensated coil design MNPQ-01 is presented. It has bore diameter of 140mm and at height of 286.5mm. Data of the field profile $\mu_0 H_z/I$ measured with a high precision fluxgate sensor in coil axis direction (z-direction) and perpendicular to the z-direction (r-direction) are shown in Fig.3(a) and Fig.3(b), respectively.

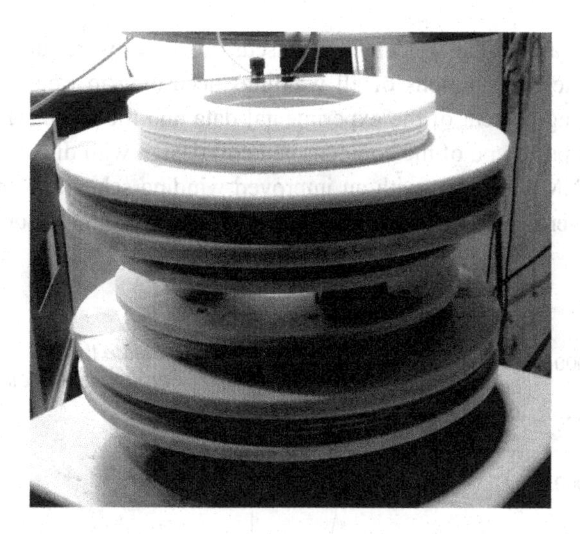

Fig. 2. Picture of the prototype MNPQ-01 of the compensated coil with 1170 windings for each individual coil. (Alternating 33, 32, 33 … windings in 36 layers; wires with 0.8mm diameter – including insulating varnish).

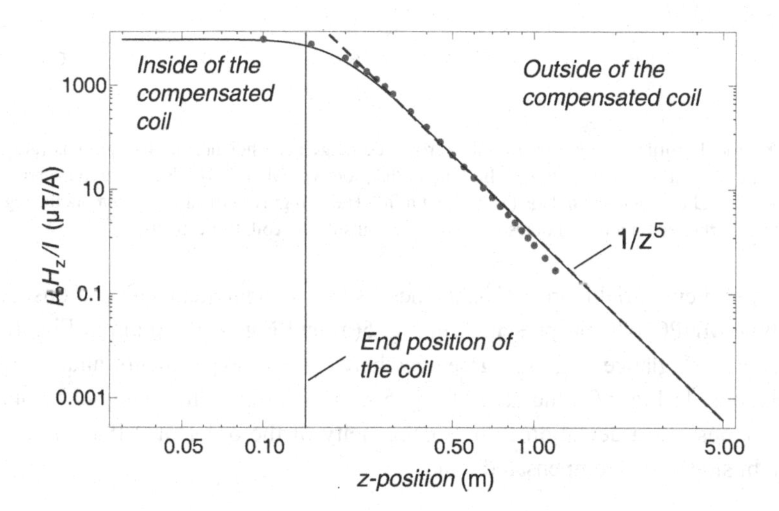

Fig. 3(a). Field profile $\mu_o H_z/I(z)$ measured over a wide range on the coil axis (gray dots) and data of the analytical calculation (solid line) of the prototype MNPQ-01. The decay of $\mu_o H_z/I(z)$ for large z-positions with z^{-5} is indicated by the straight dashed line. The end position of the coil is denoted by the gray vertical line, separating the regions inside and outside of the compensated coil .

The field amplitude calculations discussed here were all performed by summarizing the contributions of all windings according to Equ. (4.2) of Ref. 2. Note the good agreement of the experimental data and the calculated field profile. Fig. 4 shows a prototype of the compensated coil design with dimensions similar to the prototype NMPQ-01 but with an improved winding scheme: Here 36 layers of 32 windings were separated by plastic stripes of 0.2 thickness for all individual coils.

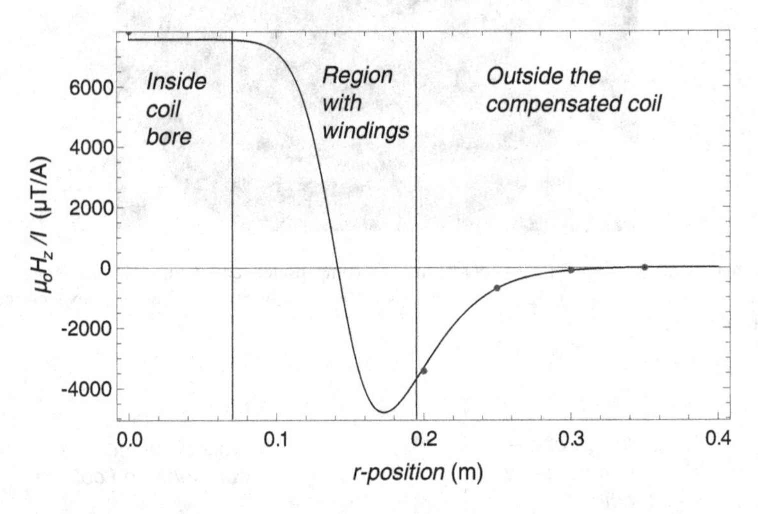

Fig. 3(b). Field profile $\mu_o H_z / I$(r) measured over a wide range perpendicular to the coil axis (gray dots) and data of the analytical calculation (solid line) of the prototype MNPQ-01. Note the good agreement of the experimental and calculated data. (This is not a fit.) The two gray vertical lines separate the region of the bore from the region with windings and the region outside the coil, respectively.

Experimental field profile data and results of analytical calculations of the prototype MNPQ-03c are presented in Fig. 5(a) and Fig. 5(b). Again in Fig.5(a) we find at a first glance a good agreement between the experiments and analytical calculations. In Fig. 5(b) the data of Fig. 5(a) are plotted with an higher resolution. Here we observe a deviation from homogeneity of the order of 0.1% between left and right side of the compensated coil.

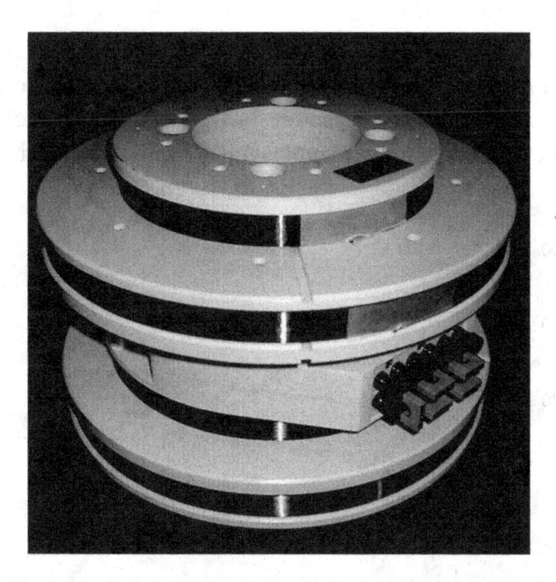

Fig. 4. Picture of the prototype MNPQ-03c of the compensated coil with 1152 windings for each individual coil (32 windings in 36 layers separated with 0.2mm thick plastic stripes; wires with 0.8mm diameter – including insulating varnish). All the six individual coils are accessible by the terminal in the middle of the coil.

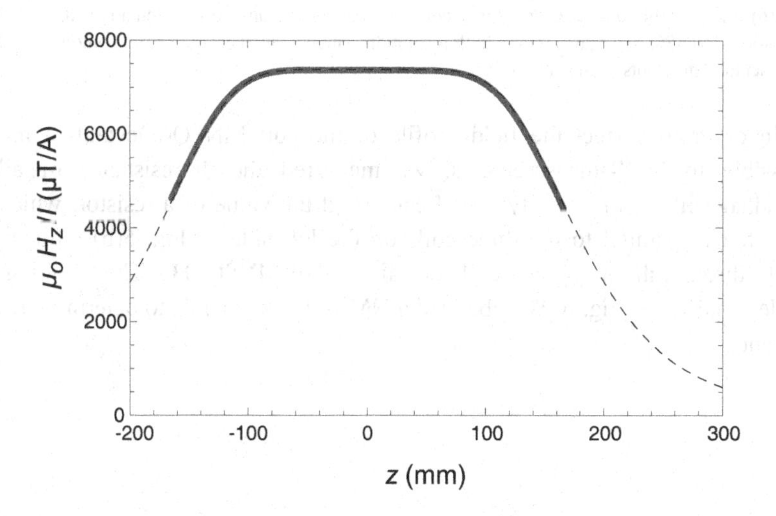

Fig. 5(a). Field profile data $\mu_o H_z/I(z)$ (gray dots) and data of the analytical calculation (dashed line) of the prototype MNPQ-03c. Note the good agreement of the experimental and calculated data.

This lack of homogeneity of the field profile makes it impossible to measure the coil constant of this prototype by Nuclear Magnet Resonance (NMR) using a water sample, since this technique requires a field homogeneity of the order of at least 10^{-5} over the dimension of the sample with 40 mm in diameter.

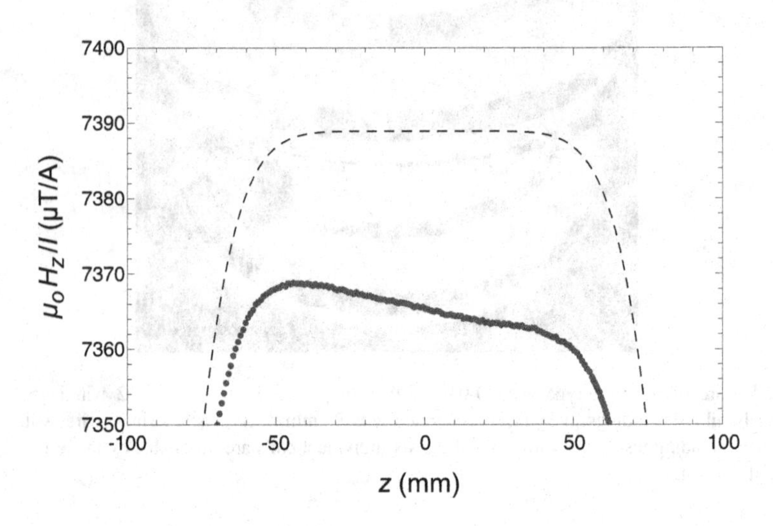

Fig. 5(b). Field profile data $\mu_o H_z/I(z)$ (gray dots) and data of the analytical calculation (dashed line) of the prototype MNPQ-03c drawn with a high resolution. There is an aberration from homogeneity for the experimental data points of the order of 0.1%.

In order to correct the field profile of the coil MNPQ-03c and to make it accessible to NMR-measurements, we measured the dc-resistance of all the individual coils of the prototype and calculated the value of a resistor, which was connected in parallel to the three coils on the left side of Fig. 5(b) reducing the current through the individual coils on this side of MNPQ-03c. The resulting field profile is shown in Fig. 6. We obtained a NMR-signal suitable to determine the coil constant.

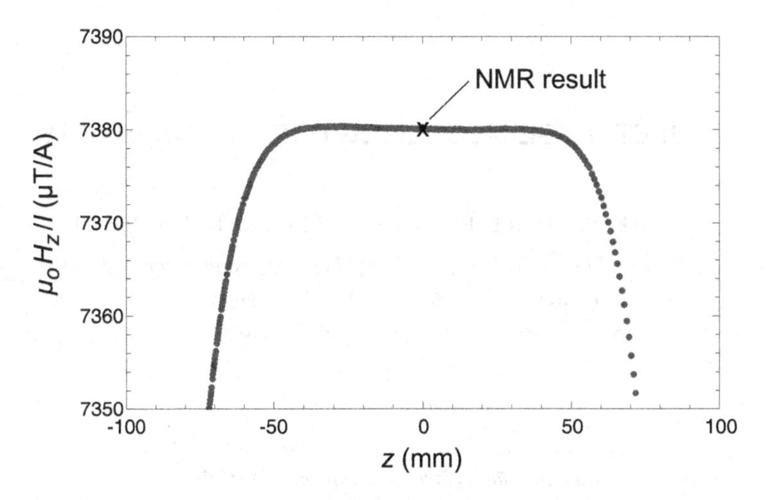

Fig. 6. Field profile data $\mu_o H_z/I$(z) (gray dots) after correction of the left side of the prototype MNPQ-03c by a resistor of 56859Ω. (Resistance values of the individual coils are of the order of 37.79Ω up to 60.53Ω) As a consequence of this correction NMR-measurements were made possible. The profile measured with the high precision fluxgate was rescaled with the value of the coil constant measured by NMR (as indicated by the black cross in the plot at z = 0)

ACKNOWLEDGMENTS

R.H. wishes to acknowledge the support by the MNPQ-Project "Ein innovatives Spulensystem zur störfeldunempfindlichen Messung magnetischen Momente oder streufeldarmen Erzeugung magnetischer Felder" funded by the BMWI.

REFERENCES

1 Lüdke J, Ahlers H, Albrecht M. Novel Compensated Moment Detection Coil. *IEEE Trans. Magn.* 2007; **43**: 3567.
2 Fiorillo, F Measurement and Chracterization of Magnetic Materials. Amsterdam: Elsevier, 2004
3 Schilling M, Hempel D.C, Jahn D, „Vom Gen zum Produkt - aber mit System" Spektrum der Wissenschaft, Oktober 2009, 34-41
4 Ludwig F, "Fluxgate-Magnetorelaxometry", Workshop "Biomedical Applications of Magnetic Nanoparticles", 2006, September 15, TU Braunschweig, Germany.

JFET NOISE MODELLING FOR MPI RECEIVERS

INGO SCHMALE, BERNHARD GLEICH, JÖRN BORGERT

Philips Technologie GmbH Forschungslaboratorien
Röntgenstraße 24, 22335 Hamburg, Germany
Email: ingo.schmale@philips.com

JÜRGEN WEIZENECKER

Hochschule Karlsruhe – Technik und Wirtschaft
Fakultät für Elektro- und Informationstechnik
Moltkestraße 30, 76133 Karlsruhe

Within MPI, very weak signals need to be detected in the frequency range of 50kHz-1MHz. In order to do so, a low-noise receiver based on low-noise transistors is required. In this paper, after motivation the choice of junction field-effect transistors, the modelling of their noise behaviour is presented. Various forms of models are contrasted and a new form is proposed. The noise model is essential for the development of an optimized receiver circuit for MPI.

1. TRANSISTOR TECHNOLOGY COMPARISON

The choice of a suitable transistor technology for a low-noise MPI receive amplifier has to be based primarily upon its noise performance. The two basic types of transistors, unipolar field-effect transistors (FET) vs. bipolar junction transistors (BJT), have minimum noise figures F_{min}, which can be achieved in case of optimal noise matching. For the FET, F_{min} is given by[1]:

$$\text{FET:} \qquad F_{\min} = 1 + \frac{4}{3}\frac{f}{f_T} \qquad (1)$$

The minimum noise figure is a function of frequency f. As the frequencies of interest within MPI are low, typically less than 1MHz, very low noise figures could be obtained according to the above formula, especially for fast devices with high transit frequencies f_T. However, the planar FET technologies such as Si-MOSFETs, GaAs-MESFETs as well as InP-HEMTs, with f_T beyond 100GHz, suffer from high flicker noise which is not included in the above formula. This type of noise is subject to a 1/f-law. Technologically, it is related to impurities at semiconductor surfaces. The junction-field effect transistor (JFET), made e.g. from silicon, is a device where the drain current flows through the bulk of the semiconductor, where it is less affected by surface effects. The frequency, at which the flicker noise has the same noise power density as the device's noise floor, is called the 1/f-knee. For JFETs, it is very low, in the kHz range, making JFETs suitable for MPI receivers.

For BJTs, the minimum noise figure is described by[1]:

$$\text{BJT:} \qquad F_{\min} = 1 + \frac{R_b}{R_{gen}} + \frac{1}{\sqrt{\beta}} \tag{2}$$

Here, F_{min} is not frequency dependent. In order to minimize it, a low base resistance R_b is desired, whilst the generator resistance R_{gen} needs to be high. But even if R_b were zero, there remains the term with the current amplification factor β. So even for the best transistors with β approaching 400, F_{min} is

$$\text{BJT:} \quad F_{\min} > 1 + \frac{1}{\sqrt{\beta}} = 1 + \frac{1}{\sqrt{400}} = 1.05 = 1 + \frac{14.5K}{290K} \tag{3}$$

As stated above, an optimal JFET, therefore, needs to have a very high f_T and a low 1/f-knee. As an example of a representative JFET, the BF862 from NXP has

$$\text{BF862:} \quad f_T = \frac{1}{2\pi}\frac{g_m}{C_{iss}} = \frac{1}{2\pi}\frac{40mS}{10pF} = 640MHz \tag{4}$$

with the values for trans-conductance g_m and the input capacitance C_{iss} taken from the transistor's datasheet. Therefore, for MPI frequencies $f < 1MHz$, one obtains

$$\text{BF862:} \qquad F_{\min} < 1 + \frac{4}{3}\frac{1MHz}{640MHz} = 1.0016 = 1 + \frac{0.45K}{290K} \tag{5}$$

As this value is much lower than the BJT-value from eqn. 3, even at the highest receive frequency of 1MHz, JFETs offer the best noise performance for an MPI low-noise amplifier. Expressed as equivalent noise temperatures, there is an improvement by a factor of approximately 30 between 14.5K and 0.45K.

2. JFET NOISE MODELLING

The modeling of FET noise can be done in various ways. Some are more physics-based, and look into the details of noise generation and to what element it is attributed to in a small-signal equivalent circuit. Others just regard the JFET as a two-port, with noise sources attached to the outside. Fig 1 shows a general small-signal equivalent circuit for the intrinsic part of the JFET (i.e. ignoring access resistances and inductances as well as parasitic capacitances).

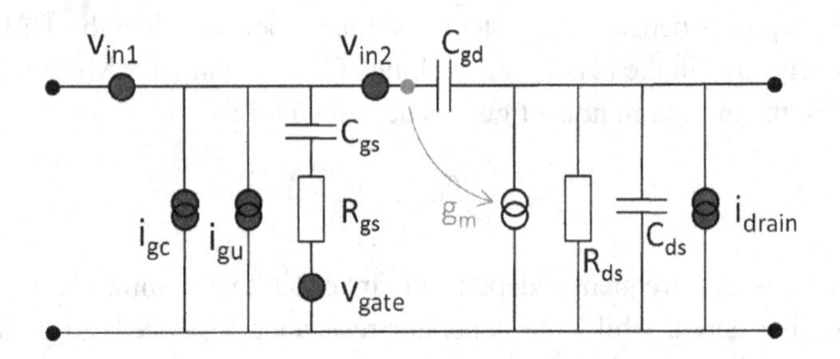

Fig. 1. Equivalent small-signal circuit of a single JFET with various noise source locations.

Various noise sources, either voltage noise sources or current noise sources, are included in the circuit, but not all of them are employed in each model. One standard way of representing the noise of a two-port is in the form of admittances, where two currents i_{gu} and i_{drain} are added at the input (port 1, gate, left) and the output (port 2, drain, right), respectively. Table 1 shows the equations for the current noise densities of these sources in the column 'Y-form'. They are valid for bias points with insignificant gate leakage. The correlation of the two currents i_{gu} and i_{drain} is imaginary; its value j0.4 is typically neglected[2].

For the purpose of calculating the noise figure, it is convenient to relate all noise sources to the input. This is called a chain-form. In order to have a situation identical to the Y-form, a voltage source v_{in1} and a current source i_{gc} become effective at the input in order to replace i_{drain} at the output. When omitting the gate-drain capacitance C_{gd}, which, typically, is much less than the gate-source capacitance C_{gs}, the noise terms become quite simple, as shown in the column 'chain form 1'. The current i_{gc} is directly correlated to the voltage noise v_{in} and cannot be identically included in the uncorrelated gate noise current source i_{gu}. Nevertheless, some authors add up these terms and come to a combined gate noise current of $g_m(f/f_T)^2$.

Table 1. Noise terms in various alternative models.

	Y-form	Chain-form 1	Chain-form 2	Posp.-form	Mixed form
$i_{drain}^2/4kT_j\Delta f$	$\frac{2}{3}g_m$			$\frac{T_d}{T_j}\frac{1}{R_{ds}}$	$\frac{2}{3}g_m$
$v_{in1}^2/4kT_j\Delta f$		$\frac{2}{3}\frac{1}{g_m}$			
$v_{in2}^2/4kT_j\Delta f$			$\frac{2}{3}\frac{1}{g_m}$		
$i_{gc}^2/4kT_j\Delta f$		$\lvert j\omega C_{gs}\rvert^2 v_{in1}^2$			
$i_{gu}^2/4kT_j\Delta f$	$\frac{1}{3}\frac{\omega^2(C_{gs}+C_{gd})^2}{g_m}=\frac{1}{3}g_m\left(\frac{\omega}{\omega_T}\right)^2$				
$v_{gate}^2/4kT_j\Delta f$				$\frac{T_g}{T_j}R_{gs}$	$\frac{1}{3}\frac{1}{g_m}$

A better way is to abandon the idea of having noise sources only at the outside terminals of an otherwise noise-free two-port. This is what happens if the correlation admittance $j\omega C_{gs}$ is integrated as a component into the equivalent circuit. It effectively shifts the input voltage noise v_{in1} to a new position v_{in2}, which is inside the two-port. The correlated current noise i_{gc} then disappears. For a junction temperature T_j=300K, and Boltzman's constant k=1.38*10^{-23} J/K, the input voltage noise density for a single JFET equates to

$$\frac{v_{in2}}{\sqrt{\Delta f}}=\sqrt{4kT_j\frac{2}{3}\frac{1}{g_m}}=0.52\frac{nV}{\sqrt{Hz}} \qquad (6)$$

The minimum noise figure is the noise figure achieved when the source impedance has the value Z_{opt}, which is a function of the transistor. The theory behind is well laid out by Fukui[3]. Ignoring for a while the input capacitance, the resistive part of the source impedance can be calculated as follows:

$$\mathrm{Re}(Z_{opt})=\sqrt{\frac{v_{in2}^2}{i_{gu}^2}}=\sqrt{\frac{\frac{2}{3}\frac{1}{g_m}}{\frac{1}{3}g_m\left(\frac{f}{f_T}\right)^2}}=\frac{\sqrt{2}}{g_m}\left(\frac{f}{f_T}\right)^{-1} \qquad (7)$$

For the BF862 at a frequency f = 1MHz, the optimal source resistance is around 20kΩ, and is still higher for lower frequencies. Compared to the very low source resistance of the coil, which is in the order of 10-100mΩ (frequency dependent!), it becomes clear that either some matching network is required or a very high number of parallel transistors has to be employed. On the other hand, the matching of the input capacitance to the coil's inductance limits the maximum number of parallel devices, and hence, the minimum noise figure. Fortunately, there is ample room for mismatch, as the noise temperature does not need to be as cold as 0.45K. In established imaging modalities such as MRI, 40K is a widely accepted value, corresponding to a noise figure of $10 * \log_{10}(1+40K/290K)=0.55dB$.

The drawback of the models presented so far is that they all have one frequency-dependent noise current at the gate. Opposed to the other noise sources, which have a flat 'white' spectrum, this current would go to infinity for very high frequencies. From RF MESFET modeling, a number of noise models are known which have intrinsic noise sources that are fitted to experimental noise data. There are various models, with 1 to 3 fitting parameters/temperatures, but, according to a comprehensive comparison[4], the model from Pospiezalski[5] is best. It has two uncorrelated noise sources: one drain current i_{drain}, and one gate voltage v_{gate} in series with the gate capacitance. As listed in table 1, the drain noise current is related to the output resistance R_{ds}, which requires introducing the drain temperature T_d as a fitting variable. On the gate side, the voltage noise is attributed to R_{gs}, which has a gate temperature T_g as a fitting variable.

Within Pospiezalski's model, however, T_d is unphysically high (~10000K), whilst T_g is somewhat arbitrary due to the difficulty of precisely knowing the value of the gate-source resistance R_{gs}. So, in order to obtain a model which is both simple and physically sound, it is suggested here to take the best parts of two models. The result is shown in the last column in table 1, the 'mixed form'. The model for the drain current noise is taken from the Y-form, whilst the gate noise is modeled in form of a voltage source in series with C_{gs}. Instead of struggling with the determination of R_{gs}, which is not typically provided in data sheets, this resistance is postulated to have the value $R_{gs} := 1/(3g_m)$ and to generate noise at the junction temperature T_j. This is effectively identical to i_{gu} from the Y- and Chain-models, as long as $f < f_T$.

3. CONCLUSION

JFETs were shown to be the best transistor technology for MPI receivers, since they have a very low minimum noise figure and no 1/f-noise in the MPI frequency range. In order to achieve the lowest noise figure, a JFET with a high transit frequency needs to be chosen. This is equivalent to saying that the input capacitance needs to be low, so more devices can be operated in parallel. Various noise models have been presented and compared, and a new 'mixed form', which is notably simple, has been derived. This model will be taken as the base of more complete MPI noise analyses.

ACKNOWLEDGMENTS

This work was financially supported by the German Federal Ministry of Education and Research (BMBF) under the grant number FKZ 13N9079.

REFERENCES

1 Tietze U, Schenk C. *Halbleiter-Schaltungstechnik*. Berlin, Heidelberg: Springer, 1999: 245-252
2 Müller R. *Halbleiter-Elektronik, Band 15, Rauschen*. Berlin, Heidelberg: Springer, 1979: 141-156
3 Fukui H. Available Power Gain, Noise Figure, and Noise Measure of Two-Ports and their Graphical Representation. *IEEE T. on CT* 1966; **2**: 137-142
4 Heyman P et al. Experimental Evaluation of Microwave FET Noise Models. *IEEE T on MTT* 1999; **2**: 156-163
5 Pospieszalski MW. Modeling of Noise Parameters of MESFETs and MODFETs and their Frequency and Temperature Dependence. *IEEE T. on MTT* 1989; **9**: 1340-1350.

NOISE WITHIN MAGNETIC PARTICLE IMAGING

INGO SCHMALE, BERNHARD GLEICH JÖRN BORGERT
Philips Technologie GmbH Forschungslaboratorien
Röntgenstraße 24, 22335 Hamburg, Germany
Email: ingo.schmale@philips.com

JÜRGEN WEIZENECKER
Hochschule Karlsruhe – Technik und Wirtschaft
Fakultät für Elektro- und Informationstechnik
Moltkestraße 30, 76133 Karlsruhe

This paper identifies and quantifies the noise sources in the receive chain of an MPI scanner. A small-signal equivalent circuit model is derived that includes all noise sources. From this, for the first time, precise calculations of the system noise factor referenced to patient body noise are presented, including frequency dependency, both of the receive coil resistance and of the patient induced noise. Conclusions are drawn with respect to the optimal count and type of JFETs. Finally, the path towards body noise limitation in human size scanners is outlined.

1. INTRODUCTION

In magnetic particle imaging (MPI), the non-linear response of magnetic nano-particles to a sinusoidal excitation is measured and, via reconstruction algorithms, expressed as a concentration map of these particles. The fundamental set-up, therefore, consists of a drive chain, where an extremely pure sinusoidal magnetic field is applied, and a receive chain that captures the very weak response at the harmonic and mixing frequencies[1]. The receive chain (fig. 1) has a high-Q receive coil followed by a band-stop filter to suppress the very dominant excitation frequency. Thereafter, either a narrowband-LNA is applied, which can give very good noise performance at and near the design frequency[2].

Alternatively, a broadband LNA is used, which permits reception in a wide frequency band (50kHz-1MHz). Such a broadband approach permits to acquire much more data in parallel and therefore enables real-time MPI, outweighing by far the slightly increased noise factor. Such broadband topology, based on many (*n*) JFET-type transistors in parallel, has been adopted for our current pre-clinical MPI demonstrator and will be the focus of this paper.

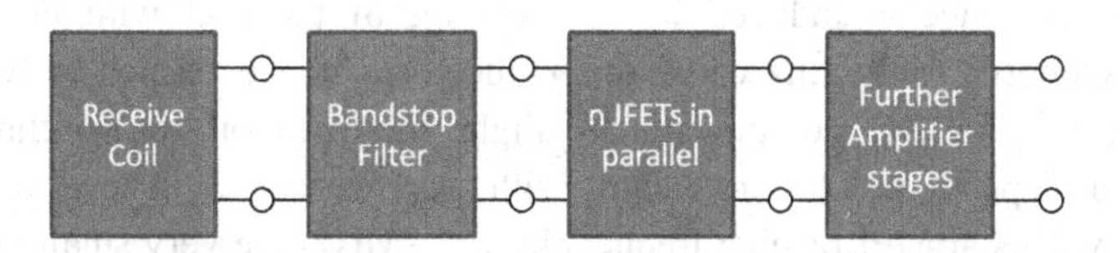

Fig. 1. Block diagram of the MPI receive chain.

Both approaches are subject to the general limitations of broadband matching of lossy reactive elements as described by Fano[3]. They basically state that a perfect broadband matching of a single receiver to a high-Q coil can never be realized, no matter how complex a network might be conceived.

For our pre-clinical demonstrator, three orthogonal receive coils surround the 12cm bore, which is intended for research on small animals. Whilst the coil geometries are very different (pairs of saddle coils for the transversal axis and a solenoid for the longitudinal axis), the electrical parameters are comparable. Fig. 2 shows coil reactance X_{coil} and resistance R_{coil} as a function of frequency. The drive-field frequencies are around 25 kHz, whilst the detectable mixing and harmonic frequencies extend from 50 kHz to approximately 1 MHz, which is represented as an inset on the bottom right of fig 2. The reactance of the coil is dominant over its resistance, with a frequency-dependent Q factor of between 50 and 200.

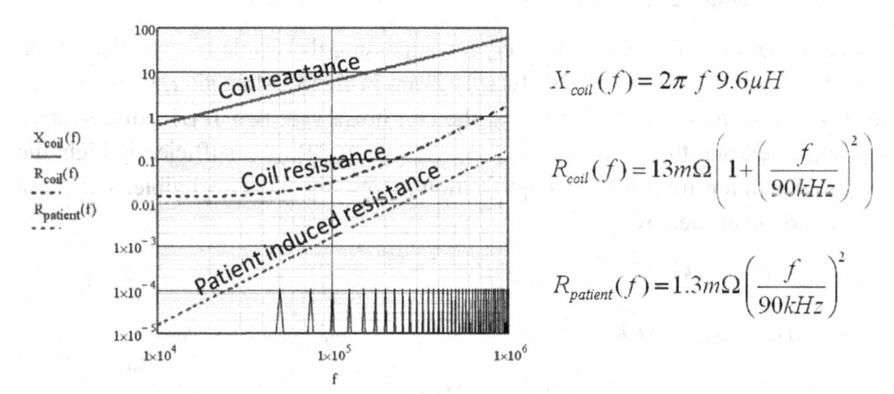

Fig. 2. Reactances and resistances (in Ohm) as a function of frequency f (in Hz). Towards higher frequencies, the gap between coil resistance and patient induced resistance approaches a constant.

The resistance of the Litz-wires used in the receive coil is frequency dependent due to skin and proximity effects[4]. Experimental data is approximated here as the sum of its DC resistance plus a term proportional to the square of the frequency. An additional resistance is induced by the loading of the coil with an animal or phantom. Opposed to the Litz wires, this induced resistance, termed body or patient resistance, has no DC component. In slight modification to Röschmann[5], we postulate a dependency on frequency with a power of 2 instead of 2.1. The resistance values at MPI receive frequencies (< 1MHz) are very small and, for the current coil technology, always lower than the coil resistance. Therefore, body noise limitation is not achieved yet in the current pre-clinical demonstrator. Neither can the body resistance reliably be measured with the existing apparatus. Therefore, the body-induced losses were characterized in a separate experiment with a coil made resonant at 20MHz. The values from this network analyzer based measurement, with the coil having about 10cm diameter and a 2.5cm distance to a volunteer, were scaled according to the inductance ratio and extrapolated down to the MPI frequency range[6].

The scaling with frequency of patient and coil resistance (fig. 2) is 'parallel' at high frequencies, whilst diverging towards low frequencies. So, if the coil is improved (better Litz wire having strands with smaller diameter, altogether larger amount of copper, cooling) such that body noise limitation is achieved at one frequency, then body noise limitation will also be achieved at all frequencies above that frequency.

2. NOISE MODELLING

The equivalent circuit for the receiver, encompassing the whole receive chain from patient via coil to the *n* parallel JFETs, is given in fig. 3. Altogether, there are five noise sources: the patient noise $v_{patient}$, the coil noise v_{coil}, two JFET noise sources v_{gate} and i_{drain}[7], and the load noise i_{load}. As the gain $g_m * R_{load}$ is sufficiently high, the noise contribution from further amplification stages (fig. 1) is negligible. The noise sources are quantified by:

$$v_{patient}^2(\omega) = 4kT_{patient}\Delta f\, R_{patient}(\omega) \qquad i_{drain}^2 = 4kT_{junction}\Delta f \frac{2}{3} n\, g_m$$

$$v_{coil}^2(\omega) = 4kT_{coil}\Delta f\, R_{coil}(\omega) \qquad i_{load}^2 = 4kT_{load}\Delta f \frac{n}{R_{load}}$$

$$v_{gate}^2 = 4kT_{junction}\Delta f \frac{R_{gs}}{n} = 4kT_{junction}\Delta f \frac{1}{3n\, g_m}$$

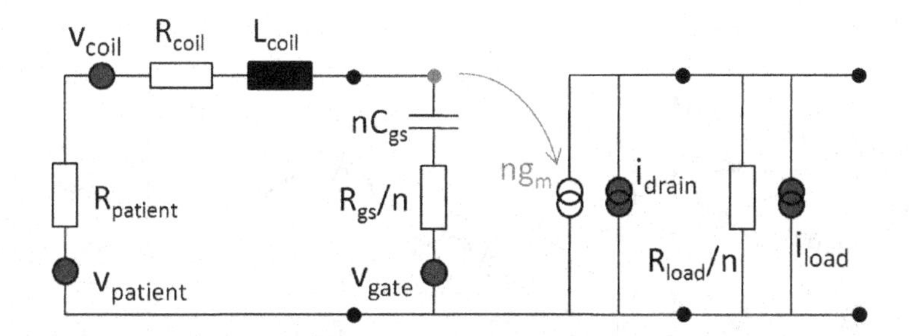

Fig. 3. Simplified equivalent small-signal model of the MPI receive chain, containing the signal source L_{coil} together with its corresponding resistances R_{coil} and $R_{patient}$, as well as n parallel JFETs including their load resistance R_{load}. C_{gd} and R_{ds} are neglected. The JFET's noise is represented in a newly proposed mixed form[7].

The response of the nano-particles to the drive-field excitation is induced within the coil and cannot be separated from the patient noise $v_{patient}$. In order to calculate the noise factor, all voltage noise sources are transferred to the output, where they become effective as parallel noise current sources. Fig. 4 shows the equivalent topology.

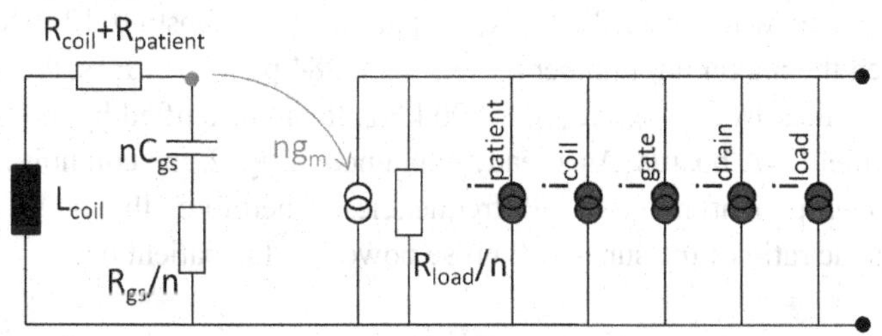

Fig. 4. Simplified equivalent small-circuit circuit of the MPI receive chain, identical to fig. 3. All noise sources are referred the output.

The governing equations are:

$$Z_{source}(\omega) = R_{coil}(\omega) + R_{patient}(\omega) + j\omega L_{coil}$$

$$Z_{sink}(\omega) = \frac{1}{n}\left(R_{gs} + \frac{1}{j\omega C_{gs}}\right)$$

$$T(\omega) = \frac{Z_{sink}(\omega)}{Z_{source}(\omega) + Z_{sink}(\omega)}$$

$$i^2_{patient}(\omega) = 4kT_{patient}\Delta f\, R_{patient}(\omega)\, \left|T(\omega)\, n\, g_m\right|^2$$

$$i^2_{coil}(\omega) = 4kT_{coil}\Delta f\, R_{coil}(\omega)\, \left|T(\omega)\, n\, g_m\right|^2$$

$$i^2_{gate}(\omega) = 4kT_{junction}\Delta f\, \frac{1}{3 n g_m}\, \left|(1 - T(\omega))\, n\, g_m\right|^2$$

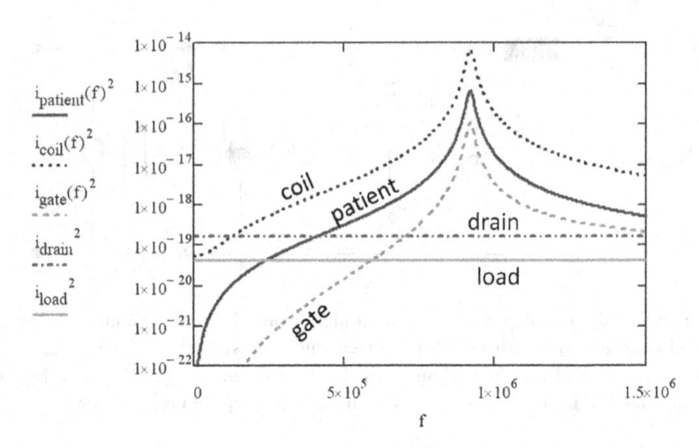

Fig. 5. Output referred current noise (in A^2, Δf=1Hz) as a function of frequency f (in Hz). The coil noise dominates at all frequencies over patient noise. The resonance at ~900kHz is from L_{coil} with nC_{gs}.

Fig. 5 quantitatively shows the contributions of the five noise sources (topology from fig. 4) as a function of frequency. A resonance becomes visible, which is due to the input circuit. The receiver from the pre-clinical demonstrator is based on a modular approach with up to 32 LNAs in parallel, each hosting 12 NXP BF862 JFETS. Given the maximum number n = 32*12 = 384 parallel JFETs, the resonance frequency becomes $1/(2\pi\sqrt{(L_{coil}nC_{gs})})$ ~ 900 kHz. It can be shifted by modifying the count of parallel LNA boards. As already explained in fig. 2, the coil noise currently dominates over patient noise at all frequencies. Therefore, the noise factor F, calculated as the ratio of the sum of all noise powers to the patient noise

$$F(\omega) = 1 + \frac{i_{coil}^2(\omega) + i_{gate}^2(\omega) + i_{drain}^2 + i_{load}^2}{i_{patient}^2(\omega)}$$

is not yet optimal. For frequencies from about 500kHz upwards, when drain noise becomes insignificant compared to body noise, the noise factor is mainly governed by the ratio of coil resistance to patient resistance, and their temperatures, and becomes

$$F(\omega) \approx 1 + \frac{i_{coil}^2(\omega)}{i_{patient}^2(\omega)} = 1 + \frac{T_{coil}}{T_{patient}} \frac{R_{coil}(\omega)}{R_{patient}(\omega)} = 1 + \frac{290K}{310K} \frac{13m\Omega}{1.3m\Omega} \approx 10$$

As already discussed above, the frequency dependency of R_{coil} and $R_{patient}$ is assumed to be identical, and hence, cancels. Therefore, the noise factor becomes frequency independent for frequencies above 500 kHz. The improvement of the Q-factor of the coil, therefore, is essential on the way towards body noise limitation. For a future human size scanner, this will be feasible, as more copper cross section will be available in the wider bore.

3. AMPLIFIER IMPROVEMENTS

In addition to the receive coil, the LNA will need to be optimized. Aside from cooling, which is promising, but not further discussed here, two parameters directly influence the noise factor: the number *n* of parallel JFETs and the JFET's transit frequency f_T. Figure 6 shows how much can be gained, even for the existing coil, starting from the current standard situation (red top curve) of 384 parallel BF862 JFET, which have a transit frequency of 640MHz[7].

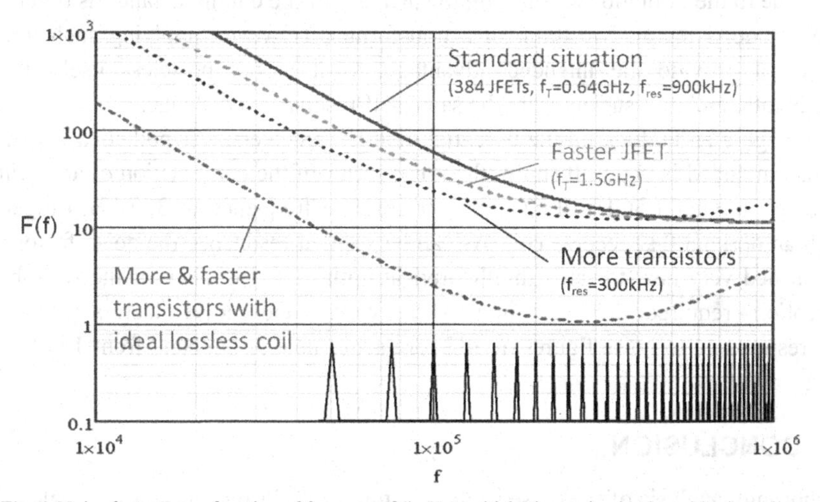

Fig. 6. Noise factor F as a function of frequency f (in Hz), with both axes having logarithmic scaling. The standard situation (from fig. 5), a situation with more (3500) transistors hence a lower resonance frequency, a situation with a faster transistor (f_T=1.5GHz), and the combination of an optimal receiver and an ideal noise-free receive coil.

By placing more transistors in parallel, the frequency of minimum noise can be shifted to lower frequencies, improving thus the noise factor at the center of the MPI receive band (50kHz-1MHz, see inset). Fig. 6 shows such a situation with the minimum shifted to 300 kHz, for which n = 3500 transistors need to be operated in parallel. However, with the current coil, this approach is impractical, as the power consumption of the receiver rises strongly. Each JFET has about 3V*15mA=45mW power consumption, and together with DC power consumption in R_{load} and in the following amplification stages, this amounts to 0.1W per JFET. This would lead to undesirable power consumption requirements in the order of several 100W per receive channel. In order to reduce transistor count, the resonance frequency shall, therefore, rather be lowered by increasing the coil inductance (whilst keeping its Q-factor constant). As this approach finds its limit with the coil's intrinsic resonance frequency, special low-C winding techniques will have to be employed.

The situation with a faster transistor (f_T = 1.5GHz) as shown in fig. 6 basically means that there is less gate-source capacitance C_{gs}[7]. In such case, more transistors can be deployed in parallel, whilst the resonance frequency remains unchanged. The benefit is a reduction of noise factor at all frequencies. But also in this case, more current flows in order to take advantage of the increase of effective trans-conductance $n*g_m$.

Due to the limitations restricting the increase of the coil inductance as described above, one is tempted to think of a transformer. However, applying such device does not provide the intended advantage, as it is not noiseless itself, limits bandwidth, and as it suffers from the same self-resonance challenge.

To give an outlook on the potential of JFET receivers, a hypothetical situation is also included in fig. 6. It shows the noise factor of the combination of an optimal receiver (having 1.5GHz JFETs and a resonance frequency at 300 kHz) together with an optimal 0 Ω receive coil. As can be seen, at resonance the noise factor can be pushed very near towards the theoretical limit of 1. But also for the wide-band reception required for real-time MPI, very good noise factors below 2 (corresponding to noise figures of 3dB) are achievable in the band from 125 to 650 kHz.

4. CONCLUSION

A thorough analysis of the noise sources within the MPI receive chain revealed that the coil resistance is the dominant noise source in the current pre-clinical scanner. Body noise limitation is expected to be reached in a future human size scanner, where more copper cross section can be provided. Further improvements in the coil winding technique will permit to reduce the count of parallel high-f_T JFETs in order to limit power consumption and to allow for miniaturization.

ACKNOWLEDGMENTS

This work was financially supported by the German Federal Ministry of Education and Research (BMBF) under the grant number FKZ 13N9079.

REFERENCES

1 Schmale I et al. An Introduction to the Hardware of MPI. *IFMBE Proc.* 2009; **25/II**: 450-453.
2 Goodwill PW et al. Narrowband Magnetic Particle Imaging. *IEEE T. on Med. Imag.* 2009; **28**: 1231-1237
3 Fano R. Theoretical limitations on the broadband matching of arbitrary impedances. *MIT research lab techn. rep.* 1948: **41**
4 Kaden H. Wirbelströme und Schirmung in der Nachrichtentechnik. Berlin: Springer, 1959/2006
5 Röschmann P. Radiofrequency penetration and absorption in the human body: limitations to high-field whole body nuclear MRI. *Med Phys.* 1987; **14**: 922-931
6 Weizenecker J et al. A Simulation Study on the Resolution and Sensitivity of MPI. *Phys. Med. Biol.* 2007, **52**: 6363-6374
7 Schmale I et al. JFET Noise Modelling for MPI Receivers. *Proceedings of IWMPI* 2010

CALCULATION AND EVALUATION OF CURRENT DENSITIES AND THERMAL HEATING IN THE BODY DURING MPI*

JULIA BOHNERT

Institute of Biomedical Engineering, Karlsruhe Institute of Technology (KIT), Kaiserstr. 12, 76131 Karlsruhe, Germany
Email: Julia.Bohnert@kit.edu

OLAF DÖSSEL

Institute of Biomedical Engineering, Karlsruhe Institute of Technology (KIT), Kaiserstr. 12, 76131 Karlsruhe, Germany
Email: Olaf.Doessel@kit.edu

In Magnetic Particle Imaging (MPI) the human body is exposed to magnetic fields of the lower kHz-range. The effects of those fields to biological tissue are yet to be determined. According to Faraday's Law, time-varying magnetic fields induce rotating electric fields. In body tissues, the induced electric field may cause an electric current, the formation of electric dipoles or the reorientation of present dipoles, depending on the strength of the magnetic field, the frequency and the properties of the body tissue, i.e. electrical conductivity and permittivity. Both electrical conductivity and permittivity vary with the frequency of the applied field. In case of a circular loop, the induced current density is proportional to the radius, the rate of change of the magnetic flux density and the conductivity of the tissue. Low frequency electric currents are able to stimulate skeletal muscles. Because of the capacitive characteristic of the cell membrane, the stimulating effect decreases with rising frequency. Furthermore, very short impulses ($t \ll 1$ ms) cannot open the Na-ion channels involved in nerve stimulation as effectively as longer ones. At higher frequencies, energy absorption becomes an issue. Exposure to electro-magnetic fields can lead to local temperature increase. The amount of absorbed energy per tissue weight is expressed by the specific absorption rate (SAR). The aim of this work is to calculate and evaluate the effects of the magnetic fields applied in MPI and propose ways to minimize them. At the same time, the risk of painful muscle stimulation should be minimized, even if MPI satisfies the requirements related to patient safety. In order to fulfill this task, simulation studies as well as experiments are being carried out. The following sections give an overview about the projects that are running or will be started in the near future.

* This work is supported by grant 13N9079 of the German Federal Ministry of Education and Research.

1. SIMULATION STUDIES

1.1. Numerical Simulations

In the numerical simulations the torso of the 'Visible Man' data set[a] is exposed to magnetic fields induced by current coil pairs. The data set contains 17 different body tissues, all of which were assigned the electrophysiological properties published by Gabriel et al[1]. The simulation software[2] solves the quasi-static Biot-Savart equation using the Finite-Elements-Method. In initial simulations the torso was exposed to a magnetic flux density of 10 mT (25 – 100 kHz), which is a reasonable MPI field strength, pointing in x-, y- and z-direction, produced by three respective 'drive field' coil pairs of 600 mm diameter and distance (fig. 1). The overall voxel model added up to $7.8 \cdot 10^6$ grid elements. The results[3] have shown that the induced current densities exceed current restrictions of the International Commission of Non-Ionizing Radiation Protection (ICNIRP)[4], while specific absorption rates (SAR) fulfill the respective limits for MRI, especially when taking into account that MPI examination times will be much shorter than those for MRI. Table 1 summarizes the relevant ICNIRP figures.

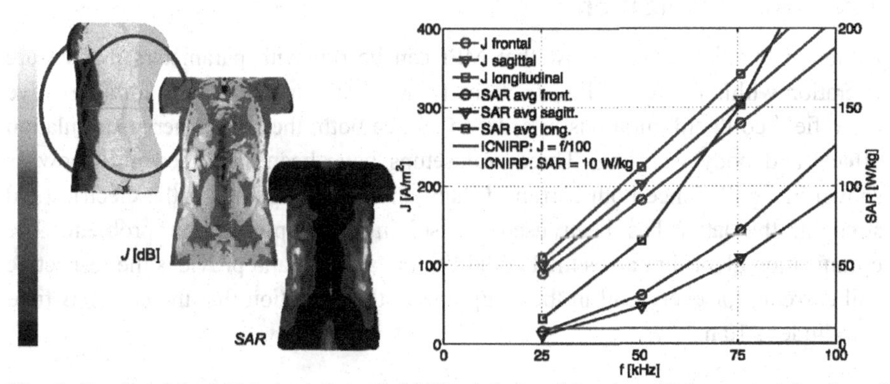

Fig. 1: Results of the initial simulations. (left:) Simulation model and qualitative current density and SAR distributions at 25.25 kHz, which is the current MPI frequency of the Philips MPI system[6]. As expected, peak values appear at the body's periphery. (right:) Values of current densities and SAR for all three drive field configurations at 10 mT central B-field and various frequencies

[a]Visible Human Project, National Library of Medicine, Bethesda, Maryland, USA

Table 1: Extraction of ICNIRP recommendations and simulated values.

	Quantity	Value
Occupational exposure[4]	J (effective) (1 – 100 kHz)	f [kHz]/100 A/m^2
	SAR (whole body) (100 kHz)	0.4 W/kg
	SAR local (10g) (head, trunk) (100 kHz)	10 W/kg
MRI restrictions[5]	SAR (whole body)	1 W/kg for 1 h
	SAR x time	120 W min/kg
	SAR instantaneous (trunk)	8 W/kg
	SAR local (10 g)	10 W/kg
Simulation results (B_{Amp} = 10 mT, f = 25.25 kHz)	J (effective)	89-110 A/m^2
	SAR local (10 g)	8 - 16 W/kg
	SAR (trunk)	0.7 – 1.1 W/kg

1.2. Coil Optimization

Although the simulations show that MPI can be run with parameters that ensure operation within the ICNIRP restrictions for MRI, it is useful to look for alternative drive field coil configurations in order to reduce both, the risk of nerve stimulation effects and body warming. Three coil setups have been simulated until now as shown in fig. 2. Since both current density and SAR originate in the electric field strength, the latter has been used for solving the optimization problem. The optimization algorithm takes the E-field vectors as input and provides the respective coil currents for every coil in the setup, under the condition that the center B-field amplitude is 10 mT.

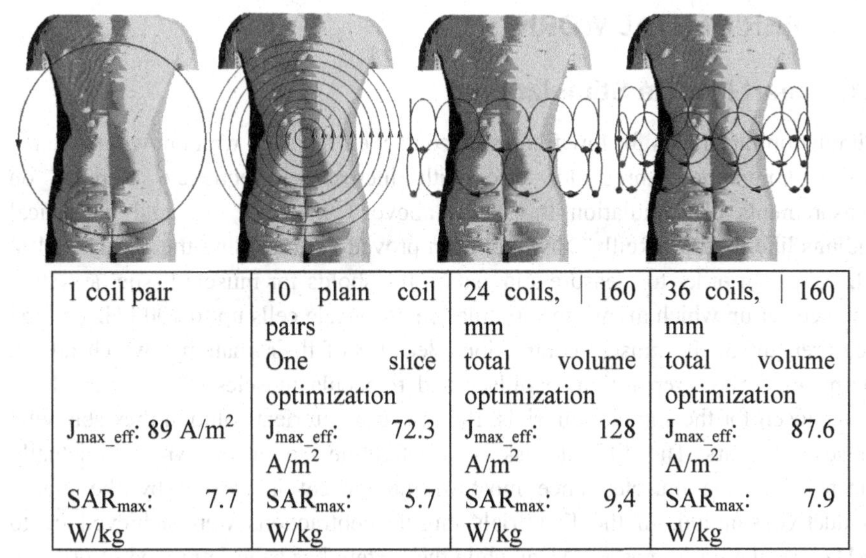

1 coil pair	10 plain coil pairs One slice optimization	24 coils, | 160 mm total volume optimization	36 coils, | 160 mm total volume optimization
J_{max_eff}: 89 A/m^2	J_{max_eff}: 72.3 A/m^2	J_{max_eff}: 128 A/m^2	J_{max_eff}: 87.6 A/m^2
SAR_{max}: 7.7 W/kg	SAR_{max}: 5.7 W/kg	SAR_{max}: 9,4 W/kg	SAR_{max}: 7.9 W/kg

Fig. 2: Three different drive field coil configurations and resulting field values (25.25 kHz).

While decreasing coil diameters leads to higher field values, an increasing number of coils reduces field values. This becomes clear when considering that higher coil currents are needed in smaller coils in order to reach 10 mT magnetic flux density in the center of the body. Future work will be needed to find the optimum coil setup.

1.3. Cell Model Simulations

In the past many mathematical models have been designed which reproduce the electric activity of single cells by a complex set of differential equations. These models are based on mammalian myocardial cells. These cell models can be stimulated by current pulse trains of various amplitudes, frequencies and lengths. The model computes the states of every ion channel of the cell membrane and subsequently the ion concentrations which are responsible for the actual membrane potential. If the membrane potential reaches a threshold, an action potential is generated. For ongoing and future work towards determinging stimulation thresholds for impulses of frequencies from 1 kHz up to 1 MHz, the cell model of Luo and Rudy[7] is favored..

2. EXPERIMENTAL WORK

2.1. Heart Muscle Stimulations

Stimulation thresholds for low frequency contact currents are well known. As stated earlier, stimulation thresholds rise with increasing frequency. Reports on measurements of stimulation thresholds above 1 kHz are rare and theoretical findings like those of Reilly[8] have not been proved yet regarding the 10 kHz – 100 kHz range. In order to measure stimulation thresholds for muscle tissue, a system has been set up which allows the stimulation of muscle cells up to 100 kHz and the measurement of the muscle contraction. Because of their anatomy, which allows comparably easy preparation, papillary and trabecula muscles of rat hearts have been chosen for the stimulation trials. Being kept in nutrient solution they stay vital for several hours. The difficult task is to determine the current which is actually injected into the muscle, since most of the current is carried by the highly conductive solution. In the first trials muscle contractions were achieved up to 5 kHz stimulation frequency. Meanwhile the system has been improved in order to enable stimulation by currents of higher frequencies.

2.2. Temperature Measurements

Besides the calculation of the absorbed power, which leads to local thermal heating in the body, temperature measurements have been carried out in a real MPI system, using a Plexiglas cylinder filled with highly concentrated saline solution.

A fiber optic temperature probe was placed at the cylinder's periphery. The vertically oriented coils of the MPI system were driven up to a magnetic flux density of 30 mT being switched on and off for defined periods of time. The results are shown in fig. 4. In future work, these findings will be reproduced through simulations in order to derive predictions for a system scaled up to a human-size MPI scanner.

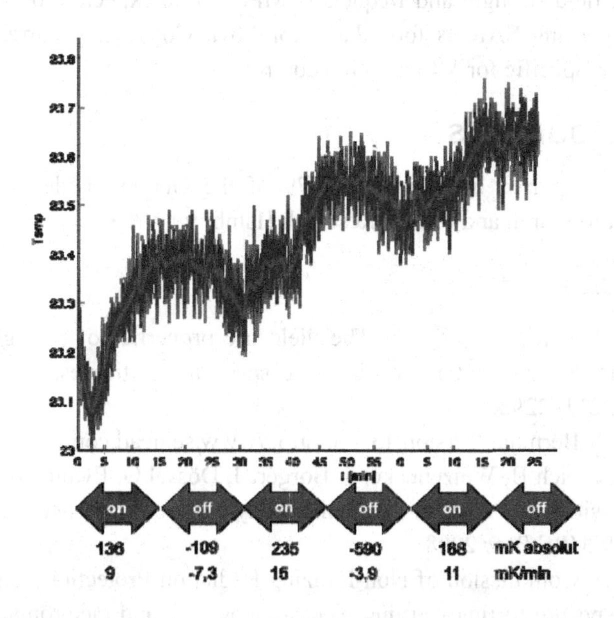

Fig. 4: Temperature variation in the saline solution (180 g/l) while switching the drive field on and off. The initial drop in temperature is caused by introducing the saline solution from room temperature into a well cooled system

2.3. Coil System Design for Inductive Muscle Stimulation

The aim of another stimulation experiment is to find out the thresholds of inductive muscle stimulation. Therefore, a figure-8, or butterfly-shaped coil is being built that induces well-localized current densities in peripheral muscles. Simulations in order to approximate necessary coil currents on the one hand and to optimize circuit element properties to reach stimulating field strengths on the other hand have been carried out already. The system is designed as a resonating circuit, with all its elements matching 25 kHz stimulation frequency, ensuring high electrical stability and safety.

3. CONCLUSION AND OUTLOOK

Magnetic Particle Imaging is a promising technique that enables fast imaging of nanoparticle concentrations at high resolution. Since MPI can be associated with peripheral nerve stimulation and/or local tissue warming, these effects have to be carefully evaluated. This paper summarizes our current approaches in order to tackle this task. Based on a careful design and control of the setup, i.e. coil configuration, field strength and frequency, MPI can be expected to meet ICNIRP regulations regarding SAR as formulated for MRI. Concerning current densities, new restrictions specific for MPI may be required.

ACKNOWLEDGMENTS

This work is supported by grant 13N9079 of the German Federal Ministry of Education and Research and Philips Research Hamburg.

REFERENCES

1 Gabriel S, Lau RW, Gabriel C. The dielectric properties of biological tissues: III. Parametric models for the dielectric spectrum of tissues. *Phys Med Biol* 1996; **41**: 2271–2293.
2 SEMCAD X Bernina, Version 13.4 at http://www.semcad.com.
3 Bohnert J, Gleich B, Weizenecker J, Borgert J, Dössel O. Evaluation of induced current densities and SAR in the human body by strong magnetic fields around 100 kHz. *IFMBE Proc* 2008.
4 International Commission of Non-Ionizing Radiation Protection. Guidelines for limiting exposure to time-varying electric, magnetic and electromagnetic fields (up to 300 GHz). *Health Phys.* 1998.
5 International Non-Ionizing Radiation Committee of the International Radiation Protection Associatin. Protection of the patient undergoing a magnetic resonance examination. *Health Phys.*1991; **61.6:** 923-928.
6 Gleich B, Weizenecker J, Borgert J. Experimental results on fast 2D-encoded magnetic particle imaging. *Phys Med Biol* 2008; **53 (6):** N81-N84.
7 Luo CH, Rudy Y. A dynamic model of the cardiac ventricular action potential. I. Simulations of ionic currents and concentraion changes. *Circulation Research* 1994; **74 (4):** 1071–1096.
8 Reilly JP, Bauer RH. Application of a neuroelectric model to electrocutaneous sensory sensitivity: parameter variation study. *IEEE Transactions on bio-Medical Engineering* 1987; **34 (9):** 752–754.

A SURVEILLANCE UNIT FOR MAGNETIC PARTICLE IMAGING SYSTEMS

STEFFEN KAUFMANN, SVEN BIEDERER, TIMO F. SATTEL,
TOBIAS KNOPP, THORSTEN M. BUZUG

Institute of Medical Engineering, University of Lübeck, Lübeck, Germany
email: kaufmann@imt.uni-luebeck.de, buzug@imt.uni-luebeck.de

Magnetic Particle Imaging (MPI) is a new tomographic imaging technique. The idea of MPI is to exploit the nonlinear magnetization curve of superparamagnetic nanoparticles for imaging their spatial distribution. To achieve this, a complex hardware setup is necessary. This paper introduces a surveillance unit to monitor and secure the operation of high power MPI systems, to ensure system safety and accuracy.

1. INTRODUCTION

Magnetic Particle Imaging (MPI) is a new tomographic imaging technique introduced in 2005[1]. The idea of MPI is to exploit the nonlinear magnetization curve of superparamagnetic nanoparticles for imaging their spatial distribution. In various works[2-4], the imaging performance has been proven. An MPI system is comprised of various technical components. Each of these components has to be monitored to ensure proper and safe operation. Potential risks are overheating of transmitting coils, voltage breakdowns, or exceeding of maximum field strengths.

To ensure automated monitoring, a surveillance unit (SU) is needed, which can detect failures and react to these failures. An SU may also ensure an improvement of imaging quality through better system estimation, in addition to safety issues. The imaging improvement may be achieved by a permanent monitoring of the MPI system. For example, temperature drifts can be monitored and changes in system function, which can lead to artifacts and lower the imaging quality, may be corrected.

This paper describes an SU, which enables monitoring of system parameters to ensure safe operation and to compensate for parameter drifts. The SU is build up as an independent dedicated hardware with real-time behavior. In case of a crash of the

MPI control system the SU can shut down the system safely. A system logbook provides a possibility for subsequent failure analysis.

2. MPI SCANNER

The principle of MPI scanners in general is described along the simplified block diagram in figure 1 (a detailed description is given by Schmale et al.[5]).

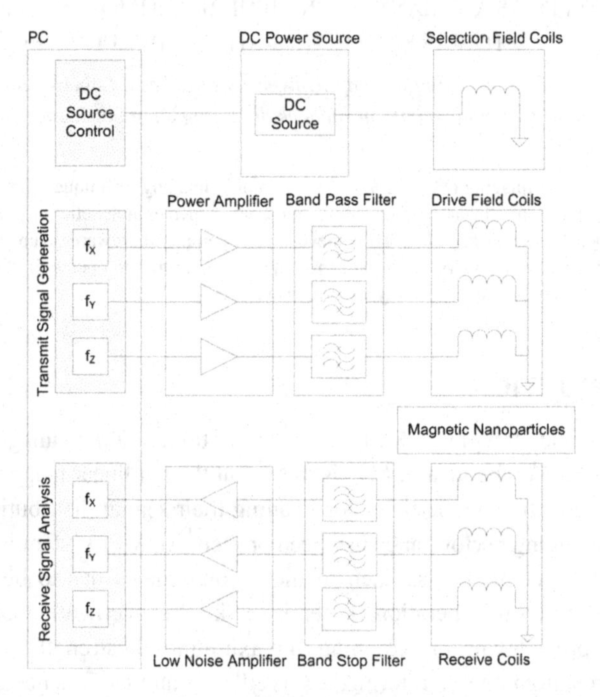

Fig. 1. Block diagram of an MPI Scanner

A PC controls the signal generation and reception. A high power DC source supplies the current for the selection field generation. Digital-to-analog converters generate the signals for the drive field. The generated signals are amplified by power amplifiers, filtered by band pass filters (BPF) and then applied to the transmit coils (TxC) to generate the drive field. The transmitted signals are non-linearly transformed by the nanoparticles. These signals induce voltages in the receive coils (RxC). A subsequent filtering of the base transmit signal by band stop filters (BSF) ensures a clipping free amplification by low noise amplifiers (LNA). The output signals of the LNA are digitalized and processed in the PC. It is obvious that the power-path parts are exposed to the highest stress level in the system and, therefore, surveillance is necessary.

3. METHODS

To detect possible system error cases, a common way is to carry out a fault tree analysis (FTA) combined with a failure mode and effect analysis (FMEA)[6]. The outcomes of these analysis lead to the parameters, which should be monitored, i.e.

1. temperature of the transmit coil,
2. temperature and pressure of the cooling circuit,
3. voltages and currents of the DC power supplies and
4. voltages and currents of the AC power amplifiers (amplitude and phase).

The currents and voltages can be acquired using different methods given by the demands. Possible values which can be acquired are the rectified, peak or effective value. All these values have in common that the unnecessary wave form information is lost. Data acquisition is done through high speed low noise analog-to-digital converters. Temperatures are acquired through standardized temperature sensors (PT100).

The magnetic field generated by the TxC is controlled by the current in the TxC. It is important to ensure that the field strength does not exceed 20 mT/μ_0, for not harming the patient through heating caused by tissue absorption of the electric field[7].

The data acquisition rates depend on the measures itself e.g. a temperature rise is maybe much slower than a voltage or current rise. This means that it is likely that measurements of the cooling circuit temperature have to be done less often than the measurement of the TxC voltage.

In addition to the acquisition of data, an appropriate method to detect system failures and react to system failures is needed. This evaluation is done by judging the acquired data with respect to their time-changing characteristics against given limits. Given limits could be static values as well as gradients or a combination of both. A subsequently build running-mean reduces the impact of outliers during the measurement process.

Failures are classified into two groups: severe failures which are compromising the system or patient safety and warnings. Therefore, two different reaction alternatives are implemented: A hard reaction and a soft reaction. A hard reaction causes the system or a part of the system to shut down immediately. The soft reaction implies a warning will be generated or a message to the system control can be send to terminate or adapt the actual measurement.

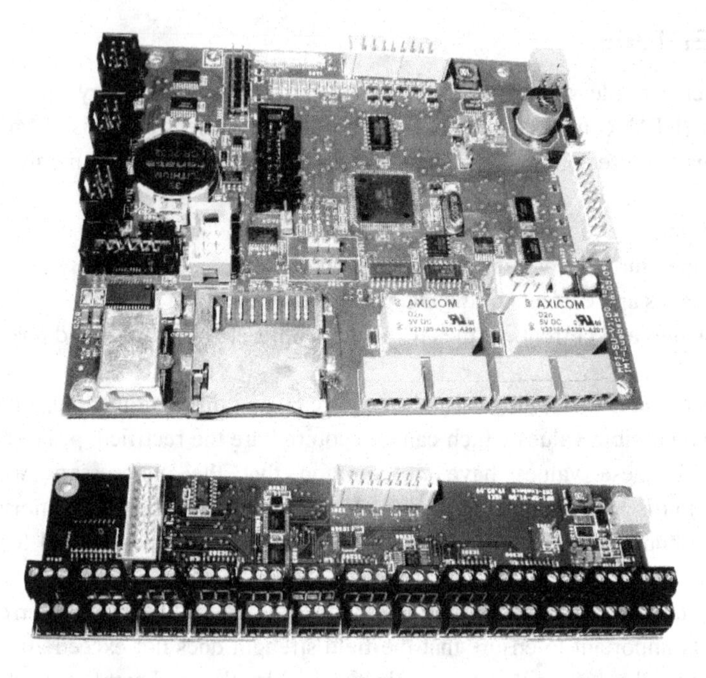

Fig. 2. Pictures of the surveillance unit and the sensor PCB

Figure 2 shows the hardware setup of the SU. As it is shown, the unit is separated into two parts: a main PCB and an expansion PCB. The main PCB contains a microcontroller, which handles the whole surveillance logic. The expansion PCB contains the data acquisition components and is cascadable for further extensions. This approach enables an easy adaption and scalability to new system demands.

4. EVALUATION AND RESULTS

To show the basic functionality of the SU, an example test case is performed. Figure 3 shows a resistor heated up by a DC source, whereby a warning is generated after exceeding the soft limit and a system shutdown is executed after reaching the hard limit. Thereby, the measurement was performed without running-mean; the impact of a positive outlier caused in this case a undesired shutdown of the system.

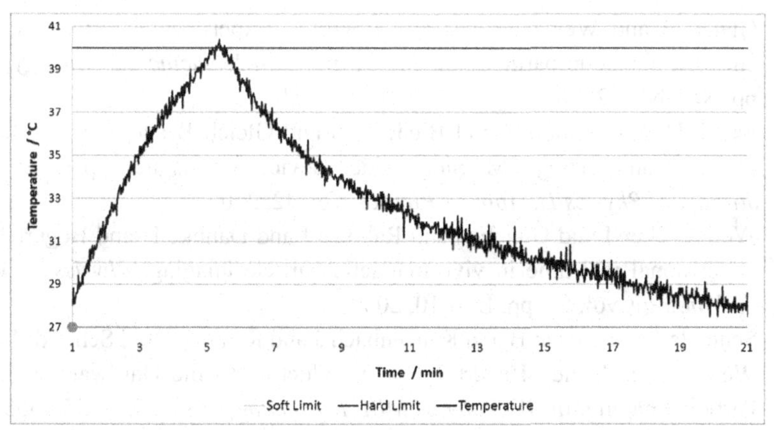

Fig. 3. Basic test case: a heated resistor

5. DISCUSSIONS

It could be shown that the SU is able to detect and react in cases of system failures to ensure the system safety. It is also shown that the SU can be used to record measurements. It is likely that the acquired measurements are helpful for further development and improvement of the imaging quality of an MPI scanner.

A future application of the SU is use as control and discriminating element in the closed loop of the TxC current regulation. A temperature rise in the TxC leads to a decrease of current und therefore to a drop of the magnetic field. This can lead to imaging artifacts, caused by a changed trajectory. Due to the fact that the SU already controls the DC source the adaption seems to be uncomplicated. Another possible improvement is the measurement of the complex impedance of the TxC. The current-voltage phase contains useful information about the system status.

6. CONCLUSIONS

In this paper, an SU for MPI systems was presented. The SU will be a helpful tool during the development of new scanner designs and within the improvement of current setups. The SU ensures system safety and the SU logbook provides a helpful tool for bug tracking. In future, the SU will be used to improve the reproducibility of the measurement trajectories and for subsequent data corrections.

REFERENCES

1 Gleich B and Weizenecker J. Tomographic imaging using the nonlinear response of magnetic particles. *Nature*, vol. 435, pp. 1214–1217, 2005.

2 Gleich B and Weizenecker J and Bogert J. Experimental results on fast 2D-encoded magnetic particle imaging. *Physics in Medicine and Biology*, vol. 53, pp. N81-N84, 2008.
3 Sattel TF and Knopp T and Biederer S and Gleich B and Weizenecker J and Bogert J and Buzug TM. Single-sided device for magnetic particle imaging. *Journal of Physics D: Applied Physics*, vol. 42, 2009.
4 Weizenecker J and Gleich B and Rahmer J and Dahnke H and Bogert J, Three-dimensional real-time in vivo magnetic particle imaging. *Physics in Medicine and Biology*, vol. 54, pp. L1-L10, 2009.
5 Schmale I and Gleich B and Kanzenbach J and Rahmer J and Schmidt J and Weizenecker J and Bogert J. An introduction to the Hardware of Magnetic Particle Imaging. In: *WC2009, IFMBE Proceedings*, vol. 25, pp 450-453, 2009.
6 Krasich M. Can FMEA assure a reliable product?. In: *Reliability and Maintainability Symposium, 2007*, Orlando, FL: IEEE, 2007: 277–281.
7 Bohnert J and Gleich B and Weizenecker J and Borgert J and Doessel O. Evaluation of Induced Current Densities and SAR in Human Body by Strong Magnetic Fields around 100kHz. In: *IFMBE Proceedings*, 2008.

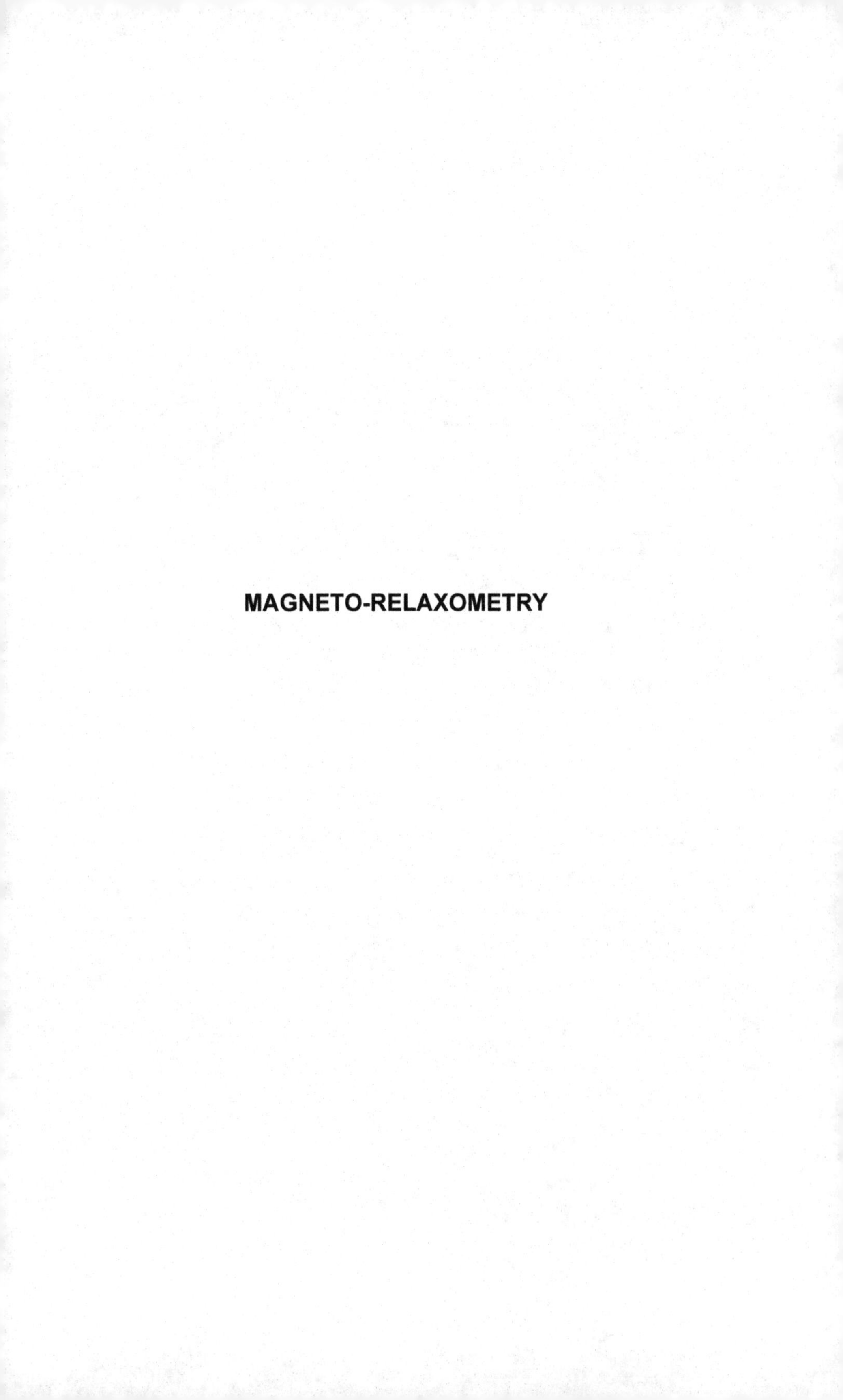

MAGNETO-RELAXOMETRY

CANCER THERAPY WITH MAGNETIC NANOPARTICLES VISUALIZED WITH MRI, X-RAY-TOMOGRAPHY, MAGNETORELAXOMETRY AND HISTOLOGY

STEFAN LYER,
RAINER TIETZE

Section for Experimental Oncology and Nanomedicine (Else Kröner-Fresenius-Foundation-Professorship) at the ENT-Department of the University Erlangen-Nürnberg, Waldstr. 1, 91054 Erlangen, Germany

LUTZ TRAHMS

PTB, Abbestr. 2-12, Berlin, Germany, Email:lutz.trahms@ptb.de

HELENE RAHN,
STEFAN ODENBACH

Institute of Fluid Mechanics, Technische Universität Dresden, 01062, Dresden, Germany
Email: stefan.odenbach@tu-dresden.de

CHRISTOPH ALEXIOU*

Section for Experimental Oncology and Nanomedicine (Else Kröner-Fresenius-Foundation-Professorship) at the ENT-Department of the University Erlangen-Nürnberg, Waldstr. 1, 91054 Erlangen, Germany
Email: c.alexiou@web.de*

Magnetic Drug Targeting (MDT) is a new approach for chemotherapy heading for a higher drug amount in the tumor and simultaneously a reduced overall dose. The aim of the present study was to investigate the distribution of the particles with common imaging techniques. Tumor bearing rabbits were examined with a 4.7 Tesla MRI before and after MDT. The biodistribution of magnetic nanoparticles after MDT was investigated with a high resolution 3-dimensional x-ray-tomography (CCD Camera, 1024x1024 pixels) of the extracted tumor with corresponding histological cross sections. Moreover quantitative analysis was performed with a multichannel SQUID system based on magnetrelaxometry. All methods show a significant enrichment of magnetic nanoparticles in the tumor region.

1. INTRODUCTION

The development of biocompatible nano sized drug delivery systems for specific targeting of therapeutics is imminent in medical research, especially for treating cancer and vascular diseases. Magnetically targeted drug delivery is a promising approach in medicine to apply a more site specific effect of administered drugs and to reduce the overall distribution in the body and subsequently drug associated negative side effects.[1, 2] Magnetic nanoparticles can be bound to therapeutic agents and targeted to the region of interest by an external magnetic field after intravascular administration.[3-5] Frequently used in medical research are superparamagnetic iron oxide nanoparticles (Fe_3O_4). These particles are biodegradable[6, 7] and they are still in use as contrast agent in magnetic resonance imaging (MRI) for lymphography.[8] Crucial for the effectiveness of Magnetic Drug Targeting (MDT) is the achieved enrichment in the targeted area. In pilot studies with radioactive labeled nanoparticles we could quantitatively analyze the distribution and the considerable nanoparticle enrichment in the targeted region Furthermore these results were confirmed by quantitative determination of the chemotherapeutic agent which was bound to the magnetic nanoparticles.[9-12] This article is to show different possibilities for imaging the magnetic iron oxide nanoparticles by different techniques *in vitro* and *in vivo.*

2. MATERIALS AND METHODS

2.1. Nanoparticles

The nanoparticles consist of iron oxides covered by phosphated starch polymers for colloidal stabilization in deionised water. Dynamic laser scattering (DLS, Nicomp 380 ZLS, Santa Barbara, CA, USA) measurements show the hydrodynamic diameter of the particles (magnetite cores embedded in the polymer coating) with an average size of about 100-200 nm.

2.2. Chemotherapeutic Agent

In our experiments drug loading was realized with Mitoxantrone (Novantron®; Wyeth-Pharma, Germany), an anthracendion derivative which inhibits the DNA and RNA synthesis and causes DNA-strand breaks by intercalation.

2.3. *In vivo* experiments

For the *in-vivo* experiments we implanted VX2-squamous cell carcinomas at the left hind limb of New Zealand White Rabbits to ensure that it is in the supplying area of the femoral artery. After development of solid tumors (2-3 weeks) the nanoparticles were injected into the femoral artery close to the tumor which was placed under the tip of the pole shoe of an electromagnet. The animals were investigated for magnetic iron oxide enrichment *in vivo* and sacrificed for further investigation afterwards. The animal experiments were used in accordance by the responsible authority (District Government of Mittelfranken, Germany, request: 54-2531.31-27/06).

2.4. Magnetic field

For the experiments we used a powerful electromagnet (Siemens AG) with a maximum magnetic field strength of 1.0 Tesla and a maximum magnetic field gradient of 70 T/m.

2.5. Magnetic Resonance Imaging

Tumor bearing animals were examined before and after MDT with a 4.7 Tesla MRI. A 4.7 T Bruker Biospec scanner with a free bore of 40 cm, equipped with an actively RF-decoupled coil system was used for these measurements.

2.6. X-Ray-Tomography

X-ray tomography experiments have been carried out with a laboratory setup based on a commercial cone beam x-ray source (Apogee 5000) with 40 μm focus size and a maximal acceleration voltage of 50 kV. The x-ray beam passes the sample, which is mounted on a high-precision rotation stage and produces an absorption image of the sample on a phosphor screen with a sensitive area of 10×10 cm^2. By means of a macrolens system as used in this case, the images are transmitted to a low-noise 1024×1024 pixel (Marconi 47-10) CCD detector. Paraffin imbedded tumor samples were measured to show the distribution of nanoparticles after MDT.

2.7. Histology

For corresponding histological cross sections, slices of 5 μm thickness were used. The slices were stained with Prussian Blue. Trivalent iron is visible as blue pigment while the remaining structures appear in red color, due to nuclear fast red counterstaining.

2.8. Magnetorelaxometry

The relaxation signal of the nanoparticles was measured using a single-channel superconducting quantum interference device (SQUID) gradiometer at a detection limit of 1ng iron. The magnetic field application leads to an aligning of the magnetic moments. Helium cooled low Tc-SQUID sensors detect the time-dependent alteration of the magnetic induction generated by the relaxing magnetization of iron oxide after the magnetic field is switched of. The measured signal amplitudes are in direct ratio to the iron oxide amount. Measurements of reference samples with a defined iron-oxide-content allow the quantitative analysis of the magnetic nanoparticles. The animals were examined by SQUID before and after MDT.

3. RESULTS

Tumor bearing rabbits were examined with MRI before and after MDT. The morphology and position of the tumor is clearly visible (fig. 1 a). Unfortunately, after MDT (fig. 1 b) nanoparticles lead to signal deletion due to their high concentration in the tumor. The appropriate image could be achieved in dependence of the particle concentration, which showed an optimum in a dilution of 1:500.

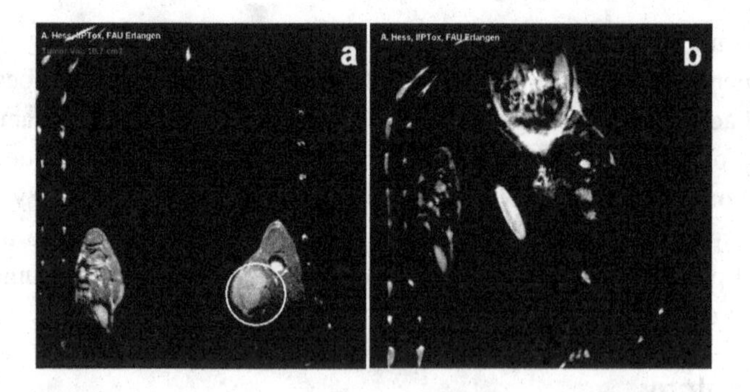

Fig. 1 a.: MRI of the VX2 tumor (white circle) at the rabbits hind limp before MDT. **b**.: Signal deletion after MDT.

Tumor tissue was removed from the animals and examined via X-ray tomography. The x-ray images of the VX2-tumor tissue samples embedded in paraffin after Magnetic Drug Targeting (MDT) showed the iron oxide nanoparticles in the vascular system of the tumor (fig. 2a). The corresponding histological cross sections displayed the nanoparticles in the vascular system of the tumor (fig. 2b,c). Sections were stained with Prussian blue for visualization of the iron oxide nanoparticles. The nanoparticles are visible as dark pigment in the vessels of the tumor.[13]

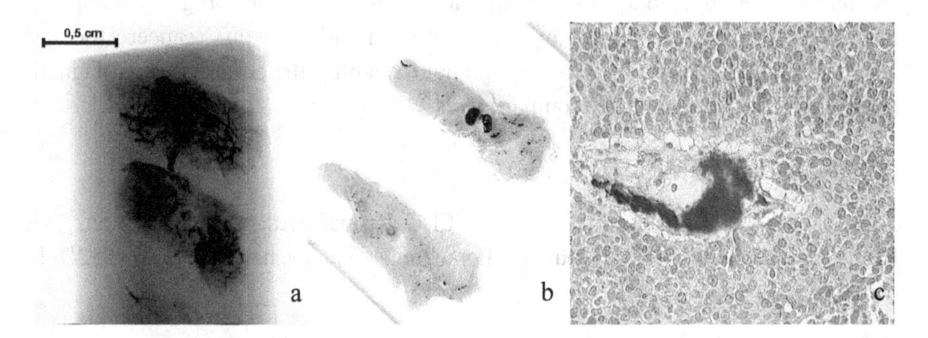

Fig. 2 .: paraffin embedded tumor. **a**: x-ray images of nanoparticles inside the tumor vessels. **b**: Histological overview of Prussian blue stained cross section of VX2 tumor tissue **c:** magnification 400 x

SQUID measurements after MDT proved non-invasively that a high amount of magnetic nanoparticles (~85%) was accumulated in the tumor region, together with a much smaller accumulation in the liver region[14, 15]. The centre of the circular-shaped field distribution corresponds to the tumor position (Fig. 3).

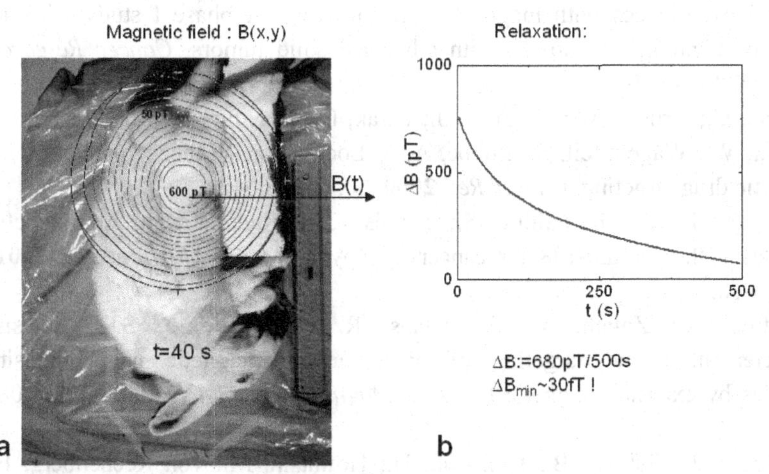

Fig. 3: **a**: Magnetic field distribution of magnetic nanoparticles relaxation after magnetization. The center of the circular shaped field distribution corresponds to the tumor position. **b**: Single channel relaxation signal of the magnetic nanoparticles.

4. CONCLUSION

Imaging techniques (x-ray, MRI) offer the opportunity to achieve information about the biodistribution of magnetic nanoparticles after Magnetic Drug Targeting and this could be very important to control non-invasively cancer therapy. Magnetorelaxometry is a sensitive technique to quantify the enrichment of magnetic nanoparticles in specific body compartments.

ACKNOWLEDGMENTS

These studies were supported by the Else Kröner-Fresenius-Foundation, Bad Homburg, Germany and the Deutsche Forschungsgemeinschaft (DFG-AL 552/3-1), Germany.

REFERENCES

1 Torchilin, V. P. Drug targeting. *Eur J Pharm Sci* **2000,** 11, S81-S91.
2 Collins, J. M. Pharmacological rationale for regional drug delivery. *J. Clin. Oncol* **1984,** 2, 498-505.
3 Lubbe, A. S.; Bergemann, C.; Riess, H.; Schriever, F.; Reichardt, P.; Possinger, K.; Matthias, M.; Dorken, B.; Herrmann, F.; Gurtler, R.; Hohenberger, P.; Haas, N.; Sohr, R.; Sander, B.; Lemke, A. J.; Ohlendorf, D.; Huhnt, W.; Huhn, D. Clinical experiences with magnetic drag targeting: A phase I study with 4'-epidoxorubicin in 14 patients with advanced solid tumors. *Cancer Research* **1996,** 56, 4686-4693.
4 Alexiou, C.; Arnold, W.; Klein, R. J.; Parak, F. G.; Hulin, P.; Bergemann, C.; Erhardt, W.; Wagenpfeil, S.; Lubbe, A. S. Locoregional cancer treatment with magnetic drug targeting. *Cancer Res.* **2000,** 60, 6641-6648.
5 Hafeli, U.; Pauer, G.; Failing, S.; Tapolsky, G. Radiolabeling of magnetic particles with rhenium-188 for cancer therapy. *J. Magn. Magn. Mater.* **2001,** 225, 73-78.
6 Asmatulu, R.; Zalich, M. A.; Claus, R. O.; Riffle, J. S. Synthesis, characterization and targeting of biodegradable magnetic nanocomposite particles by external magnetic fields. *J. Magn. Magn. Mater.* **2005,** 292, 108-119.
7 Neuberger, T.; Schopf, B.; Hofmann, H.; Hofmann, M.; von Rechenberg, B. Superparamagnetic nanoparticles for biomedical applications: Possibilities and limitations of a new drug delivery system. *J. Magn. Magn. Mater.* **2005,** 293, 483-496.

8 Taupitz, M., Wagner, S., Hamm, B., Dienemann, D., Lawaczeck, R., Wolf, K. J. MR Lymphography using iron oxide particles. Detection of lymph node metastases in the VX2 rabbit tumour model. *Acta Radiologica* **1993,** 34, 10-15.

9 Alexiou, C.; Jurgons, R.; Schmid, R. J.; Bergemann, C.; Henke, J.; Erhardt, W.; Huenges, E.; Parak, F. Magnetic drug targeting - Biodistribution of the magnetic carrier and the chemotherapeutic agent mitoxantrone after locoregional cancer treatment. *J Drug Target* **2003,** 11, 139-149.

10 Alexiou, C.; Jurgons, R.; Seliger, C.; Kolb, S.; Heubeck, B.; Iro, H. Distribution of mitoxantrone after magnetic drug targeting: Fluorescence microscopic investigations on VX2 squamous cell carcinoma cells. *Z Phys Chem* **2006,** 220, 235-240.

11 Storm, G.; Belliot, S. O.; Daemen, T.; Lasic, D. D. Surface Modification of Nanoparticles to Oppose Uptake by the Mononuclear Phagocyte System. *Adv Drug Deliver Rev* **1995,** 17, 31-48.

12 Alexiou, C.; Jurgons, R.; Schmid, R.; Hilpert, A.; Bergemann, C.; Parak, F.; Iro, H. In vitro and in vivo investigations of targeted chemotherapy with magnetic nanoparticles. *J. Magn. Magn. Mater.* **2005,** 293, 389-393.

13 Alexiou, C.; Jurgons, R.; Seliger, C.; Brunke, O.; Iro, H.; Odenbach, S. Delivery of superparamagnetic nanoparticles for local chemotherapy after intraarterial infusion and magnetic drug targeting. *Anticancer Res.* **2007,** 27, 2019-2022.

14 Wiekhorst, F.; Seliger, C.; Jurgons, R.; Steinhoff, U.; Eberbeck, D.; Trahms, L.; Alexiou, C. Quantification of magnetic nanoparticles by magnetorelaxometry and comparison to histology after magnetic drug targeting. *J. Nanosci. Nanotechnol.* **2006,** 6, 3222-3225.

15 Jurgons, R.; Seliger, C.; Hilpert, A.; Trahms, L.; Odenbach, S.; Alexiou, C. Drug loaded magnetic nanoparticles for cancer therapy. *Journal of Physics-Condensed Matter* **2006,** 18, S2893-S2902.

LOCALIZATION AND QUANTIFICATION OF MAGNETIC NANOPARTICLES BY MULTICHANNEL MAGNETORELAXOMETRY FOR THERMAL ABLATION STUDIES

HEIKE RICHTER, FRANK WIEKHORST, UWE STEINHOFF, LUTZ TRAHMS

Physikalisch-Technische Bundesanstalt, Abbestrasse 2-12,
10587 Berlin, Germany
Email: heike.richter@ptb.de

MELANIE KETTERING, WERNER A KAISER, INGRIG HILGER

Institute of Diagnostic and Interventional Radiology,
University Hospital Jena, Jena, Germany

For thermal ablation application the quantity of magnetic nanoparticles (MNP) needs to be thoroughly controlled to govern adequate heat production in the carcinoma region. Here, we demonstrate the capability of magnetorelaxometry (MRX) for the non-invasive monitoring of total MNP amount in mice after intratumoral injection of MNP prior to thermal ablation. Modelling a MNP accumulation by a single magnetic point dipole, the dipole parameters corresponding to location and total amount of the accumulation are obtained by non-linear least square fitting of the magnetic field pattern caused by the MNP and measured by multichannel MRX. Normalizing to the moment of a reference sample of known MNP content enables a robust and reliable quantification of the amount of MNP in the defined region of the mouse.

1. INTRODUCTION

Localized magnetic heating treatments (hyperthermia[12,13], thermal ablation[2,5]) using superparamagnetic iron oxide nanoparticles (MNP) continue to be an active area of cancer research and therapy[7], where cancer cells are inactivated by high temperatures with minimal side effects in healthy tissues. One of the critical parameters is the accumulation of adequate amounts of MNP in cancer cells or in the tumor region that generate lethal doses of 55 to 60 °C[4]. In vitro, magnetic heating treatment studies[6] already indicate the advantage of an effective MNP labelling over 24 hours before magnetic heating. But little is known about the efficiency of intratumoral MNP accumulation *in vivo*. Here we suggest MRX[3,15,8,9] as a proper tool for the contactless, quantitative monitoring of the MNP biodistribution. Our proof of principle presents the localization and quantification of the total amount of MNP in two carcinoma mice with intratumoral MNP injection at the actual point of time where thermal ablation would be applied.

2. MATERIALS AND METHODS

2.1. In vivo carcinoma models

Two female SCID (Severe Combined Immune-Deficient) mice were obtained from the Institute of Animal Research of the Clinics of Friedrich Schiller University, Jena. The animals were adequately housed (controlled bedding, room temperature, dark cycle) and feed (adequate diet and water). Experimental tumors were grown after an injection of 200 µl of BD Matrigel™ Basement Membrane Matrix (Becton Dickinson GmbH, Heidelberg) subcutaneously between the shoulder blades containing 10^7 9L/lacZ cells (mouse 1) or 10^7 MDA-MB-435S cells (mouse 2), respectively. All experiments were approved by the regional animal care committee and were in accordance with international guidelines on the ethical use of animals. Experiments were started approximately 6 weeks after tumor implantation. Prior to the experiments, the animals received an anesthetic gas then 200 µl (= 40 mg total iron amount) of an MNP suspension (fluidMAG-D of chemicell GmbH, Berlin, with solids content β = 200 mg/ml, hydrodynamic diameter d_{hydr} = 200 nm) was injected into the tumor. After 24 hours, the mice were sacrificed by CO_2 in order to keep the condition of the onset of thermal ablation treatments. Subsequently, the mice were fixed in 96 % ethanol.

2.2. Multichannel Magnetorelaxometry

In our multichannel MRX measurements, the magnetic relaxation of the MNP was measured by a biomagnetic 304-channel SQUID-system[10] (Superconductive Quantum Interference Device) operating in the magnetically shielded room BMSR-2, which enables the detection of magnetic fields down to a few fT[11]. During the measurement, the mouse was fixed in a plastic foil, attached in an abdominal position on a non-magnetic table with a slide-in tray. An external static magnetic field generated by a Helmholtz coil ($d = 2r \approx 85$ cm) with homogenous magnetic flux density B = 1 mT was applied in z-direction to the sample for about 60 s outside the magnetically shielded room. Due to the superparamagnetic behaviour of the particles, the magnetic moments of the MNP in the sample align along the applied magnetic field direction. After switching off the magnetic field, the sample was rapidly transferred underneath the measurement device (delay of about 6 s) and the decaying magnetic induction $B_z(t)$ was measured for 70 s at a sampling rate of

250 Hz. During the measurement the door of the magnetically shielded room was kept open.

By multichannel MRX we obtained a magnetic field pattern at each time point of the MNP relaxation with slowly decreasing amplitude. By non-linear least square fitting (Levenberg-Marquardt algorithm) of the magnetic field data, using a single magnetic point dipole model, the center $\vec{r} = (x, y, z)$ and the magnetic moment $\vec{m}$ of the MNP accumulation were determined as a function of time. Strictly speaking this fit is valid for a point-like dipole. However, in our case the extension of the MNP accumulation in the tumor was small compared to the distance of the source to the sensor (~ 7 cm), hence the dipole fit is yet a valid approximation. The reconstructed dipole position (center of gravity of MNP accumulation) was then related to a reference point, which was obtained by measuring a cylindrical calibration coil with a known magnetic moment of 17 nAm^2. For the accuracy in spatial resolution we obtained $\Delta x = \Delta y = 0.5$ mm, dependent on the reproducibility of the measurement position.

For quantification, reference samples were prepared from originally administered MNP, immobilizing 200 µl of the original suspension in plaster (commercially available). Additionally, corresponding quality checks were performed of the reference solution and the immobilized reference samples in different dilution steps. We found good scaling for the fluid and immobilized samples. For quantification the reconstructed magnetic moment dipole of the mouse was related to the reference sample, which was measured under the same experimental setup and reconstructed utilizing magnetic dipole fitting. Note, that a MNP-specific quantification is practicable because any remanent magnetization solely contributes to the offset in MRX-signals and hence the amplitude of the relaxation curve scales with the MNP amount in the sample. Curve shapes of the reference and mouse sample were thoroughly checked to be the same.

3. RESULTS AND DISCUSSION

Figure 1 illustrates the results for mouse 1 and 2, respectively, in a schematic plot of the mouse in prone position. The tumor region is indicated by a orange circle and the determined location is therein marked as a black dot. As can be seen, in both measured carcinoma mice, the localization of the center of mass of the MNP accumulation was explicitly obtained in the tumor region by MRX. Table 1 lists the details of the obtained lateral dipole positions from the magnetic dipole fit and the central tumor positions in the *x-y*-plane in relation to the reference point, as well as the tumor. The *z*-position of the dipole was determined to be well above the base of the sample tray for both mice, i.e. 1.3(1) cm for mouse 1 and 1.7(1) cm for mouse 2.

The MNP quantification in the localized regions of the two mice was obtained using the immobilized reference sample, measured under the same conditions. We yield 39.8(4) mg total iron amount in the tumor region of mouse 1, i.e., the full amount of applied magnetic nanoparticles. For mouse 2, however, we obtained 30.2(4) mg total iron amount, 25% less than applied.

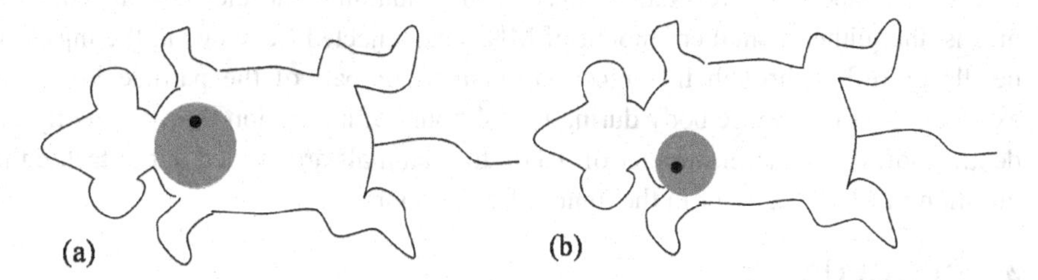

Fig. 1. Sketch of mouse 1 (a) and mouse 2 (b) with tumor region marked as orange circle. Localization result of the MNP accumulations are denoted by a black dot.

Table 1. Localization result in comparison to central tumor position

Sample	*x,y* dipole position /mm	Central tumor position /mm	Tumor diameter /mm
mouse1	13.4(5), -13.3(5)	12.0(5), -18.0(5)	16.0(5)
mouse2	-14.5(5), -5.7 (5)	-14.0(5), -5.0(5)	9.0(5)

Additional x-ray images (Mobilett II, Siemens AG, Erlangen) taken of the native mouse 1, right after intratumoral injection of the MNP and after 24 hours (the latter see Fig. 2) indicate, that a small fraction of the MNP suspension may also be lost into the surrounding tissue (dashed orange oval).

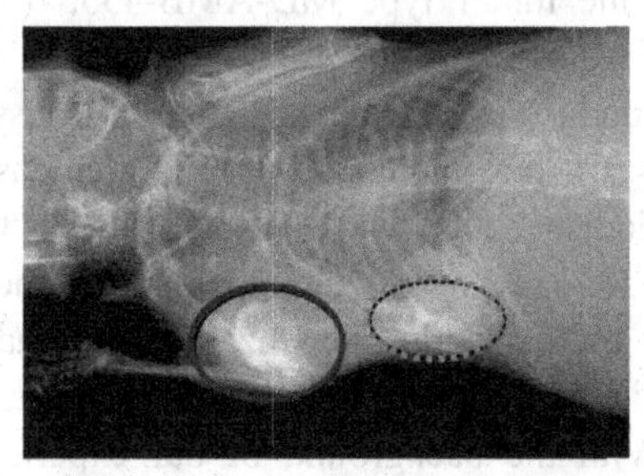

Fig. 2. X-ray image of mouse 2, 24 hours after intratumoral MNP injection. Tumor region (solid blue oval) and MNP leakage into surrounding tissue (dashed orange oval) are indicated.

However, the apparent loss of MNP in mouse 2 cannot be explained by a possible leakage of MNPs from the tumor to the surrounding tissue, because this would not change the net magnetic moment of the particles in the whole animal, which MRX as an integral method measures. Also a degradation of the particles that destroys their magnetic moment can be ruled out, because it is very unlikely that this process leaves the shape of the relaxation curve of the remaining particles unchanged. This means, that either a smaller amount of MNP was injected (leavings in the injection needle or reflux through the injection channel) or part of the particle load was excreted from the mouse body during the 24 hours of incubation time. Currently in-depth studies on a larger number of laboratory animals are carried out to tackle the question of MNP behavior in the tumor after 24 hours.

4. CONCLUSION

Using multichannel MRX with magnetic dipole fitting employing a Levenberg-Marquardt algorithm, we were able to localize and moreover quantify MNP accumulation in the tumor region of mice. Complementary to x-ray imaging, MRX offers an integral and quantitative method to detect the total MNP amount being present in the mouse, so all MNP accumulations in the animals contribute to the signal. In all measurements, the shape of the relaxation curve did not differ from the reference measurement. This is a clear indication that the magnetic properties of the individual MNP as well as of their composition did not change due to the biomedical application. The center of mass of MNP accumulations was clearly determined in the tumor regions of both mice. The quantification results show that 24 hours after intratumoral MNP injection all applied MNP were found in the tumor type 9L/lacZ (mouse 1) while only three quarters of the administered MNP were retrieved by MRX in the tumor type MD-AMB-435S (mouse 2). This finding emphasizes the need of a quantitative control of the magnetic ablation therapy, even though we do not fully understand the mechanism of this loss at present.

The first findings of our methodical study demonstrate that quantitative monitoring of MNP biodistribution via MRX is a useful tool for monitoring the particle distribution for magnetic thermoablation therapy. We employed multichannel MRX for the contactless localization and quantification of magnetic nanoparticle accumulations post mortem, and there is no reason why this should not be possible *in vivo*. With the background of our experience with the magnetic marker monitoring[14] and quantification of MNP for magnetic drug targeting[1,15,8] we envision that MRX monitoring of MNP accumulations in tumors can be measured even without anesthesia.

ACKNOWLEDGMENTS

This work was supported by DFG research programs "Magnetische Nanopartikel für die Krebstherapie" TR408/4-1 and HI689/7-1. The technical assistance of Susann Burgold, Yvonne Heyne and Brigitte Maron, Wolfgang Müller and Kay Schwarz is gratefully acknowledged. Thanks to Dietmar Eberbeck for fruitful discussions.

REFERENCES

1 Dames P, Gleich B, Flemmer A. Targeted delivery of magnetic aerosol droplets to the lung. *Nature Nanotech* 2007; **2:** 495-499.

2 Diederich CJ. Thermal ablation and high-temperature thermal therapy: overview of technology and clinical implementation. *Int J Hyperthermia* 2005; **21**: 745-753.

3 Eberbeck D, Wiekhorst F, Steinhoff U. Aggregation behaviour of magnetic nanoparticle suspensions investigated by magnetorelaxometry. *J Phys: Cond. Matter* 2006; **18**: 2829-2846.

4 Hilger I, Rapp A, Greulich KO. Assessment of DNA damage in target tumor cells after thermoablation in mice. *Radiology* 2005; **237**: 500-506.

5 Hilger I, Hergt R, Kaiser WA. Effects of magnetic thermoablation in muscle tissue using iron oxide particles: an *in vitro* study. *Invest Radiol.* 2000; **35:** 170-179.

6 Kettering M, Winter J, Zeisberger M. Magnetic nanoparticles as bimodal tools in magnetically induced labelling and magnetic heating of tumour cells: an *in vitro* study. *Nanotechnology* 2007; **18**: 175101.

7 Pankhurst Q, Connolly J, Jones S. Application of magnetic nanoparticles in biomedicine. *J Phys Appl Phys* 2003; **36**: R167-181.

8 Richter H, Wiekhorst F, Schwarz K. Magnetorelaxometric quantification of magnetic nanoparticles in an artery model after *ex vivo* magnetic drug targeting. *Phys Med Biol* 2009; **54**: N417-N424.

9 Richter H, Kettering M, Wiekhorst F. Magnetorelaxometry for localization and quantification of magnetic nanoparticles for thermal ablation studies. *Phys Med Biol* 2010; **55**: 623-633.

10 Schnabel A, Burghoff M, Hartwig S. A sensor configuration for 304 SQUID vector magnetometer. *Neurol Clin Neurophysiol* 2004; **70**: 1-5.

11 Thiel F, Schnabel A, Knappe-Grüneberg S. Demagnetizing of magnetically shielded rooms. *Rev Sci Instrum* 2007; **78**: 35106.

12 van der Zee J. Heating the patient: a promising approach? *Ann Oncol* 2002; **13**: 1173-1184.

13 van Landeghem FKH, Maier-Hauff K, Jordan A. Post-mortem studies in glioblastoma patients treated with thermotherapy using magnetic nanoparticles. *Biomaterials* 2008; **30**: 52-57.

14 Weitschies W, Kosch O, Moennikes H. Magnetic Marker Monitoring: An application of biomagnetic measurement instrumentation and principles for the determination of the gastrointestinal behaviour of magnetically marked solid dosage forms. *Adv Drug Deliv Rev* 2005; **57**: 1210-1222.

15 Wiekhorst F, Selinger C, Jurgons R. Quantification of magnetic nanoparticles by magnetorelaxometry and comparison to histology after magnetic drug targeting. *J Nanosci Nanotech* 2006; **6**: 3222-3225.

IMAGING OF MAGNETIC NANOPARTICLES BASED ON MAGNETORELAXATION AND MINIMUM NORM ESTIMATIONS

DANIEL BAUMGARTEN AND JENS HAUEISEN

Institute of Biomedical Engineering and Informatics, Ilmenau University of Technology; POB 100 565; D-98694 Ilmenau, Germany

and

Biomagnetic Centre, Clinic of Neurology, University Hospital Jena; Erlanger Allee 101; D-07747 Jena, Germany

Email: daniel.baumgarten@tu-ilmenau.de

A novel approach to the quantitative imaging of magnetic nanoparticles is presented. The distributions are reconstructed by minimum norm estimations of multiple dipoles from multichannel magnetorelaxometry measurements. In computer simulations and experimental studies the feasibility of this approach is investigated. The results demonstrate that the approach is promising, though the spatial resolution has yet to be improved.

1. INTRODUCTION

For nearly all medical applications of magnetic nanoparticles, a quantitative knowledge about the distribution of the nanoparticles is essential. Today, MRI is widely used for the imaging of magnetic nanoparticle distributions. A novel technique to determine these distributions is Magnetic Particle Imaging which is based on the nonlinear magnetization of the particles in an oscillating field[1]. However, these approaches have the drawbacks of limited quantification ability (MRI) and high demands on the involved nanoparticles (MPI).

We propose a complementary approach for the quantitative imaging of magnetic nanoparticles. Essentially, the particle distribution is reconstructed by minimum norm estimation from multichannel magnetorelaxometry measurements, determining the magnitudes of multiple magnetic dipoles in the region of interest[2]. In this paper, both measurement and source reconstruction aspects of the approach are illuminated. Reconstruction results from simulated and measured data are presented that demonstrate the feasibility of the approach.

2. METHODS

2.1. Magnetorelaxometry

The proposed imaging approach is based on magnetorelaxometry (MRX). In an MRX experiment[3], an ensemble of magnetic nanoparticles is magnetized by an externally applied magnetic field. During this excitation, the moments of the particles orientate towards the direction of the external field. After switching off the excitation field, the particles relaxate to their original state following two different relaxation processes, depending on their binding state and resulting in different relaxation times. The magnetization of unbound particles decays by Brownian motion of the particles themselves (Brown relaxation). Particles that are bound, e. g. to a target substance, show Néel relaxation. In this process, only the magnetic moments flip within the particles. If the relaxation behavior or magnetic remanence, respectively, is measured in multiple locations, the distribution of the particles can be reconstructed by means of inverse methods.

2.2. Minimum Norm Based Imaging Techniques

2.2.1. *Forward model*

The source space for the minimum-norm estimation is formed by a regular grid in the plane or volume of interest. At each grid point, a dipole is defined as source. Considering only the relaxation amplitude or remanence, respectively, these sources can be modeled by a magneto-static dipole. The magnetic field $\vec{b}$ at position $\vec{r}$ that is produced by a magnetic dipole at position $\vec{r}_0$ with moment $\vec{m}$ is computed according to (μ_0 is the permeability of free space):

$$\vec{b}(\vec{r}) = \frac{\mu_0}{4\pi}\left(\frac{3\vec{m}\cdot(\vec{r}-\vec{r}\,')}{\left|\vec{r}-\vec{r}\,'\right|^5}(\vec{r}-\vec{r}\,') - \frac{\vec{m}}{\left|\vec{r}-\vec{r}\,'\right|^3}\right) \tag{1}$$

For a more sophisticated forward model, the temporal characteristic of the particles' relaxation that is known from calculations or reference measurements can be incorporated. A simple and widely used approximation for this relaxation is the logarithmic decay[4], with the amplitude B_0 and the relaxation time constant τ:

$$f_b(t) = B_o \cdot \ln\left(1+\frac{\tau}{t}\right) \tag{2}$$

2.2.2. *Minimum norm estimation*

The information of the source locations and the sensor positions is represented in the lead field matrix L. With respect to the relaxation amplitude, the magnetic field $\vec{b}$ in the sensor positions can be calculated by multiplying the lead field matrix with the dipole magnitudes $\vec{m}$:

$$\vec{b} = L \cdot \vec{m} \tag{3}$$

Minimizing the least squares difference between measured and calculated field, the dipole magnitudes can be estimated using the pseudoinverse lead field matrix L^+:

$$\vec{m}_{est} = L^+ \cdot \vec{b} \tag{4}$$

Different regularization methods are applied to ensure numerical stability and improve the robustness of the solution. One approach uses the *truncated singular value decomposition* (TSVD) of the lead field matrix, neglecting singular values of L^+ that are smaller than the parameter σ_r:

$$\vec{m}_{est} = L_r^+ \cdot \vec{b} = \left(U \Sigma V^T\right)_r^+ \cdot \vec{b} = \sum_{i=0}^{r} \frac{\vec{u}_i^T \vec{b}}{\sigma_i} \vec{v}_i \tag{5}$$

Employing *Tichonow* regularization[2], the dipole parameters are estimated as:

$$\vec{m}_{est} = \left(L^T L + \lambda W^T W\right)^+ \cdot L^T \cdot \vec{b} \tag{6}$$

For the integration the temporal relaxation behavior f the static forward model is expanded[5]. The spatio-temporal lead field matrix L_T is computed as the Kronecker product of $f_T = \left(f(t_1), f(t_2), ..., f(t_T)\right)^T$ and L:

$$L_T = f_T \otimes L \tag{7}$$

The relaxation amplitudes of the dipoles are estimated by replacing L by L_T and $\vec{b}$ by $b_T = \left(b(t_1), b(t_2), ..., b(t_T)\right)^T$ in (3) and applying the same regularization methods.

3. COMPUTER SIMULATIONS

3.1. Remanence Data

In first computer simulations, the fields of two-dimensionally distributed static sources were computed involving realistic sensor positions from the setups described in the experimental data section below. The sources were reconstructed employing the static imaging approaches with the reconstruction grid positioned in the plane of interest. Prior to the computation, the depth of this plane below the sensor system is determined by non-linear dipole localization. As can be seen from Fig. 1 (left), the reconstruction quality increases with larger signal-to-noise ratios (SNRs). Our simulations reveal that also the sensor source distance and the source grid spacing influence the reconstruction quality.

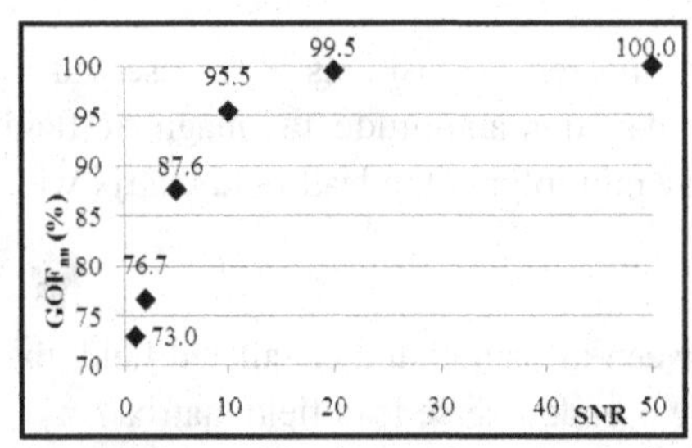

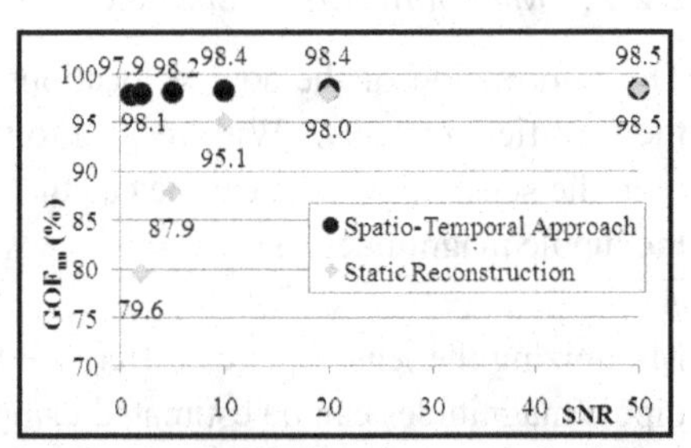

Fig. 1. Influence of noise on the reconstruction quality: Goodness-of-fit (based on normalized mean squared errors) between field of the simulated source, not superimposed by noise, and field computed from the reconstructed distribution for the remanence data (l) and spatio-temporal relaxation data (r).

3.2. Relaxation Data

To evaluate the effects of integrating the temporal characteristic in the reconstruction, computer simulations of spatio-temporal sources were performed utilizing the sensor positions of the 16 channel system (see below). With respect to the low spatial resolution of the sensor setup, the simulated source was formed by a single dipole with its magnitude decaying as described by (2). The sources were reconstructed employing both the static and the spatio-temporal approach.

Fig. 1 (right) illustrates the considerably improved robustness against noise of the spatio-temporal approach as compared to the static method. Additionally, our simulations show that even with small deviations between the relaxation constants of the model function and the data, the spatio-temporal approach shows better results. Moreover, the novel spatio-temporal approach proved to be less sensitive towards the choice of the regularization parameter r in the applied TSVD method.

4. EXPERIMENTAL RESULTS

4.1. Sensor Setups

For the experimental investigations described in the following paragraphs, different multichannel SQUID systems have been employed. In the Biomagnetic Centre Jena a 195 channel Vector-Biomagnetometer ATB Argos 200[6] with its sensors arranged in triplets in four planes as well as a micro SQUID system[7] with 16 first order gradiometer sensors positioned within a rectangular plane were used. Both systems are installed in a magnetically shielded room. Besides, a 304 channel Vector-Magnetometer[8] in the strongly magnetically shielded room BMSR-2 was used at the Physikalisch-Technische Bundesanstalt Berlin (PTB). Here, the SQUIDs are grouped in 19 modules, each module containing four planes.

4.2. Phantom Measurements

Polyethylene filter columns served as probes for the phantom measurements (Fig. 2 left). Magnetic nanoparticles bound to the filters by biotin-streptavidin binding reactions known from immunofiltration assays to detect Streptococcus sobrinus antigen. Similar measurements were performed with the Argos and PTB system, respectively: After magnetizing the columns in a static field, their magnetic remanence after the relaxation process was measured. From those data, the nanoparticle distributions were reconstructed using the static approach (Fig. 2 r.).

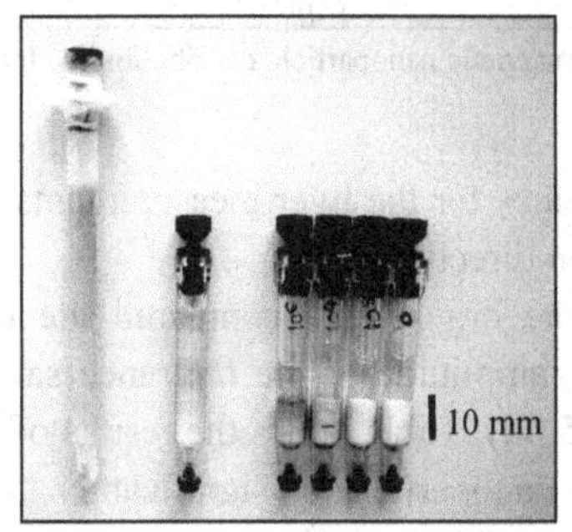

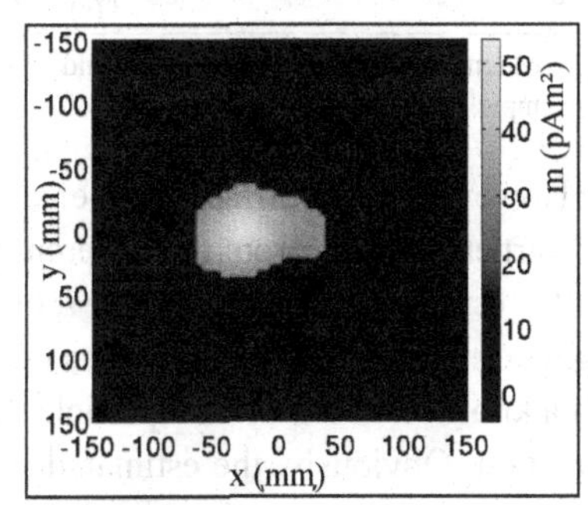

Fig. 2. Column phantoms (left) and reconstructed distribution of the 35 mm phantom (right)

4.3. In-Vitro Measurements

For the in-vitro validation of our imaging approach, rat organ samples were prepared by injecting a defined amount of magnetic nanoparticles into the tail vein of rats. After one hour, the organs were extracted. A reference sample was prepared by fixing sample nanoparticle solution in Agarose gel. The prepared samples were magnetized in a homogenous excitation field emitted by a Helmholtz coil outside the magnetically shielded room. Subsequently, the samples were positioned below the 16 channel system and their relaxation behavior was measured[5]. Fig. 3 shows the

signals measured by the different channels (left) as well as the reconstructed nanoparticle distribution (right), both for the liver sample. The position and the dimension of the sample could be reconstructed properly, while the shape reconstruction and therewith the spatial resolution lacks from the low number of channels of the measurement system. To evaluate our approach's ability to quantify magnetic nanoparticle distributions, the total magnetic moments of the reconstructions were compared to the strongest signal amplitudes in the relaxation measurements. Table 1 shows this comparison together with the ratio of the amplitudes. The relaxation-reconstruction ratio is comparable for all three samples.

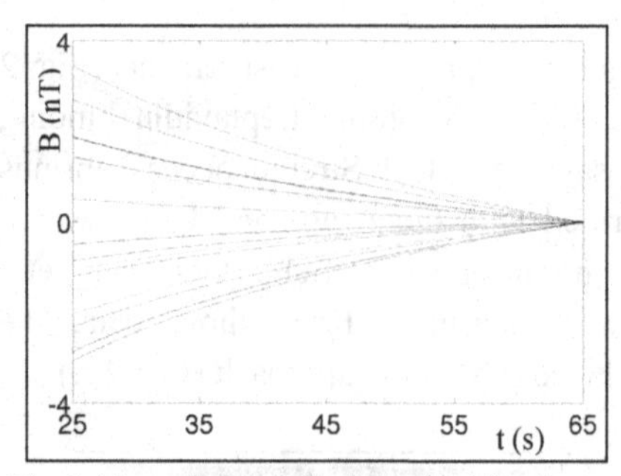

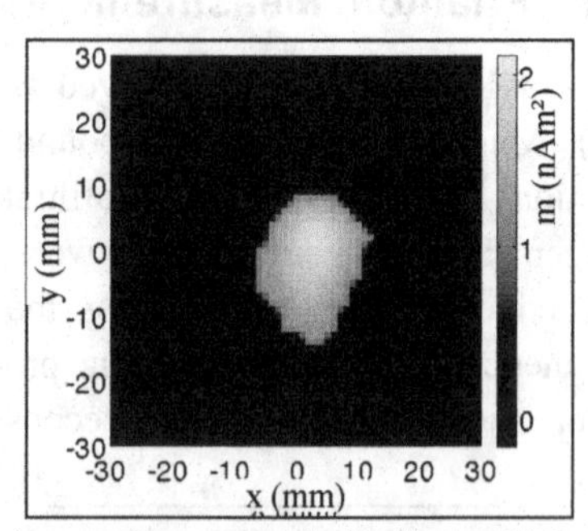

Fig. 3. Magnetic relaxation behavior (a) and reconstructed magnetic nanoparticle distribution (b) for the liver sample magnetized in vertical direction.

However, slight differences between the values for the liver measurements and reconstructions arise from the different excitation directions.

To estimate the nanoparticle content in the organs, we compared the total magnetic moment of the reconstructions to the amplitude of the reference sample with a known amount of nanoparticle fluid (0.05 ml). Table 2 lists the results of this estimation. Obviously, the estimated amount of nanoparticles is significantly larger in the liver than in the milt which is in congruence with a-priori expectations.

Table 1: Comparison of relaxation signal amplitude and total magnetic moment of the reconstruction for different samples with different magnetization directions.

Sample	Measured relaxation amplitude	Total magnetic moment of the reconstruction	Ratio (T/Am^2)
Liver, vertical magnetization	6.57 nT	116.00 nAm^2	0.056
Liver, horizontal magnetization	5.59 nT	90.48 nAm^2	0.062
Milt, vertical magnetization	0.72 nT	13.43 nAm^2	0.053

5. CONCLUSION

Our results show that the proposed approach provides a promising technique for the non-invasive, quantitative and specific determination of biodistributions of magnetic nanoparticles. However, the spatial resolution of the technique, limited both by the spatial resolution of the measurement system and the inverse method itself, is not competitive to qualitative imaging methods such as MRI.

Table 2: Estimation of nanoparticle content in the different organs (all vertical magnetization).

Sample	Total magnetic moment	Estimated nanoparticle content
Reference sample	*55.50* nAm^2	*0.050 ml*
Liver	116.00 nAm^2	0.105 ml
Milt	13.43 nAm^2	0.012 ml

The promising results of our approach strongly suggest the application of the method to MRX measurement data in further studies. Improvements in spatial distribution and reconstruction quality are expected from involving inhomogeneous excitation fields and the combination of the multiple dipole forward model with the multipole expansion approach.

ACKNOWLEDGMENTS

The authors would like to thank Mario Liehr, Frank Gießler (Biomagnetic Centre Jena), Frank Wiekhorst, Uwe Steinhoff (PTB Berlin), Christian Bergemann (Chemicell GmbH), Peter Münster (Senova GmbH), and Peter Miethe (fzmb GmbH – Research Centre of Medical Technology and Biotechnology).

This work was funded by the E. C. Sixth Framework Programme (STREP project "Biodiagnostics", contract no. NMP4-CT-2005-017002) and in part supported by the state of Thuringia under participation of the European Funds for Regional Development (TAB projects 2006FE0096 and 2008FE9048).

REFERENCES

1 Gleich B, Weizenecker J. Tomographic imaging using the nonlinear response of magnetic particles. *Nature* 2005; **435(7046)**: 1214–1217.
2 Baumgarten D, Liehr M, Wiekhorst F, et al. Magnetic nanoparticle imaging by means of minimum norm estimates from remanence measurements. *Med Biol Eng Comp* 2008; **46**: 1177–1185.
3 Wiekhorst F, Jurgons R, Eberbeck D, et al. Quantification of magnetic nanoparticles by magnetorelaxometry after local cancer therapy with magnetic drug targeting. *J Nanosci Nanotechnol* 1996; **6(9–10)**: 3222–3225.
4 Berkov DV, Kötitz R. Irreversible relaxation behaviour of a general class of magnetic systems. *J Phys Condens Matter* 1996; **8**: 1257-1266.
5 Baumgarten D, Haueisen J. A spatio-temporal approach for the solution of the inverse problem in the reconstruction of magnetic nanoparticle distributions. *IEEE Trans Magn*; to be published.
6 Di Rienzo L, Haueisen J. Theoretical lower error bound for comparative evaluation of sensor arrays in magnetostatic linear inverse problems. *IEEE Trans Magn* 2006; **42(11)**: 3669–3673.
7 Nowak H, Gießler F, et al. A 16-channel SQUID-device for biomagnetic investigations of small objects. *Med Eng Phys 1999;* **21(8)**: 563–568.
8 Schnabel A, Burghoff M, Hartwig S, et al. A sensor configuration for a 304 SQUID vector magnetometer. *Neurol Clin Neurophysiol* 2004; **70**.

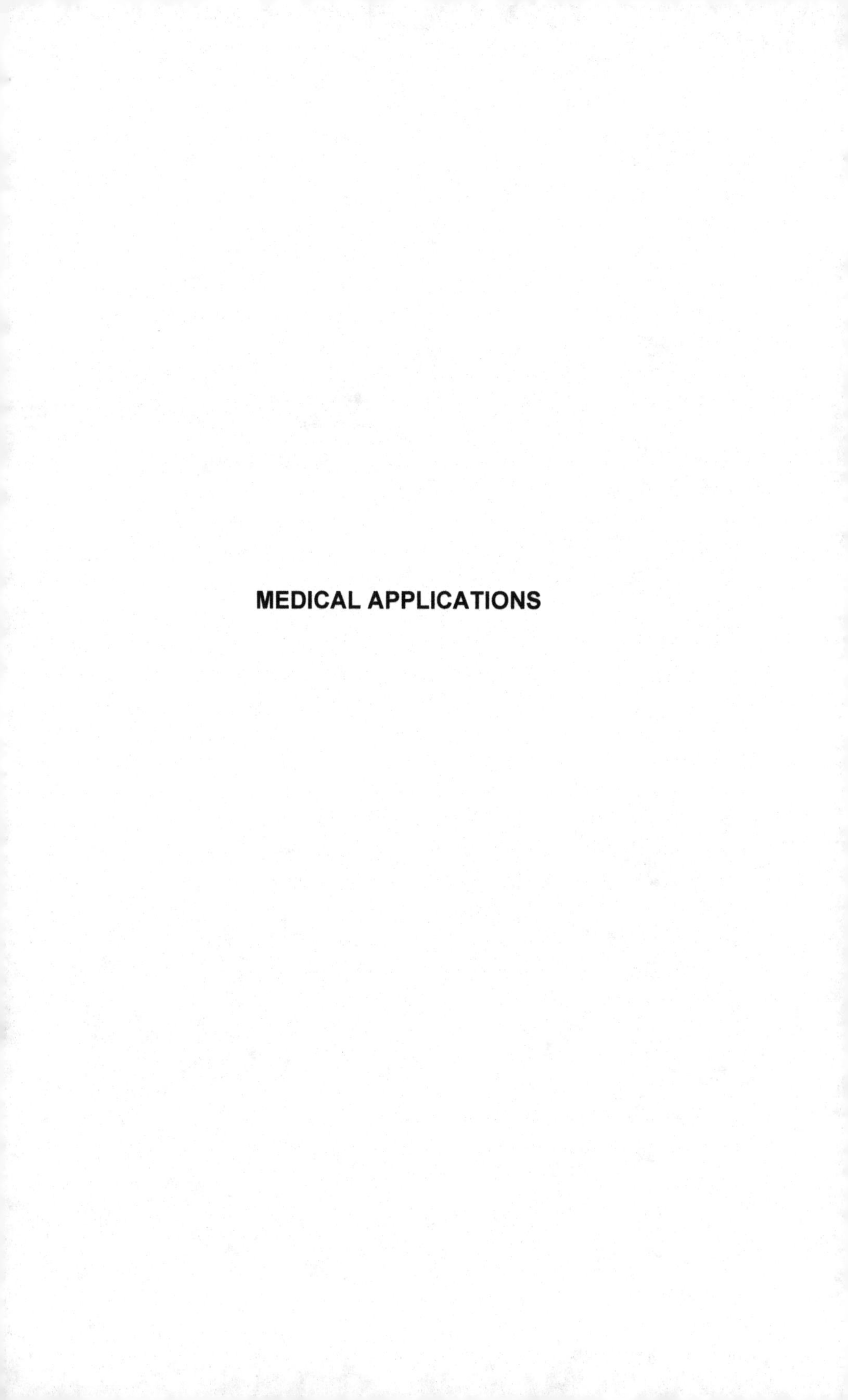

MEDICAL APPLICATIONS

DEVELOPING CELLULAR MPI: INITIAL EXPERIENCE

J.W.M. BULTE, P. WALCZAK, S. BERNARD
Departments of Radiology, Biomedical Engineering, and Chemical & Biomolecular Engineering; Cellular Imaging Section, Institute for Cell Engineering, Johns Hopkins University School of Medicine, Baltimore, MD. Email: jwmbulte@mri.jhu.edu

B. GLEICH, J. WEIZENECKER, J. BORGERT
Philips Research Europe, Hamburg, Germany

H. AERTS, H. BOEVE
Philips Research Europe and Philips Medical Systems-, Eindhoven, The Netherlands

Using clinical formulations of SPIO particles used as MRI contrast agents, we investigated the potential of magnetic particle imaging (MPI) for quantitative stem cell tracking. We observed a linear correlation between MPI signal and iron content, representative for the total cell number over a wide range of concentrations, independent of the particle state as free or intracellular entity. Unlike in MRI, Resovist had a 4–fold higher efficacy per unit Fe than Feridex for two different stem cell types tested. MPI has potential for non-invasive quantitative cell tracking and deserves further exploration with or without the use of MRI in parallel.

1. INTRODUCTION

MRI cell tracking using superparamagnetic iron oxide particles (SPIO) has found many applications in understanding cell biology and developing cell therapy. However, due to its indirect detection of cells through the SPIO effect on proton relaxation, there are several limitations that prevent its full exploitation. These include 1) the difficulty to absolutely quantify cell concentration and iron content - part of the difficulty relies in the existence of different relaxation regimes (dependent on the agglomeration state and size of SPIO cluster); 2) the difficulty of discriminating SPIO-labeled cells in areas of hemorrhage and traumatic injury (which are often present in targets of cell therapy), as caused by the proton dephasing effects of methemoglobin, ferritin, and hemosiderin (especially at higher fields); 3) the occasional misinterpretation of isolated "black spots" due to differences in magnetic susceptibility effects around blood vessels and air-tissue interfaces (i.e. stomach and GI tract); and 4) the inability to track cells in areas devoid of proton signal (i.e., the lungs). ^{19}F MRI cell tracking can overcome several of these limitations[1] but suffers from inherent lack of sensitivity. In the present study, we have determined the feasibility of developing cellular magnetic particle imaging (MPI). MPI relies on the non-linear response of magnetic material as a direct manner for detecting the presence of an iron oxide nanoparticle agent in an oscillating magnetic field[2]. Spatial encoding can be realized by a static, inhomogeneous magnetic field, saturating the magnetic material almost everywhere except in the vicinity of a special point, the field free point.

2. METHODS

C17.2 neural stem cells (NSCs) and rat mesenchymal stem cells (MSCs) were labeled with the clinical SPIO formulations Resovist (R) or Feridex (F) combined with poly-L-lysine (48 hr incubation at 62.5 - 25 μg Fe/ml culture medium). These two cell types were chosen in order to assess the MPI dependence on cell size and cytoplasmic iron content for smaller cells (NSCs, ~10 μm) and larger cells (MSCs, ~25 μm). Cells were washed, counted, and 50 μl gelatin samples were prepared containing between 2.5×10^3 and 1×10^6 cells. The mean cellular iron content was determined using a Ferrozin-based spectrophotometric assay. For MPI analysis, the non-linear magnetic response of labeled and reference (free iron oxide particles in solution) samples was measured in a spectrometer using an oscillating magnetic field (10 mT amplitude, 25 kHz frequency, 30 sec sampling time). After Fourier transformation the intensity of the harmonic signals, i.e. 3rd and 11th, was monitored.

3. RESULTS

The mean iron content was determined as 13.67 pg Fe/cell for MSCs+R, 4.21 pg Fe/cell for MSCs+F, 1.97 pg Fe/cell for NSCs+R, and 0.84 pg Fe/cell for NSCs+F. Figure 1 shows the MPI signal plots as function of iron content (A,B) and corresponding cell number (C,D). Reference gelatin samples are included for reference (A,B). Except for the lowest amount of the smaller NSCs, which had < 1pg Fe/cell, there was a linear relation between the MPI signal and iron content. Slope values for the 3rd harmonic were 1.2×10^{-3} Am^2/g Fe for MSCs+R, which is equivalent to 1.7×10^{-14} Am^2 per cell; 2.8×10^{-4} Am^2/g Fe for MSCs+F, or 1.2×10^{-15}

Am^2 per cell; $8.6x10^{-4}$ Am^2/g Fe for NSCs+R; and $1.7x10^{-4}$ Am^2/g Fe for NSCs+F. Note that for both R and F, the reference samples have the same MPI value vs. unit of iron as for the cell samples. For all samples, as compared to Feridex, Resovist had a 4-fold higher MPI efficacy (on 3rd harmonic) per unit of iron. This large difference was observed for both NSCs and MSCs. With the current equipment the efficiency for Fe oxide with infinite susceptibility is $3x10^{-2}$ Am^2/g Fe so that, for MSCs+R, the detection limit for imaging is below 100 cells.

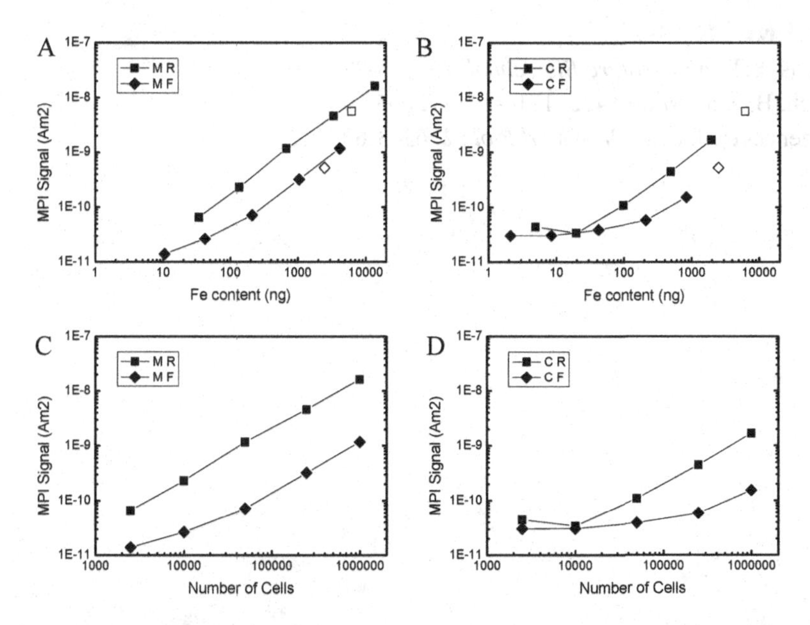

Fig. 1. MPI signal measurements of magnetically labeled stem cells. Shown are the signal amplitudes as a function of Fe content (A,B) and the corresponding number of cells (C,D) obtained for the 3rd harmonic. Data are shown for MSCs (A,C) labeled with Resovist (MR) and Feridex (MF), and NSCs (B,D) labeled with Resovist (CR) and Feridex (CF). Reference (free, non-cell bound particles) gelatin samples are included in A,B (open symbols).

4. CONCLUSIONS

Stem cells can be readily detected with MPI at biologically relevant concentrations. MPI enables a linear quantification of both cell number and iron content over a wide range of concentrations, regardless of the state of SPIO as free or intracellular entity. Unlike its use as MRI contrast agent, we found a large difference (4-fold) in MPI efficacy between Feridex and Resovist. While the underlying mechanism is not fully understood, it opens up a new rationale for synthesis and testing of novel magnetic nanoparticles. There appear to be no physical constraints towards developing a whole body human scanner[3], which should encourage further development of cellular MPI given that SPIO formulations can be used that are already in use as clinical MRI cell tracking agents.

ACKNOWLEDGMENTS

This work was supported by NIH EUREKA RO1 DA026299.

REFERENCES

1 Ahrens, E.T. et al. *Nature Biotechnol.* **23**, 983-987 (2005)
2 Gleich, B. et al. *Nature* **435**, 1214-1217 (2005)
3 Weizenecker, J. et al. *Phys Med Biol* **52**, 6363-6374 (2007).

SENTINEL LYMPHNODE DETECTION IN BREAST CANCER BY MAGNETIC PARTICLE IMAGING USING SUPERPARAMAGNETIC NANOPARTICLES

DOMINIQUE FINAS, BRITTA RUHLAND, KRISTIN BAUMANN

Department of Obstetrics and Gynecology, University Clinic of Schleswig-Holstein
University of Luebeck, Ratzeburger Allee 160
Luebeck, 23538, Germany
Email: finas.d@arcor.de, britta.ruhland@uk-sh.de, kristin.baumann@uk-sh.de

TOBIAS KNOPP, TIMO F. SATTEL, SVEN BIEDERER, KERSTIN LUEDTKE-BUZUG

Institute of Medical Engeneering
University of Luebeck, Ratzeburger Allee 160
Luebeck, 23538, Germany
Email: {knopp,biederer,sattel,luedtke-buzug}@imt.uni-luebeck.de

KLAUS DIEDRICH

Department of Obstetrics and Gynecology, University Clinic of Schleswig-Holstein
University of Luebeck, Ratzeburger Allee 160
Luebeck, 23538, Germany
Email: klaus.diedrich@uk-sh.de

THORSTEN M. BUZUG

Institute of Medical Engeneering
University of Luebeck, Ratzeburger Allee 160
Luebeck, 23538, Germany
Email: buzug@imt.uni-luebeck.de

Radical axillary lymphonodectomie (ALN) in breast cancer patients is associated with high morbidity and significant loss of quality of life. These effects can be strongly reduced by introducing the concept of sentinel lymphonodectomy (SNLB). Within this method dye and radio nuclides are injected into the breast. Super paramagnetic iron oxide nano particles (SPIOs) could replace these marker substances. By using the magnetic particle imaging (MPI)-procedure, a three-dimensional imaging and distinct localization of SPIOs (Resovist®) can be achieved. To prove the mentioned principle of SNLB by MPI a mouse model is applied. This project is part of a comprehensive test program to develop the new SNLB technique. A new MPI hand probe with unilateral solenoid arrangement designed for use in the operating theater is under construction. Intraoperative three-dimensional MPI imaging facilitates the axillary SNL detection and moreover makes it more precise. Through the avoidance of intensive surgical exploration of the axilla the morbidity is dramatically reduced. Additionally the concept of SNLB by MPI can be applied in principle in all solid tumors.

1. INTROUDUCTION

Breast cancer is the most frequent cancer of the female population worldwide in western industrialized countries.[1] Breast tumors are draining to the axillary lymph nodes. Therefore the axillary exploration is part of the surgical staging in breast cancer.[2] The individual prognosis decreases dramatically if tumor cells are present in lymph nodes. But, the radical axillary lymphonodectomy (ALN) is associated with high morbidity and significant loss of quality of life. These effects can be strongly reduced by introducing the concept of sentinel lymphonodectomy (SNLB). Within this method dye and radio nuclides are injected into the breast (Figure 1).[3]

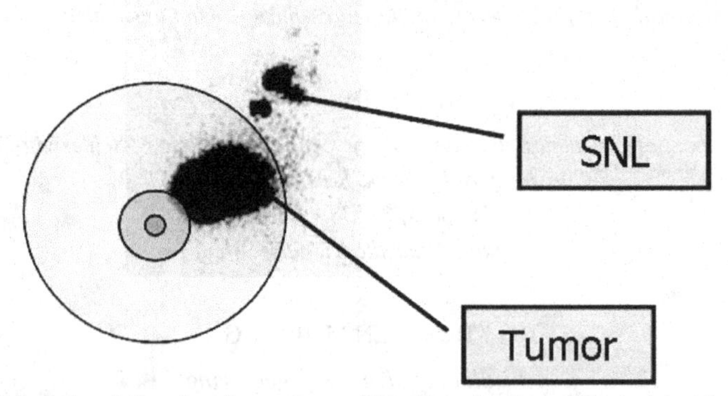

Figure 1 Lymphoscintigraphy after peritumoral injection of radio nuclides to detect the SNL.

Super paramagnetic iron oxide nano particles (SPIOs) could replace these marker substances. Through the recently developed magnetic particle imaging (MPI)-procedure, a three-dimensional imaging and distinct localization of SPIOs (Resovist®) can be achieved. Therefore detection of sentinel lymph nodes will be done by using MPI. This eliminates the exposure of patient and participating medical staff to ionizing radiation within in the SNLB process. Qualitative and quantitative enrichment of SPIOs in the axillary lymphatic tissue is unexplored until now. Moreover, the MPI procedure was not applied in vivo within this setting so far. We will generate results in the mentioned issues within a mouse model.

2. MATERIALS AND METHODS

A mouse model is applied to prove the mentioned principle of SNLB by MPI. To develop the methodology we use healthy mice.[4] After that we will proof if this works in a tumor bearing mouse model with metastasis in the axillary lymph nodes.[5,6] A previously defined amount of SPIOs will be injected into the mammary gland next to the axillary region of a healthy female Balb/c mouse. As first step we will explore how long the SPIOs take to reach the axillary lymph nodes. Therefore the mice will be treated with constant amounts of SPIOs and sacrificed after lengthened time intervals. The second step will show us if the lymph nodes who accumulates the SPIOs are sentinel lymphnodes. Therefore we will inject the same SPIO dose and a dye at the same time. After waiting the optimal delay we do the sacrifice. Our third step will explore the optimal SPIO dose we need for optimal enrichment in the axillary lymph nodes. Therefore the mice will be treated with increasing amounts of SPIOs. After the previously defined optimal time interval mice will be sacrificed. The fourth step is to try out our findings in a tumor model. Immunosuppressed SCID mice will be inoculated with breast cancer cell lines as previously published.[5,6] Taking under consideration our findings of optimal time interval and optimal axillary SPIO enrichment mice will be sacrificed.

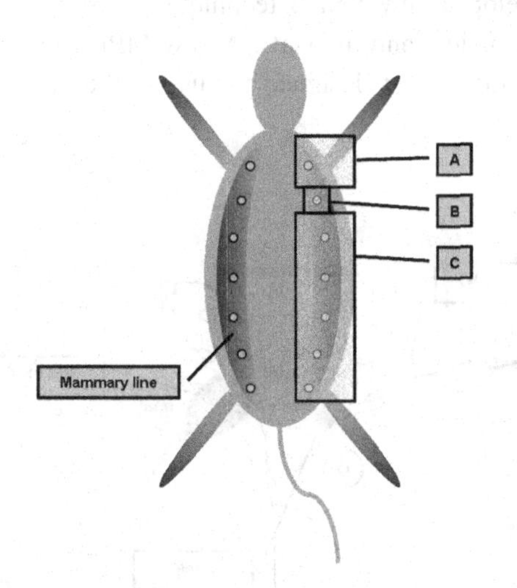

Figure 2 Axillary and environmental tissue – Resection area A-C.

We will analyze the axillary and the environmental tissue for the presence and concentration of SPIOs with different techniques (Figure 2).

Iron particles will be detected by histological examination at formalin fixed and paraffin embedded tissue, stained with iron sensitive Prussian blue stain correlated by electron microscopy.[7] For the determination of iron concentration within tissue homogenisates we will use the atomic absorption spectrometry. To define the SPIO concentration within the tissue and to prove if we can find them with MPI we will use MPI spectrometry. With the atomic absorption spectrometry we create a quantitative calibration curve to correlate the values we get by MPI spectrometry.

Nanoparticles are widely discussed as environmental toxins. To make the method sure, we will extract the inoculated SPIOs from all organs. After explantation and homogenization of brain, liver, lung, uterus, ovaries, intestines, kidneys and spleen we will explore them with the atomic absorption spectrometry whether there is any SPIO.

3. RESULTS

We aim to show that SPIOs and the MPI technique are effective to be used as SNLB tracer and finder in an in vivo mouse model. This project is part of a comprehensive test program to develop a new SNLB technique. This will be less complex and incriminating for the patient and the staff. A new MPI hand probe (Figure 3) with unilateral solenoid arrangement designed for use in the operating theater is under construction.

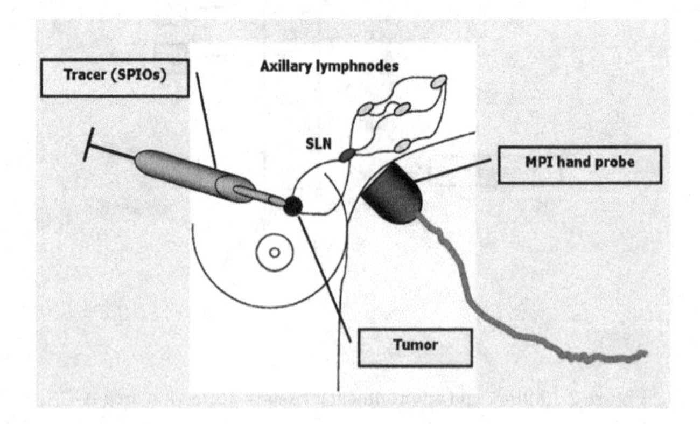

Figure 3 Intra operative peri tumoral tracer injection and axillary sentinel lymph node (SNL) detection with MPI hand probe.

Therewith the sentinel lymph node detection can be easily performed after intra operative tracer application. Furthermore the precise detection and localization of the sentinel lymph nodes with a real time three-dimensional imaging will be possible. The ultimate proof will be the use in the human model. Compared with the standard SNLB this method will be much less expensive and a less burdensome diagnostic process.

4. CONCLUSION

For conventional SNLB the axilla has to be widely explored to identify the SNL. Intra operative three-dimensional imaging with the MPI hand probe facilitates the axillary SNL detection and moreover makes it more precise.[8] Through the avoidance of intensive surgical exploration of the axilla the morbidity is dramatically reduced. The tracer for MPI is easy to obtain. This makes the method accessible to all patients. The concept of SNLB by MPI can be applied in principle in all solid tumors.

ACKNOWLEDGMENTS

This project is supported by the German Federal Ministry of Education and Research (BMBF Grant number 01EZ0912). It is also part of the University Research Program "Imaging of Disease Processes", University of Luebeck.

REFERENCES

1 Jemal A, Siegel R, Ward E, Hao Y, Xu J, Murray T, Thun MJ. Cancer statistics, 2008. *CA Cancer J Clin* 2008; **58:** (2): 71-96.

2 Kuehn T, Bembenek A, Decker T, Munz DL, Sautter-Bihl ML, Untch M, Wallwiener D. A concept for the clinical implementation of sentinel lymph node biopsy in patients with breast carcinoma with special regard to quality assurance. *Cancer* 2005; **103:** (3): 451-461.

3 Kühn T, Bembenek A, Büchels H, Decker T, Dunst J, Müllerleile U, Munz DL, Ostertag H, Sautter-Bihl ML, Schirrmeister H, Tulusan AH, Untch M, Winzer KJ, Wittekind C. Sentinel-Node-Biopsie beim Mammakarzinom: Interdisziplinär abgestimmter Konsensus der Deutschen Gesellschaft für Senologie für eine qualitätsgesicherte Anwendung in der klinischen Routine. *Geburtsh Frauenheilk* 2003; **63**: 835-840.

4 Robe A, Pic E, Lassalle HP, Bezdetnaya L, Guillemin F, Marchal F. Quantum dots in axillary lymph node mapping: biodistribution study in healthy mice. *BMC Cancer* 2008; **8**: 111.

5 Ling LJ, Wang S, Liu XA, Shen EC, Ding Q, Lu C, Xu J, Cao QH, Zhu HQ, Wang F. A novel mouse model of human breast cancer stem-like cells with high CD44+CD24-/lower phenotype metastasis to human bone. *Chin Med J (Engl)* 2008; **121:** (20): 1980-1986.

6 Tsunoda N, Kokuryo T, Oda K, Senga T, Yokoyama Y, Nagino M, Nimura Y, Hamaguchi M. Nek2 as a novel molecular target for the treatment of breast carcinoma. *Cancer Sci* 2009; **100:** (1): 111-116.

7 Weissleder R, Elizondo G, Wittenberg J, Lee AS, Josephson L, Brady TJ. Ultrasmall superparamagnetic iron oxide: an intravenous contrast agent for assessing lymph nodes with MR imaging. *Radiology* 1990; **175:** (2): 494-498.

8 Ruhland B, Baumann K, Knopp T, Sattel T, Biederer S, Lüdtke-Buzug K, Buzug TM, Diedrich K, Finas D. Magnetic Particle Imaging durch Superparamagnetische Nanopartikel zur Sentinellymphknotendetektion beim Mammakarzinom. *Geburtsh Frauenheilk* 2009; **69**: 758.

MAGNETIC SENSING METHODS AND MATERIALS FOR MEDICAL APPLICATIONS

BENNIE TEN HAKEN†, MARTIJN VISSCHER, MARTIN SOBIK
MIRA Institute for Biomedical Technology and Technical Medicine
Low Temperature Div., University of Twente, P.O. Box 217
7500 AE Enschede, The Netherlands
Email: B.tenHaken@utwente.nl

ALDRIK H. VELDERS
MESA+ Institute for Nanotechnology
Supramolecular Chemistry and Technology, University of Twente, P.O. Box 217
7500 AE Enschede, The Netherlands
Email: A.H.Velders@utwente.nl

Sensitive detection methods on magnetic nanoparticles in cells, tissue, and body liquids have a huge potential for new analysis methods both in medicine and biotechnology. Dedicated magnetic nanoparticles have been developed and approved for various medical procedures, such as angiography and liver imaging in the case of MRI technique. The combination of nanotechnology and advanced magnetic sensing routes opens a realistic perspective of magnetic methods replacing nuclear and optical detection techniques in medicine and biotechnology. Within these prospects, we focus both on sensor development and on the detection and activation of new biocompatible magnetic nanoparticles in selected clinical applications.

1. INTRODUCTION

Magnetic particles in clinical context are detectable because of the small and linear magnetic response of the human body. This is analogue to the radioactive materials applied in nuclear imaging by positron emission tomography (PET), gamma cameras and gamma probes. In both cases the "contrast" material has a unique signature and the body is transparent for the detected signal. Whole-body imaging is reserved for large and expensive scanner systems as MRI and PET. During a surgical intervention a handheld device is routinely used to localise specifically marked tissue, e.g. the sentinel lymph node (fig. 1). In the nuclear variant this

† Work partially supported by the European CARBIO Network (MRTN-CT-2006-035616).

requires a handheld gamma probe and a radioactive marker. A magnetic equivalent for this is the handheld device developed by Endomagnetics, which is basically a very advanced metal detector. In our group we are working on methods for sensing and activation of existing and new magnetic nanoparticles.

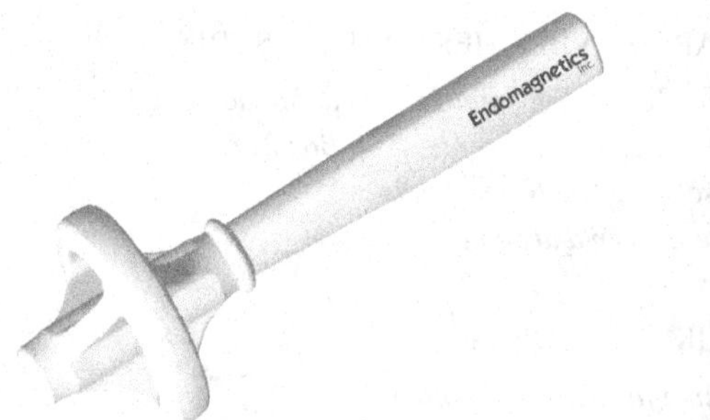

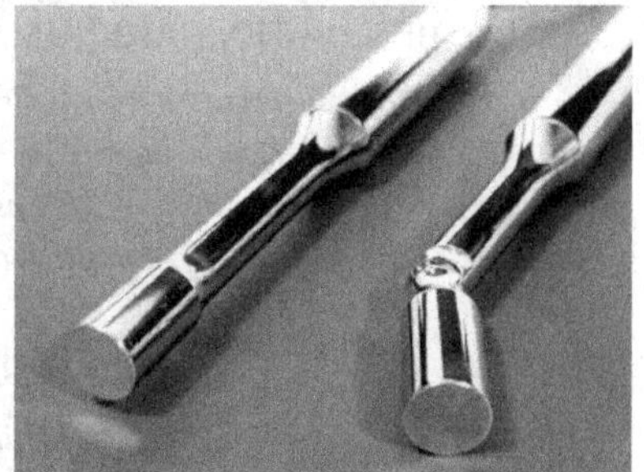

Fig. 1. Two examples of handheld probes for medical use. Left the prototype magnetic probe from Endomagnetics and two commercially available Gamma probes from Crystal Probe System at right.

2. EXPERIMENTAL METHODS

Since a few years an interesting group magnetic materials is approved for medical use. Super-Paramagnetic Iron Oxide (SPIO) nanoparticles have a large magnetic moment and a small volume. These particles can be injected in the bloodstream to enable MRI-angiography.[1] After injection these particles are transported to the liver and excreted from the body. This excretion path enables using SPIO particles for liver imaging.[2] SPIO particles are also successfully applied to treat cranial carcinoma by a novel hyperthermia technique.[3] In a different approach SPIO particles are used to localize sentinel lymph nodes in patients with a handheld device during surgery[4,5] and with MRI.[6]

In our group we started clinical experiments testing the approach for sentinel node detection in ex-vivo breast and colon tissue after tumor resection. Sentinel lymph node detection is based on the drainage pattern from the tumor area via the lymphatic system.[7] SPIO particles injected in or around the tumor pass through the lymph vessels to the first lymph node that drains the tumor area. In addition to the solution with SPIO particles, a blue dye was injected which enables visual localization of the lymph node. Lymph mapping using blue dye is one of the current methods that can be regarded as the gold standard in clinical practice. Sentinel nodes, either blue or black, were resected from the specimen and separately analyzed for the presence of SPIO with magnetometry, high field MRI (14 T) and conventional optical microscopy.

A novel class of magnetic materials which is also part of our research, are Carbon NanoTubes (CNT's), filled with magnetic materials as iron and cobalt (fig. 2). CNT's have an extremely high aspect ratio (length/diameter >100), leading to a highly non-linear anisotropic and hysteretic magnetization curve for an ensemble of aligned Fe-filled CNT's.[8] These CNT's are considered for novel hyperthermia treatments, local temperature sensing and drug delivery.[9] The individual Fe-CNT's have a strong magnetic moment with a preferred direction along their axis. The special properties of CNT's and other novel magnetic nanoparticles open the perspective of entirely new detection techniques in biomedical applications. In particular the strong magnetic moment with its preferred magnetic orientation is advantageous for the development of economical promising detection techniques, which can be combined with medical procedures as minimal-invasive interventions.

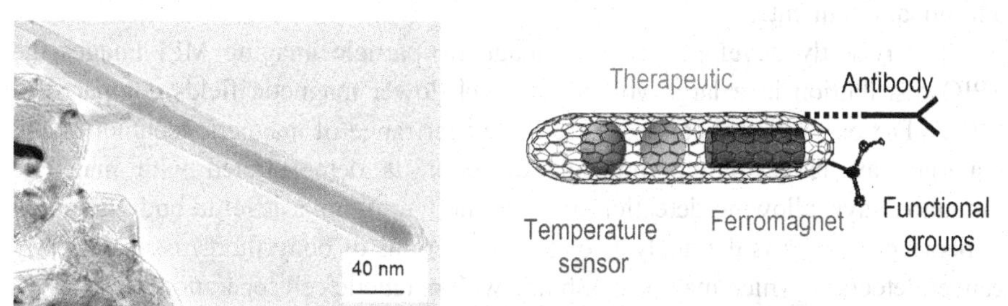

Fig. 2. SEM picture of a multi-wall CNT with a needle shaped Fe-filling produced by the IFW Dresden (left). The cartoon on the right illustrates the range of biomedical applications for these particles that is investigated in the framework of a European research network (www.carbio.eu).

3. RESULT AND DISCUSSION

Four patients with breast cancer and two patients colon cancer were included for our first ex vivo experiments. In two breast cancer patients and in both colon cancer patients SPIO uptake in lymph nodes was observed. Magnetometry, high field MRI and microscopy showed the accumulation of SPIO in lymph nodes after local administration around the tumor (fig. 3). The T2*-weighted high field MRI of single lymph nodes showed hypointense areas that are characteristic for the presence of SPIO contrast agent. Furthermore, Pearls Prussian Blue staining in conventional optical microscopy indicated the presence of iron. So, these preliminary results indicate that the concept of sentinel node detection with SPIO is promising for a more comprehensive study.

The ex-vivo experiments using SPIO nanoparticles for the detection and localization of the sentinel lymph node in colorectal cancer are now continued to prove the clinical value of magnetic detection of the sentinel node and to investigate the technical possibilities of this approach. Several aspects are to be considered. Particle size can be very important in lymph node mapping, since very small particles easily pass through the sentinel node, causing the detection of a second echelon node. On the other hand, large diameter particles cannot enter the lymphatic system and, subsequently, sentinel node detection fails. A quantitative analysis of the SPIO content in lymph nodes can be related to the clinical status of the lymph nodes with regard to metastasis.

Accumulated SPIO particles can be localized intra-operatively with a hand held probe. Development of sensitive magnetic methods will offer equipment that enables an accurate determination of the amount of SPIO in the sample. Pre-operative imaging of the SPIO containing sentinel node using high resolution techniques might be beneficial for the choice for the surgical approach and additional treatment.

The recently developed concept magnetic particle imaging MPI images the SPIO distribution in a large volume at much lower magnetic fields compared to MRI.[10] For ex-vivo applications there is broader range of magnetic techniques and materials available. Single molecule detection is demonstrated with magnetic immunoassays, allowing detection down to the femto-molar level in body liquids.[11] A perspective area is the analysis of larger fractions of body fluids/tissue for early cancer detection, which may be combined with magnetic cell separation.[12]

The preparation and application of solutions of CNT's in biological or medical context is still ongoing. Stability and iron filling of CNT's in solution was proved by spectrophotometry, magnetometry and microscopy. Towards application of CNT's, animal experiments using iron filled CNT's are in preparation.

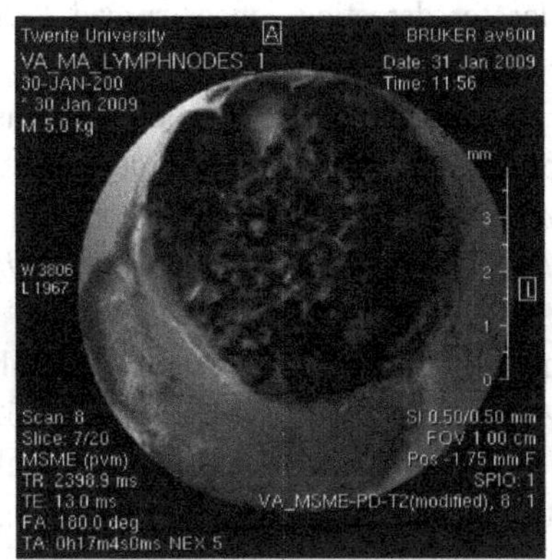

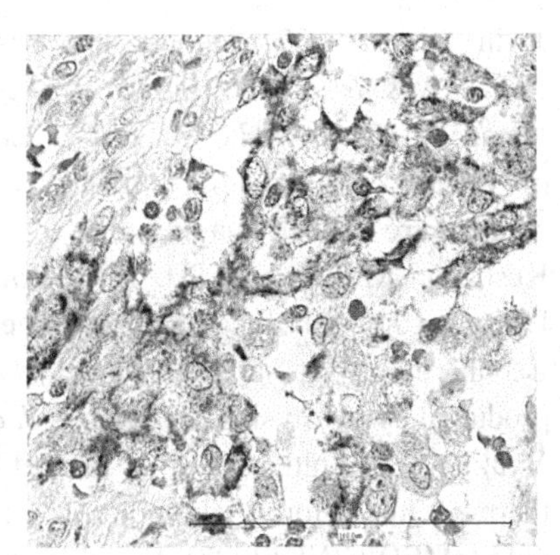

Fig. 3. Two images showing the presence of SPIO in the lymph node. Left: High field T2* MRI of a single lymph node. The diameter of the circular field is approximately 8 mm. On the right side a microscopic image with Pearls Prussian Blue staining indicating the presence of iron (scale bar 100 µm).

4. CONCLUSION

The preliminary results for clinical application of SPIO in sentinel node biopsy are promising. Even after ex-vivo administration in resected tissue the sentinel node contained SPIO particles. Additional clinical ex-vivo experiments for colorectal cancer are in preparation, extending the analysis of the content of SPIO in lymph nodes with advanced magnetic analysis. Clinical in-vivo experiments in breast cancer patients can be very helpful to solve the logistical and safety problems with sentinel node detection using radio-isotopes.

REFERENCES

1 Bjornerud A, Johansson L, The utility of superparamagnetic contrast agents in MRI: theoretical consideration and applications in the cardiovascular system, *NMR in Biomedicine* (2004) Vol. 17 (7), p465.

2 Reimer P, Balzer T, Ferucarbotran (Resovist): a new clinically approved RES-specific contrast agent for contrast-enhanced MRI of the liver: properties, clinical development, and applications, *European Radiology* (2003) Vol. 13 (6), p1266-1276.

3 Hauff K.M. et. al., Intracranial thermotherapy using magnetic nanoparticles combined with external beam radiotherapy: results of a feasibility study on patients with glioblastoma multiforme, *J. Neurooncol* (2007) Vol. 81, p53.

4 Hattersley S.R. et. al., Apparatus and method for determining magnetic properties of materials, (2006) Patent WO/2006/117530.

5 Joshi T *et al* 2007 Magnetic nanoparticles for detecting cancer spread *Breast Cancer Res. Treat.* **106** (Suppl. 1) S129
6 Harada T, Tanigawa N, Matsuki M, et al., Evaluation of lymph node metastases of breast cancer using ultrasmall superparamagnetic iron oxide-enhanced magnetic resonance imaging, *Eur. J. of Radiology* (2007) Vol.63 (3), p401.
7 Keshtgar, M.R.S. and P.J. Ell, *Sentinel lymph node detection and imaging.* European Journal of Nuclear Medicine, 1999. **26**(1): p. 57-67.
8 Leonhardt A. et. al., Enhanced magnetism in Fe-filed carbon nanotubes produced by pyrolysis of ferrocene, *J. of Appl. Phys.* (2005) Vol. 98, #074315.
9 Vyalikh A., Wolter A.U.B., Dampel S. et. al., A carbon-wrapped nanoscaled thermometer for temperature control in biological environments, *NANOMEDICINE* (2008), Vol. 3 (3), p. 321.
10 Gleich B, Weizenecker R, Tomographic imaging using the nonlinear response of magnetic particles, (2005) *NATURE* Vol. 435 (7046), p1214.
11 Megens M., Menno Prins M, Magnetic biochips: a new option for sensitive diagnostics, *J. of Mag. and Magn. Materials* (2005) Vol. 293, p702.
12 Trainer M, Horton A, Bendele TM, et al. Celltracks cytometer for rare cell detection, (2002), *Cytometry* Suppl. Vol. 11 , p129.

SUPERPARAMAGNETIC IRON OXIDES FOR MR-VISUALIZATION OF TEXTILE IMPLANTS

I. SLABU T. SCHMITZ-RODE, M. HODENIUS
Applied Medical Engineering, Medical Faculty, Helmholtz-Institute
RWTH Aachen University
52074 Aachen, Germany
slabu@hia.rwth-aachen.de

U. KLINGE, J. OTTO
Department for Surgery, Medical Faculty
RWTH Aachen University
52074 Aachen, Germany

G. A. KROMBACH, N. KRÄMER, H. DONKER
Department for Radiology, Medical Faculty
RWTH Aachen University
52074 Aachen, Germany

M. BAUMANN
Applied Medical Engineering, Medical Faculty, Helmholtz-Institute
RWTH Aachen University
52074 Aachen, Germany

The magnetic properties of superparamagnetic iron oxides (SPIOs) and their distribution within PVDF-filaments of textile implants are investigated by means of a superconducting quantum interference device (SQUID), a transmission electron microscope (TEM), a magnetic force microscope (MFM) and magnetic resonance imaging (MRI). These analyses are necessary for quality control in manufacture and the depiction of an implant in MRI.

1. INTRODUCTION

With approximately 1.5 million implantations each year worldwide, mesh repair has become the standard procedure for the treatment of hernia. However, the recurrence rate is 10 to 30% due to migration and erosion of the implant, shrinkage and deformation of the mesh area or fistula formation as a result of ingrowths or integration of the mesh into scar tissue. These consequences of the biological response to the foreign material are noticeably influenced by the properties of the mesh.[1] A non-invasive visualization of the mesh facilitates a safer diagnosis, providing the ability to spare redundant surgeries. For this purpose, superparamagnetic iron oxide (SPIO) nanoparticles were implemented into textile meshes in order to monitor these with MRI. SPIOs create a hypointense signal in MRI and the caused magnetic field susceptibility can be detected as signal voids in the MR images.[2,3] Therefore, signal loss on MRI is associated with the presence of these particles. As a result, the implant can be depicted with MRI.

A homogeneous distribution of the SPIOs in the filaments of the mesh and an optimal modulation of their magnetic properties are important for the assembly and for the MR-delineation of the textile implants. Therefore, the physical properties of differently synthesized SPIOs are determined using a superconducting quantum interference device (SQUID), a transmission electron microscope (TEM), a magnetic force microscope (MFM) and magnetic resonance imaging (MRI).

2. MATERIALS AND METHODS

Superparamagnetic Fe_3O_4 nanoparticles are synthesized either as nanocolloids that are dispersed in a carrier fluid with chemically coated particles or as a powder without coating treatment.

Using the method of Shinkai[4], the nanoparticles are prevented from agglomeration by coating treatment with dodecanoic acid. In this way, two samples (S1 and S2) of ferrofluid are stabilized. With a molar ratio Fe^{2+}/NO_2^{-} of 40/1 for S1 and 3/1 for S2, and by adjacent centrifugation for 10 min with a StatSpin Microcentrifuge (StatSpin, Norwood, Massachusetts, USA) at 246 G (2000 rpm) and 984 G (4000 rpm), respectively, S1 and S2 contain different core sizes of SPIOs. The particle size distribution and the morphology of ferrofluid particles are examined using a transmission electron microscope (TEM) (EM 400 T apparatus, Philips, The Netherlands). The average particle size is listed in Table 1.

With the method of Khalafalla[5], SPIOs without any surfactant are fabricated. In this case, the ferrofluid is lyophilized and then pulverized with a pestle. These uncoated nanoparticles build clusters whose sizes are varied by grinding procedures using a ball mill (MM200, Retsch, 2004, Germany). The grain distribution of the powder is investigated utilizing a laser diffractometer (Mastersizer 2000, Malvern Instruments, Germany) (Table 1).

Table 1. Average particle and grain sizes for samples synthesized as ferrofluid and powder, respectively.

Sample	Core diameter D_{TEM} [nm]	Grain diameter D_{Laser} [μm]
S1	10.3±3.2	-
S2	5.2±1.6	-
S3	9.4±2.8	27.1±3.7
S4	9.4±2.8	12.2±3.5

After the preparation of the magnetic particles, the meshes are manufactured. Therefore, polyvinylidene fluoride (PVDF) and a small quantity of SPIOs (approx. 3 mg/g) are melted together. This mixture is extruded to filaments, which are then assembled to textile meshes (FEG Company, Aachen, Germany).

The magnetization of the nanoparticles is measured using a superconducting quantum interference device (SQUID) (MPMS-XL, Quantum Design, USA). The measurements are performed at room temperature (T = 300 K) varying the magnetic field strength between -10 kOe and 10 kOe.[6]

For a mesh of a good quality, the particles have to be homogenously distributed within its filaments. With the help of the light microscope, only bigger clusters can be identified and distinguished from material defects. Therefore, single SPIOs and their distribution within a mixed formation of several clusters are analyzed using a combined atomic force microscope (AFM) and magnetic force microscope (MFM) (DI 3100 Nanoman AFM, Veeco, USA).[7] The sample is put on a silicon wafer, dried and then, prior to the measurement, magnetized by an external magnetic field that is oriented in-plane with the surface of the substrate.

As a proof of principle, a mesh with embedded SPIOs (mean core size 9.4 nm±2.8 nm) is placed between two pieces of meat to simulate the physiological surrounding, and MRI is performed. The mesh is made of filaments with a diameter of 120 μm and its size is approx. 2 cm x 0.8 cm. The meat phantom is measured in a 1.5 Tesla scanner (Achieva, Philips, The Netherlands) using T2*-weighted sequences (TR = 285 ms, TE = 23 ms, FoV/matrix = 200 mm/248, NSA = 2, FA = 18°) and a 2-channel receiver coil.

3. RESULTS AND DISCUSSION

As shown in Figure 1, sample S1 primarily consists of single Fe_3O_4 particles in the shape of a sphere (inset Fig. 1).

The susceptibility measurements reveal a characteristic superparamagnetic behavior with immeasurable coercivity and remanence at 300 K (Fig. 2). Figure 2 shows the best fit for the Langevin function:

$$M = M_S\left(\coth\left(\frac{\mu H}{k_B T}\right) - \left(\frac{k_B T}{\mu T}\right)\right),$$

where $\mu = M_S \pi D^3/6$ is the average magnetic moment of each particle, k_B the Boltzmann constant, T the absolute temperature and M_S the saturation magnetization.[5,8] From this data fitting, the mean magnetic moment per particle is found to be $1.36 \cdot 10^{-16}$ emu and the average diameter is calculated to $D = 8.87$ nm.

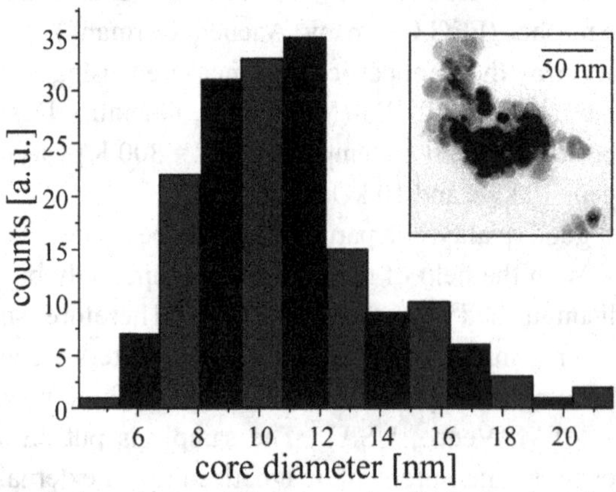

Fig. 1. TEM micrograph determination of Fe_3O_4 core size distribution (sample S1, Table 1). The inset shows the picture of separated SPIOs in shape of a sphere.

Figure 3 shows an AFM/MFM image of clusters of various sizes of SPIOs in sample S1. The particles can be identified as white structures in the MFM image (Fig. 3, right image). This corresponds to the repulsion between the particles and the MFM tip. Using this method, it is possible to distinguish between material asperities (Fig. 3, left image) and magnetic particles within the filament of the mesh.

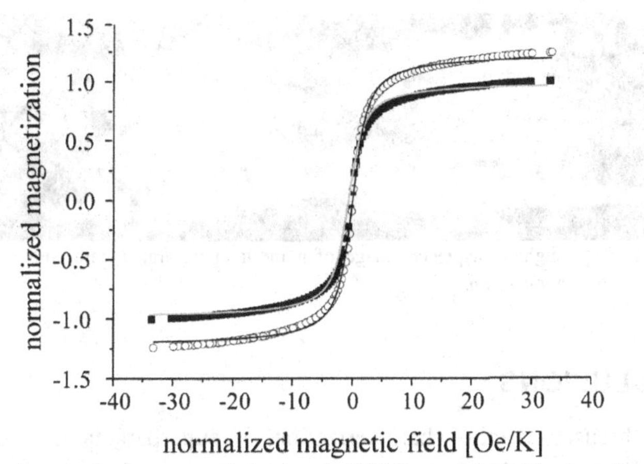

Fig. 2. Normalized magnetization vs. applied magnetic field for particles without coating: experimental data for S3 (circles) and S4 (squares) with fitted curves.

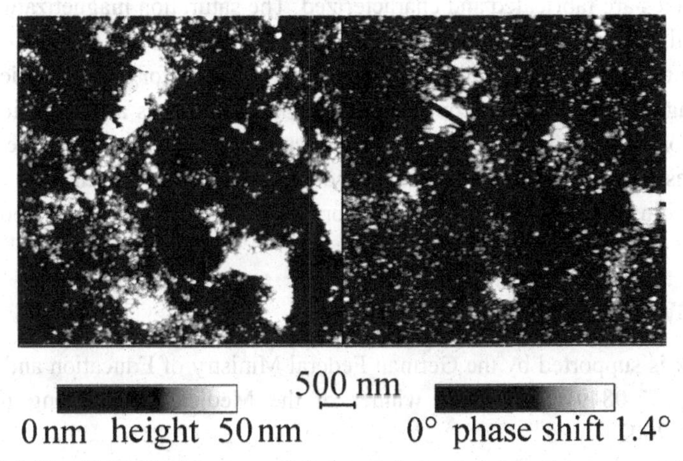

Fig. 3. AFM (left) and MFM (right) images of single and clustered particles that are magnetized in-plane with the surface of the substrate before the measurement. In the MFM image, the white color represents repulsion. The size of the marked cluster is 500 nm.

The PVDF mesh with embedded SPIOs of the meat phantom clearly shows circumscribed susceptibility artifacts on MRI. Figure 4 shows the mesh on a T2*-weighted image.

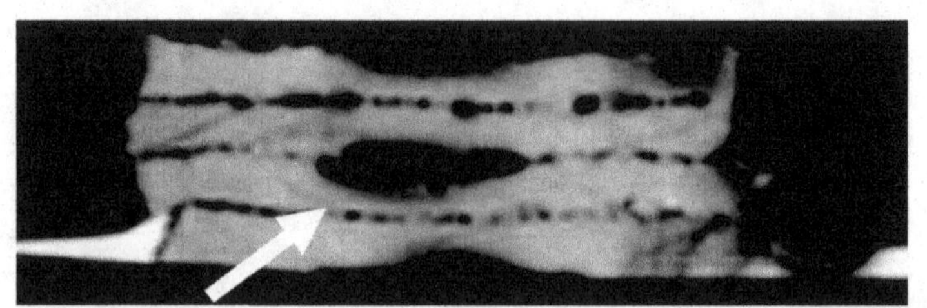

Fig. 4. T2*-weighted sequence image of a mesh incorporated with SPIOs (arrow) placed in a meat phantom.

4. CONCLUSIONS

This work focuses on the characterization of superparamagnetic nanoparticles which are integrated within textile implants in order to visualize these with MRI. Using different methods of synthesis several samples of superparamagnetic Fe_3O_4 nanoparticles are fabricated and characterized. The saturation magnetization and the susceptibility are measured using a SQUID magnetometer. All samples show a superparamagnetic behavior, though with different values for the magnetic moment. Using magnetic force microscopy, single SPIOs and clusters are identified. This is most important for quality control in manufacturing the mesh and for the depiction of the mesh with MRI, as it examines the homogeneity of the distribution of the SPIOs within the filament. As a proof of principle, a mesh with integrated SPIOs is visualized with MRI.

ACKNOWLEDGMENTS

This work is supported by the German Federal Ministry of Education and Research (Ref. 01 EZ 0849) and is the winner of the Medical Engineering Innovation Challenge 2007.

REFERENCES

1 Klinge U, Klosterhalfen B, Birkenhauer V, Junge K, Conze J, Schumpelick V. Impact of Polymer Pore Size on the Interface Scar Formation in a Rat Model. *J Surg Res* 2002; **103**: 208–214.

2 Kim DK, Zhang Y, Voit W, Rao KV, Muhammed M. Synthesis and characterization of surfactant-coated superparamagnetic monodispersed nanoparticles. *JMMM* 2001; **225**: 30–36.

3 Vlaardingerbroek MT, den Boer JA. *Magnetic Resonance Imaging*. Berlin: Springer, 2003.

4 Bulte JW, Kraitchmann DL. Iron oxide MR contrast agents for molecular and cellular imaging. *NMR Biomed* 2004; **17**: 484–499.
5 Shinkai M, Honda H, Kobayashi T. Preparation of Fine Magnetic Particles and Application for Enzyme Immobilization. *Biocatalysis* 1991; **5**: 61–69.
6 Khalafalla SE, Reimes GW. Preparation of dilution-stable aquaneous magnetic fluids. *IEEE Trans Magn* 1980; **16**: 178–183.
7 Albrecht M, Janke V, Sievers S, Siegner U, Schüler D, Heyen U. Scanning force microscopy study of biogenic nanoparticles for medical applications. *JMMM* 2005; **290-291**: 269–271.
8 Aharoni A. *Introduction to the Theory of Ferromagnetism*. Oxford: Clarendon Press, 1996.

DETECTION OF AUTOLOGOUS CHONDROCYTES AT POLYETHYLENE SCAFFOLDS IN VIVO - EXPERIMENTAL STUDY*

ILONA SCHOEN[1], FRANK ANGENSTEIN[2],
KERSTIN NEUMANN[1], ERNST ROEPKE[1,3,*]

Department of Otorhinolaryngology, Head and Neck Surgery, Martin Luther University, Halle-Wittenberg, 06907 Halle, Germany [1]
Email: ilona.schoen@medizin.uni-halle.de

Special Lab of non invasive Imaging, Leibniz Institute of Neurobiology, Brennecke Str. 6, 39118 Magdeburg, Germany [2]
Email: frank.angenstein@ifn-magdeburg.de

MRI has become an established method for the evaluation of cartilage repair in knee joints or intervertebral discs. This study used MRI to follow the integration of hybrid systems of autologous cells and porous polyethylene into the calvaria of guinea pigs. To differentiate the implanted chondrocytes from the surrounding cartilage and to monitor their location under *in vivo* conditions by MRI, cells were labeled with different ferumoxide nano particles. In addition the cells were labeled with a fluorescence marker and analyzed with in vivo and in vitro fluorescence microscopy in a time period up to 4 month after implantation. The results indicate that autologous cells tolerate the iron nano particles, which allows us to monitor the fate of the implants over time in the living animals.

1. INTRODUCTION

Autologous cells are used as substitute for filling defects or for covering porous polyethylene (PE) implants to suppress inflammatory reactions and diminish implant rejections. To follow the fate of the inserted cells it is essential to distinguish these cells from the surrounding tissue. A recently published study[1] demonstrated a good integration of the PE-implants seeded with autologous cells, by histological examination. At each observation time animals had to be decapitated, the tissue fixed, embedded, cut and stained for microscopic evaluation.

---

* This work is supported by BMBF FK 10/36 and 11/24.

[3] Present address: Klinikum Pirna GmbH Klinik für Hals-, Nasen- u. Ohrenkrankheiten, Struppener Str.13 01796 Pirna

The here presented study used MRI in order to compare the follow up of the integration of tissue-engineered cartilage in vivo and in vitro.

2. MATERIALS AND METHODS

2.1. Cell Isolation and Culture

The isolation of the chondrocytes was done as described previously[1]. Briefly, for in vitro studies 50 000 cells were seeded into six well plates or on cover slips and cultivated until confluence (5 days). Cells were incubated with Fe nano particles for 24 hours.

After carefully washing with cell culture media, the cells were further incubation for 24 hours and the vitality of the cells was estimated. DIL incubation at different concentrations was done for 48 hours followed by further 24 hour incubation to with DIL free media to remove the excess of the label. After further two weeks in vitro cultivation the specimen were implanted into the guinea pig ear or calvaria.

2.2. Animal Experiments

Animals were anesthetized with a mixture of xylazine hydrochloride (Rompun Bayervital, Leverkusen, Germany) and ketamine hydrochloride (Ketanest 50, Parke-Davis, Freiburg, Germany). After shaving the surgical area was disinfected and the skin at the ear concha was incised with a scalpel to generate a small piece of auricular cartilage. The defect was closed with a 6-0 monofil nonabsorbable stitch (Ethicon, Norderstedt, Germany) and the animal was marked by a tattoo at the opposite ear.

The implantation of the labeled cell seeded PE specimen into the ear concha (6 animals) or calvaria (8 animals) was done after a further anesthesia. After opening the skin a small whole was gouged and the specimen placed into this whole. Three specimens (control-without iron particles, Endorem and fluid MAG labeled) were placed per animal in a first test run. In a second experimental group one specimen per animal were inserted. A total number of 14 animals were analyzed.

2.3. Labeling with Iron Nanoparticles and a Fluorescence Marker

Four different iron particles were tested: first fluidMAG-D, second fluidMAG-D/Q, third target-MAG-N (chemicell) and, fourth Endorem (Guerbet). The tested particles were of equal size (about 100nm) but differed in their surface charge. While Endorem and fluidMAG-D were neutral covered with dextran, fluidMAG-D/Q positive had positive loaded quaternary ammonium groups at their surface and target-N negative charged phosphate groups. Endorem is already clinically approved as contrast agent for MRI examinations of the liver. According to the manufacturer's instruction Endorem had been applied as suspensions at a concentration of 0,075ml/kg body weight.

Cells were mixed with iron particles and brought onto the PE surface. After 2 weeks in vitro cultivation the hybrid systems became implanted according to the protocol given above.

Dialkycarbocyanine CM-DIL labeling was done as described by Studeny et al.[9] Briefly, the dye was dissolved in dimethylformamide (Sigma) to a concentration of 2.5mg/ml. In order to get a strong fluorescent signal dye concentrations from 10µg/ml to 40µg/ml had been tested in cell culture experiments.

2.4. MRI Studies

First MRI measurements were performed with specimen embedded in 1% agarose. In vivo examinations were performed one week, one, two and four month after implantation. The animals were anesthetized with xylazine/ketamine (see above) during MRI measurements in a 4.7 T animal scanner (BRUKER Biospec 4720 Bruker BioSpin MRI GmbH). MR images were obtained using a RARE T1-weighted imaging sequence (TR = 1000ms, TE 10ms, RARE factor 4, average 8, matrix 256 x 256 with field of view 8 x 8 cm and a slice thicknessof 0.8 mm. Two animals were analyzed in parallel.

2.5. Histological Examinations

The fixed samples were embedded in Technovit 7200 according to the manufacturer's recommendations, cut into sections of 4 µm and collected on super frost slides (Menzel, Braunschweig, Germany)) for histological analysis. Fe-particles were detected by Prussian blue staining as described in the literature[10].

The spreading of the cells in the scaffold was performed with laser scanning microscopy (Leica DM-IRE2 confocal microscope, Leica Microsystems, Wetzlar, Germany).

3. RESULTS

3.1. Cell Culture Experiments

MRI was used to test the efficacy of various magnetic particles to label autologous cells for in vivo detection. A summary of the viability of chondrocytes in cells culture experiments after incubation with the different particles is given in Table 1. According to these data, cells labeled with Endorem followed by fluidMAG-D/12 were the most viable. As expected, dimethyl formamide (DMF) and DIL solubilized in DMF lead to a reduction of the viability. Based on this result the following in vivo studies were performed with Endorem and fluidMAG D/12.

Table 1. Viability of cells incubated with iron nano particles.

label	c_{FE} [µg/ml]	viability[%]
control	0	100
fluidMAG-D/12	10	375
fluidMAG-D/Q	10	210
targetMAG-N	20	35
Endorem	10	465
DMF	10	84
fluorescence label DIL	10	68
Endorem+DIL	10	161
fluidMAG-D/12+DIL	10	154

3.2. MRI Studies

Before implantation with Fe-nano particles labeled cells, the specimens were imaged using a T1-weighted imaging sequence. The strongest signal depression was found with fluidMAG-D/12 particles (not shown). LSM images of PE-specimen with DIL labeled cells showed a homogeneous distribution of labeled cells (Fig.1).

First, specimens were implanted into the ear concha to test the in vivo compatibility of the hybrid system. No inflammation was observed but MRI was unable to identify the implants although the in vitro controls showed a clear signal loss. Histological staining of the specimen exhibited iron positive areas around the PE-implant.

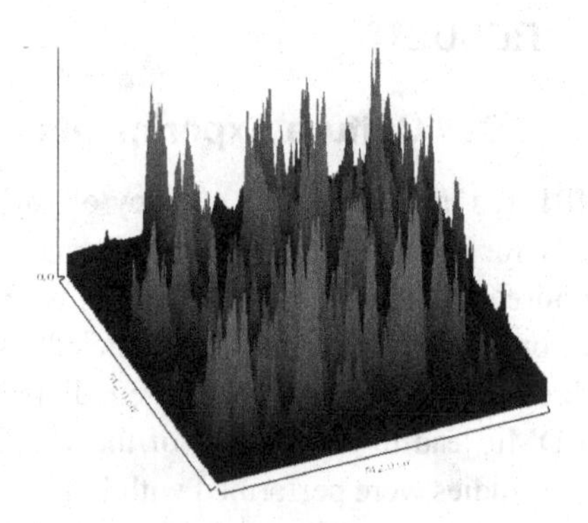

Fig. 1 LSM-image of DIL labeled cells grown on porous PE-surfaces

The ear concha as an air filled area appears dark and the implant could not be discriminated because they additionally reduce the signals. Therefore, in further experiments implants were placed onto the calvaria and forehead to avoid this problem. Figure 2 (a-b) presents the MRIs of labeled specimen one week after implantation in vivo. Under this condition the implants were easily detectable.

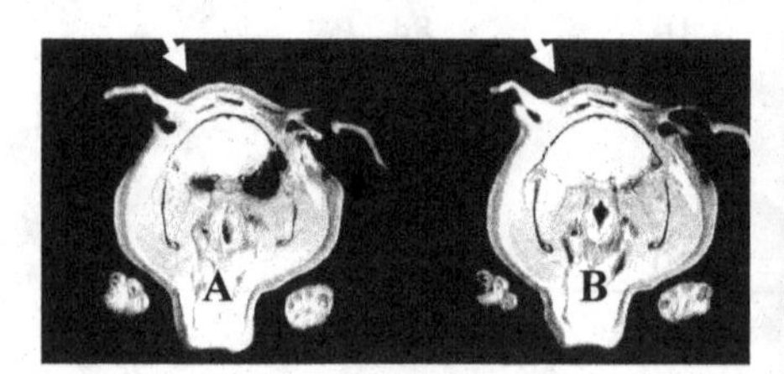

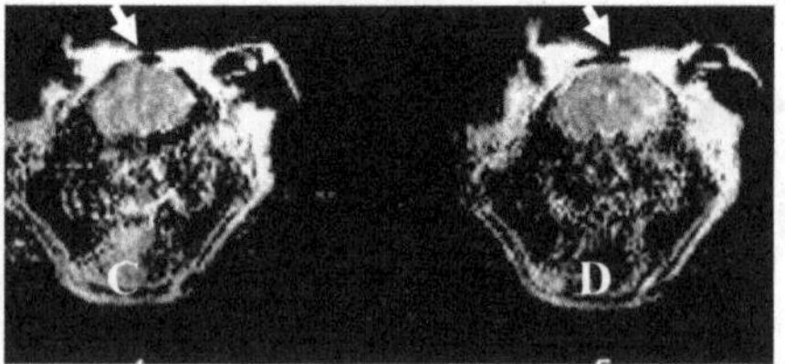

Fig. 2 MRI – control of the guinea pig one week (A;B) and 16 weeks (C,D) after implantation of the cell seeded PE – implant(arrows). Cells labeled with Endorem.

3.3. Histological Examinations

Prussian blue staining showed the FE-particles in the direct neighborhood to the implant (Fig.3a). The fluorescence signal was very weak, compared with the starting signal (Fig.3b

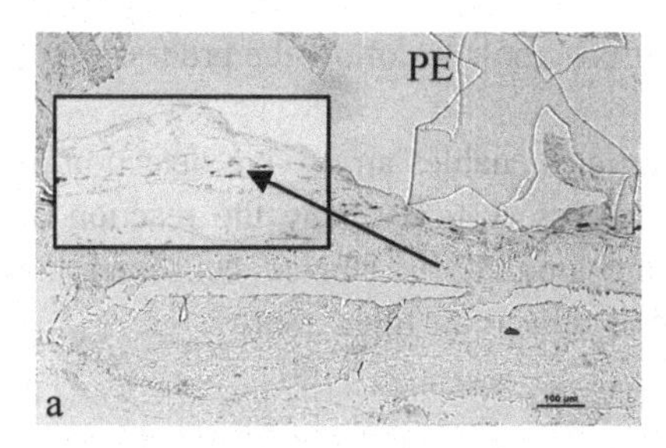

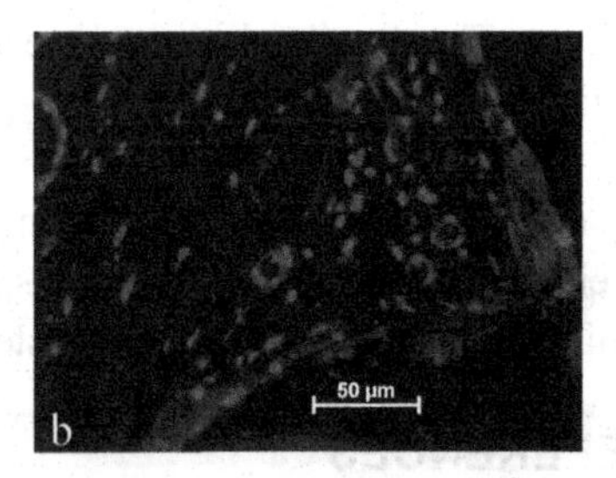

Fig. 3 Prussian blue staining of cell seeded porous PE specimen(a). Cells labeled with Fe-nano particles, after 4 month in vivo (b).

4. DISCUSSION

De Potter et al.[4] demonstrated the fibrovascularisation of PE spheres after enucleation. MRI was used for serial axial postcontrast T1 weighted images of 10 patients. A 1.5 Tesla system was used for control monitoring up to one year to. But the MRI results without histological correlation had to interpret with caution.

In 2004 a group from France[5] reported about patella cartilage repairs evaluation in an animal study 20, 40 and 60 days after implantation with T2 mapping in an 8.5T system. The analysis was performed with frozen specimen ex vivo. The results were compared with the histological analysis of the same specimen and a good correlation was found. Nevertheless the detection of cartilage repair was performed ex vivo and, therefore, the authors offered MR biopsy with the help of T 2 mapping.

Gosau et al.[6] reported the difficulties to exhibit Medpor (PE) – implants with imaging systems like ultrasound, CT or MRI.

Choi et al.[7] used Gd- enhanced T1 –weighted sequences in an animal experimental study comparable to the above mentioned clinical observations by de Potter[2]. Shapiro et al.[8] used ultra small iron oxide nano particles (USPIO dextran coated, 0.96µm-5.80µm in diameter) successfully to label single cells of different origin. Further research has been done to improve the relation of iron to particle size. Stroh et al.[9] described the use of very small super paramagnetic iron oxide particles (VSOP) with 9nm in diameter due to monomer citrate coating and detected embryonic stem cells in rat brain. The authors used a 17.6 T magnet; the highest magnetic field available for MRI of rodents. Shapiro et al.[8] utilized a 7.0 and 11.7 T devices. Another group of Hill et al.[10] labeled mesenchymal stem cells with iron fluorescent particles and detected the labeled cells after injection into the heart of mini pigs up to 3 weeks after labeling in vivo. An 1.5 T magnet was used. After explantation cells were detected by fluorescence microscopy and Prussian blue staining. The described methods seem to be useful tools to follow the processing of tissue engineered cartilage in vivo.

The additional labeling with Fe-nano particles enables an in vivo detection of the cells by MRI. Further experiments are necessary to evaluate the reaction of foreign body giant cells with respect to the amount Fe labeled cells and the exhibition of the labeled hybrid system in the concha as air filled area.

REFERENCES

1 Schoen I, Rahne T, Markwart A, Neumann K, Berhaus A, Roepke E. Cartilage replacement by use of hybrid systems of autologous cells and polyethylene: an experimental study. J Mater Sci Mater Med 2009; 20: 2145-2154.

2 Studeny M, Marini FC, Champlin RE, Zompetta C, Fidler IJ, Andreeff M. Bone marrow derived mesenchymal stem cells as vehicles for interferon ß delivery in tumors. Cancer Research 2002; **62:** 3603-3608.

3 Burck HC. Histologische Technik Stuttgart New York: Thieme 1988: 145.

4 De Potter, Duprez Th, Cosnard, G. Postcontrast imaging assessment of porous polyethylene orbital implant (Medpor). Ophthalmology 2000; **107**:1656-1660.

5 Watrin-Pinzano A, Ruaud JP, Cheli Y, Gonord P, Grossin L, Bettembourg-Brault L, Gillet P, Payan E, Guillot G, Netter P, Loeuilli D. Evaluation of cartilage repair tissue after biomaterial implantation inrat patella by using T2 mapping. MAGMA 2004; 17:219-228.

6 Gosau M, Schel S, Draenert GF, Ihrler S, Mast G, Ehernfeld M. Gesichtsschädel augmentationen mit porösen Polyethylenimplantaten (Medpor®). Mund Kiefer Gesichts Chir. 2006; 10:178-184.

7 Choi HJ, Lee JS, Park HJ, Oum BS, Kim HJ, Park DY. Magnetic resonance imaging assessment of fibrovacular ingrowth into porous polyethylene orbital implants. Clin Exp.Ophthalmol. 2006; 34: 354-359.

8 Shapiro EM, Skrtic S, Sharer K, Hill JM, Dunbar CE, Koretsky AP. Sizing it up: Cellular MRI using micron-sized iron oxide particles. Magn Reson Med. 2006; 55:242-249.

9 Stroh A, Faber C, Neuberger T, Lorenz P, Sieland K, Jakob PM, Webb A, Pilgrimm H Schober R, Pohl EE, Zimmer C. In vivo detection limits of magnetically labeled embryonic stem cells in the rat brain using high field (17.6T) magnetic resonance imaging. Neuroimage. 2005; 24:635-45 108:1009-1014.

10 Hill JM, Dick AJ, Raman VK, Thompson RB, Yu ZX, Hinds KA, Pessanha BS, GuttmanMA, Varney TR, Martin BJ, Dunbar CE, McVeigh ER, Lederman R. Serial cardic imaging of injected mesenchymal stem cells. Circulation. 2003; 26;108: 1009-1014.

CURRENT IRON OXIDE NANOPARTICLES: IMPACT ON MRI AND MPI

FLORIAN M. VOGT, JÖRG BARKHAUSEN

Clinic for Radiology and Nuclearmedicine, University Hospital Schleswig Holstein, Ratzeburger Allee 160, Luebeck, Schleswig-Holstein, 23538, Germany
Email: florian.vogt@uk-sh.de

SVEN BIEDERER, TIMO F. SATTEL, TOBIAS KNOPP, KERSTIN LÜDTKE-BUZUG, THORSTEN M. BUZUG

Institute of Medical Engineering, University of Luebeck, Ratzeburger Allee 160, Luebeck, Schleswig-Holstein, 23538, Germany
Email: {biederer,buzug}@imt.uni-luebeck.de

Superparamagnetic Iron Oxides (SPIOs) have been investigated for almost two decades and proven their usefulness as contrast agents for human MR imaging. Recently, magnetic particle Imaging (MPI) has emerged as a new technique for the visualization and quantification of SPIOs. In this contribution, different commercial SPIOs are evaluated using a magnetic particle spectrometer (MPS).

1. INTRODUCTION

SPIOs have been proven as a contrast agent for human MR lymphography and characterization of hepatosplenic tumors. Furthermore, experimental studies have been performed with SPIOs for the detection of macrophages in animal models for different disease of the central nervous system including inflammation, tumors, or ischemia, in bone marrow alterations and atherosclerotic plaques. However, for clinical applications, USPIOs still require rather high doses of the contrast agent, and lesions are only indirectly visualized by susceptibility artifacts. Therefore, although USPIOs have been used in experimental studies for almost two decades the compounds have not found their way into daily clinical routine.

Recently, magnetic particle imaging (MPI)[1] has emerged as a new technique for the visualization and quantification of iron oxide based contrast agents ex-vivo as well as in-vivo. Whereas in MRI the pharmacokinetic properties of the compounds are important, in MPI the size and the isotropy of the magnetic core are most crucial. Therefore, our study aimed to characterize different USPIOs with regard to their potential as MPI contrast agents and clinical requirements are discussed.

2. MATERIAL AND METHODS

To exploit the imaging performance of MPI for different SPIOs, the nanoparticle signal excited at the FFP can be explored using magnetic particle spectroscopy.[2] The MPS can be interpreted as a zero dimensional MPI system, i.e. the gradient field is omitted and only the oscillating field is used. Thus, all particles are exposed to the same magnetic field. For the experiments, the magnetic field amplitude was set to be between 10 mT and 30 mT, while the oscillating frequency was chosen to 25 kHz. The MPI performance of different particles can be measured by the number of harmonics that can be acquired before the signals spectrum drops below the noise level.

To characterize their potential with regard to the detection of harmonics four different SPIOS are investigated in this study: Resovist® (Bayer Schering Pharma AG, Berlin, Germany), Endorem™ (Guerbert S.A., Villepinte, France), Lumirem® (Guerbert S.A., Villepinte, France) and Sinerem® (Guerbert S.A., Villepinte, France). The application in MRI of the SPIOs differs.

Whereas Resovist and Endorem are approved MRI contrast agents for the liver, Sinerem is used for detection of metastatic disease in lymph nodes and Lumirem for examinations of the bowel. Lumirem is for oral ingesting, while the others are delivered by infusion. The coating of Sinerem and Endorem is based on dextran and the one of Resovist is carboxydextran. Lumirem is the only one, with a coating based on modified silane. All of these USPIOs have a superparamagnetic iron-oxide core (Fe_3O_4) but with different core sizes. An explicit overview of the properties of the different SPIOS is given in Tab. 1.

To measure the SPIOs in the MPS, they are separately filled with Eppendorf pipettes in tubes of volume 10 μl. For comparison, the presented signals are normalized to an iron concentration of 500 mmol/L. In all measurements, the total acquisition time is set to 10 s providing a high signal-to-noise ratio.

Tab. 1 Overview of the properties of the different SPIOs.

USPIO	Coating	Hydrodyn. diameter (nm)	Iron-core diameter (nm)	Concentration (mmol/l)
Resovist	Carboxydextran	60	5-20	500
Endorem	Dextran	80-150	4-6	200
Sinerem	Dextran	20	4-6	377
Lumirem	Silane	300	8-10	3.1

3. RESULTS AND DISCUSSION

Resovist, an approved T2* contrast agent for MRI, is the most important benchmark material as it exhibits some and so far the best MPI performance. However, even though Resovist is superior to the other tested SPIOs and thus is a good choice for imaging with MPI today, there is still considerable room for improvement in the tracer material. The reasoning behind this is that Resovist consists of particles with different sizes following a log-normal distribution.

The majority of particles is smaller than 20 nm and contributes a signal to only some of the lower harmonics, whereas a small fraction of the particles has 20 nm core diameters and determines the slope of all higher harmonics. Furthermore, Resovist deviates for different on the market available batches with regard to the distribution of nanoparticle sizes. Due to a wide distribution of sizes within the batches, especially within the desired particle size range of 20 nm, different magnetic spectra can be measured by MPS.

Finally, due to the hydrodynamic diameter larger than 50 nm, Resovist is classified as a SPIO rather than an USPIO; thus Resovist is predominantly concentrated in the liver and spleen, with reduced or minimal uptake in the macrophages of the deep compartments. Hence, Resovist might be the best commercial available contrast agent for MPI yet but would demonstrate several drawbacks in clinical routine.

Only particles with a hydrodynamic diameter of 50 nm and less (USPIOs) will enable the potential use as a long circulation contrast agent, which allow blood pool imaging or the detection and treatment of inflammatory or degenerative disorders. Thus, there is a strong interest in synthesizing monodisperse nanoparticles of minimum size 30 nm potentially allowing for an increase in sensitivity by a factor of 100 using MPI.

4. CONCLUSION

Superparamagnetic iron oxide particles (SPIOs) have been widely used experimentally for numerous in vivo applications such as magnetic resonance imaging contrast enhancement but only a few scientific investigations and developments have been carried out in improving the quality of magnetic particles, their size distribution, their shape and surface. MPI, as a potential technique allowing new radiation-free applications in molecular diagnostics, image guide therapy and therapy monitoring, demands to focus on these issues. The diameter of the core and types of specific coating for these nanoparticles influence not only the performance of this new technique but rather the end application and should be chosen by keeping a particular application in mind, whether it be aimed at i.e. inflammation response or anti-cancer agents.

ACKNOWLEDGMENTS

This work was financially supported by the Innovation Foundation (ISH) of the state of Schleswig-Holstein, Germany (project id 2007-60). It is also part of the University Research Program “Imaging of Disease Processes", University of Luebeck.

REFERENCES

1 Gleich B, Weizenecker J, Tomographic imaging using the nonlinear response of magnetic particles. *Nature* 2005; **435**: 1214-1217.

2 Biederer S, Knopp T, Sattel T F, Lüdtke-Buzug K, Gleich B, Weizenecker J, Borgert J, Buzug T M: Magnetization Response Spectroscopy of Superparamagnetic Nanoparticles for Magnetic Particle Imaging, *Journal of Physics D: Applied Physics*, 2009, **42(20)**: 1-7.

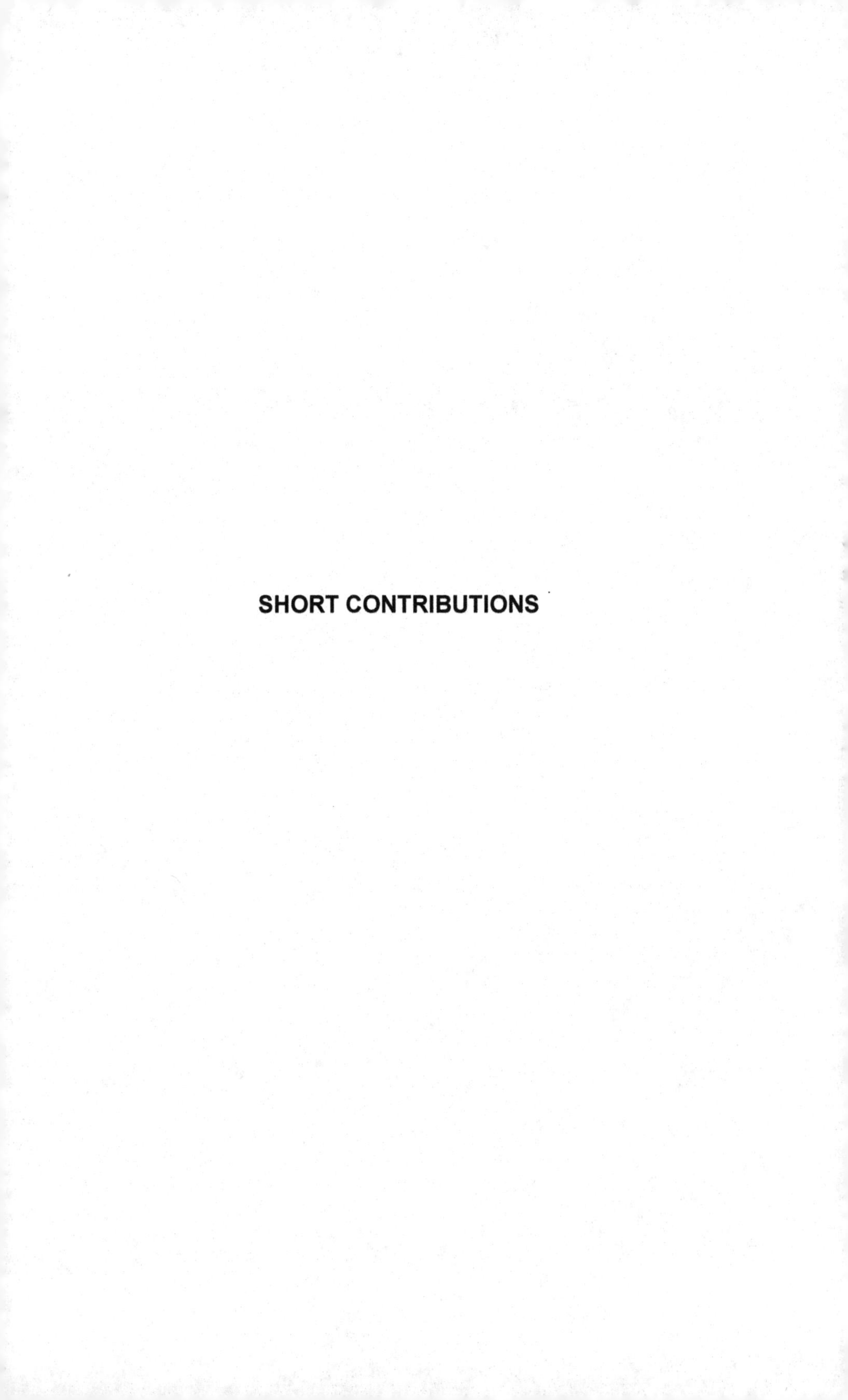

SHORT CONTRIBUTIONS

COLLOIDAL STABILITY OF WATER BASED DISPERSIONS CONTAINING LARGE SINGLE DOMAIN PARTICLES OF MAGNETITE

N. BUSKE

Magnetic Fluids,
Köpenicker Landstr. 203, 12437 Berlin, Germany

S. DUTZ

Department of Bio NanoPhotonics, Institute of Photonic Technologies,
Albert-Einstein-Straße 9, Jena, 07745, Germany
Email: silvio.dutz@ipht-jena.de

The crystal size of Large Single Domain Particles (LSDP) of magnetite is assumed to range between 20 und 100 nm. In this region the particles show increasing coercivity and relative remanence with increasing particle diameter [1].

The extraordinary magnetic properties of these particles and the corresponding dispersions can be used in magnetorelaxometry (MRX), magnetic resonance imaging (MRI), magnetic particle imaging (MPI), hyperthermia, drug targeting, and magnetofection.

The preparation problem is to establish a sufficient colloidal stability. This problem will be discussed here from the point of the DLVO-theory as well as with some experimental test results.

THE LACK OF A MUCOSAL GLYCOCALYX AS A POTENTIAL MARKER FOR THE DETECTION OF COLORECTAL NEOPLASIA BY MAGNETIC PARTICLE IMAGING

KATRIN RAMAKER, NIELS RÖCKENDORF, ANDREAS FREY

Division of Mucosal Immunology,
Research Center Borstel,
23845 Borstel, Germany

Colorectal cancer (CRC) is one of the most commonly diagnosed cancers and shows one of the highest mortality rates. This need not be the case as the disease is readily curable if recognized and treated early. Unfortunately, only 39% of CRCs are detected at such an early stage, mostly due to the reluctance of patients to undergo the recommended invasive diagnostical tests such as flexible sigmoidoscopy or colonoscopy. Thus, there is a need for less embarassing, non-invasive diagnostic tests for CRC.

We set out to develop such a diagnostic procedure. For this purpose we make use of our finding that the so-called glycocalyx, a dense network of highly glycosylated proteins and lipids that are anchored in the apical cell membrane of the healthy mucosal epithelium, is lacking on colorectal neoplasia. The absence of such a cell coat on the dedifferentiated cells should allow specific binding of particulate ligands to membrane receptors which, in the healthy epithelium, are shielded by the glycocalyx and thus are inaccessible for particles.

If a contrast agent is made up of superparamagnetic iron oxide nanoparticles covered with membrane receptor ligands the highlighted neoplastic lesions should be visible by Magnetic Particle Imaging.

CLINICAL APPLICATION OF IRON OXIDE NANOPARTICLES IN MAGNETIC RESONANCE IMAGING AND RESEARCH PERSPECTIVES

MARC PORT , CLAIRE COROT, ISABELLE RAYNAL, CAROLINE ROBIC,
PHILIPPE ROBERT, JEAN MARC IDÉE, GAELLE LOUIN,
JEAN SEBASTIEN RAYNAUD, OLIVIER ROUSSEAUX

Guerbet Research BP 57400, 95943 Roissy CDG, France
Email: marc.port@guerbet-group.com

Superparamagnetic nanoparticles of iron oxides (SPIO and USPIO) have become a major tool for medical imaging with a wealth of applications. For nearly 20 years, research in the field of magnetic resonance imaging (MRI) contrast agents has been oriented towards the study and development of these iron oxide nanoparticles, because they are highly effective in MRI as strong enhancers of proton relaxation (1/T1 , 1/T2 and 1/T2*).

The multiple components which govern the efficacy of these agents require them to be characterised as accurately as possible by information such as the size of the iron oxide crystals, the charge, the nature of the coating, the hydrodynamic size of the coated particle, etc. These physico-chemical characteristics not only affect the efficacy of the superparamagnetic particles in MRI but also their stability, biodistribution and metabolism as well as their clearance from the vascular system.

The aim of this presentation is to present

1. the MRI efficacy of iron oxide nanoparticles
2. the physico-chemical characterisation of iron oxide nanoparticles
3. the clinical applications of iron oxide in MRI illustrated by new results obtained with the USPIO P904 in MR angiography, atherosclerosis and Alzheimer imaging.

AUTHOR INDEX

Aerts, H. Philips Research Europe and Philips Medical Systems, Eindhoven, The Netherlands

Albrecht, M. Magnetic Measurements, PTB Braunschweig, Bundesallee 100, D-38116 Braunschweig, Germany

Alexiou, C. Section for Experimental Oncology and Nanomedicine (Else Kröner-Fresenius-Foundation-Professorship) at the ENT-Department of the University Erlangen-Nürnberg, Waldstr. 1, D-91054 Erlangen, Germany

Angenstein, F. Special Lab of non invasive Imaging, Leibniz Institute of Neurobiology, Brennecke Str. 6, D-39118 Magdeburg, Germany

Antonelli, A. Department of Biomolecular Sciences, University of Urbino, Via Saffi 2, Urbino, 61029, Italy

Barkhausen, J. Clinic for Radiology and Nuclearmedicine, University Hospital Schleswig Holstein, Ratzeburger Allee 160, Lübeck, Schleswig-Holstein, D-23538 Lübeck, Germany

Baumann, K. Department of Obstetrics and Gynecology, University Clinic of Schleswig-Holstein, University of Lübeck, Ratzeburger Allee 160, D-23538 Lübeck, Germany

Baumann, M. Applied Medical Engineering, Medical Faculty, Helmholtz-Institute, RWTH Aachen University, D-52074 Aachen, Germany

Baumgarten, D. Institute of Biomedical Engineering and Informatics, Ilmenau University of Technology; POB 100 565; D-98694 Ilmenau, Germany

Behr, V.C. Department of Experimental Physics 5, University of Wuerzburg, Am Hubland, D-97074 Wuerzburg, Germany

Bernard, S. Departments of Radiology, Biomedical Engineering, and Chemical & Biomolecular Engineering; Cellular Imaging Section, Institute for Cell Engineering, Johns Hopkins University School of Medicine, Baltimore, MD, USA

Biederer, S. Institute of Medical Engineering, University of Lübeck, Ratzeburger Allee 160, D-23538 Lübeck, Germany

Boeve, H. Philips Research Europe, High Tech Campus 34, Eindhoven, 5656 AE, The Netherlands

Bohnert, J. Institute of Biomedical Engineering, Karlsruhe Institute of Technology (KIT), Kaiserstr. 12, D-76131 Karlsruhe, Germany

Borgert, J. Philips Research Europe, Sector Medical Imaging Systems, Röntgenstr. 24-26, D-22335 Hamburg, Germany

Brown, R. Department of Physics, Case Western Reserve University, 10900 Euclid Avenue, Cleveland, OH, 44106, USA

Bulte, J.W.M. Departments of Radiology, Biomedical Engineering, and Chemical & Biomolecular Engineering; Cellular Imaging Section, Institute for Cell Engineering, Johns Hopkins University School of Medicine, Baltimore, MD, USA

Buske, N. Magnetic Fluids, Köpenicker Landstr. 203, D-12437 Berlin, Germany

Buzug, T.M. Institute of Medical Engineering, University of Lübeck, Ratzeburger Allee 160, D-23538 Lübeck, Germany

Conolly, S. Department of Bioengineering, University of California, Berkeley, CA 94720 USA

Corot, C. Guerbet Research BP 57400, 95943 Roissy CDG, France

Diedrich, K. Department of Obstetrics and Gynecology, University Clinic of Schleswig-Holstein, University of Lübeck, Ratzeburger Allee 160 D-23538 Lübeck, Germany

Dössel, O. Institute of Biomedical Engineering, Karlsruhe Institute of Technology (KIT), Kaiserstr. 12, D-76131 Karlsruhe, Germany

Donker, H. Department for Radiology, Medical Faculty, RWTH Aachen University, D-52074 Aachen, Germany

Dutz, S. Department of Bio NanoPhotonics, Institute of Photonic Technologies, Albert-Einstein-Straße 9, Jena, D-07745, Germany

Eberbeck, D. Physikalisch-Technische Bundesanstalt, Berlin, Abbestrasse 2-12, D-10587 Berlin, Germany

Erbe, M. Institute of Medical Engineering, University of Lübeck, Ratzeburger Allee 160, D-23538 Lübeck, Germany

Farrell, D. Department of Physics, Case Western Reserve University, 10900 Euclid Avenue, Cleveland, OH, 44106, USA

Ferguson, R.M. Materials Science & Engineering Dept., University of Washington, Box 352120 Seattle, WA, 98195-2120, USA

Finas, D. Department of Obstetrics and Gynecology, University Clinic of Schleswig-Holstein, University of Lübeck, Ratzeburger Allee 160 D-23538 Lübeck, Germany

Frey, A. Division of Mucosal Immunology, Research Center Borstel, D-23845 Borstel, Germany

Gehrke, J.-P. Department of Experimental Physics 5, University of Wuerzburg, Am Hubland, D-97074 Wuerzburg, Germany

Giustini, A.J. Dartmouth Medical School, Dartmouth College Hanover, NH 03755, USA

Gleich, B. Philips Research Europe, Sector Medical Imaging Systems, Röntgenstr. 24-26, D-22335 Hamburg, Germany

Goodwill, P. UC SF / UC Berkeley Joint Graduate Group in Bioengineering, University of California, Berkeley CA 94720, USA

Griswold, M. Department of Physics, Case Western Reserve University, 10900 Euclid Avenue, Cleveland, OH, 44106, USA

Hahn, J. Institut für Elektrische Messtechnik und Grundlagen der Elektrotechnik, TU Braunschweig Hans-Sommer-Str. 66 Braunschweig, D-38106 Braunschweig, Germany

Haueisen, J. Institute of Biomedical Engineering and Informatics, Ilmenau University of Technology; POB 100 565; D-98694 Ilmenau, Germany

Hiergeist, R. Magnetic Measurements, PTB Braunschweig, Bundesallee 100, D-38116 Braunschweig, Germany

Hilger, I. Institute of Diagnostic and Interventional Radiology, University Hospital Jena, Jena, Germany

Hodenius, M. Applied Medical Engineering, Medical Faculty, Helmholtz-Institute, RWTH Aachen University, D-52074 Aachen, Germany

Hoopes, P.J. Dartmouth Medical School, Dartmouth College Hanover, NH 03755, USA

Hütter, J. Bayer Schering Pharma AG, Cardiovascular Imaging & Contrast Media Research Muellerstrasse 178, D-13353 Berlin, Germany

Idée, J.M. Guerbet Research BP 57400, 95943 Roissy CDG, France

Jakob, P.M. Department of Experimental Physics 5, University of Wuerzburg, Am Hubland, D-97074 Wuerzburg, Germany

Kafka, G. Department of Physics, Case Western Reserve University, 10900 Euclid Avenue, Cleveland, OH, 44106, USA

Kaiser, W.A. Institute of Diagnostic and Interventional Radiology, University Hospital Jena, Jena, Germany

Kampf, T. Department of Experimental Physics 5, University of Wuerzburg, Am Hubland, D-97074 Wuerzburg, Germany

Kaufmann, S. Institute of Medical Engineering, University of Lübeck, Ratzeburger Allee 160, D-23538 Lübeck, Germany

Kettering, M. Institute of Diagnostic and Interventional Radiology, University Hospital Jena, Jena, Germany

Ketzler, R. Magnetic Measurements, PTB Braunschweig, Bundesallee 100, D-38116 Braunschweig, Germany

Khandar, A.P. Materials Science & Engineering Dept., University of Washington, Box 352120 Seattle, WA, 98195-2120, USA

Klinge, U. Department for Surgery, Medical Faculty, RWTH Aachen University, D-52074 Aachen, Germany

Knopp, T. Institute of Medical Engineering, University of Lübeck, Ratzeburger Allee 160, D-23538 Lübeck, Germany

Krämer, N. Department for Radiology, Medical Faculty, RWTH Aachen University, D-52074 Aachen, Germany

Krishnan, K.M. Materials Science & Engineering Dept., University of Washington, Box 352120 Seattle, WA, 98195-2120, USA

Krombach, G.A. Department for Radiology, Medical Faculty, RWTH Aachen University, D-52074 Aachen, Germany

Kuhn, M. Philips Health Care, Philips Medical Systems DMC GmbH, Röntgenstr. 24-26, D-22335 Hamburg, Germany

Kullmann, W.H. University of Applied Sciences Wuerzburg-Schweinfurt, Ignaz-Schön-Straße 11, D-97421 Schweinfurt, Germany

Loef, C. Philips Research Laboratories Aachen, Weißhausstraße 2, D-52066 Aachen, Germany

Lohrke, J. Bayer Schering Pharma AG, Cardiovascular Imaging & Contrast Media Research Muellerstrasse 178, D-13353 Berlin, Germany

Louin, G.	Guerbet Research BP 57400, 95943 Roissy CDG, France
Lüdke, J.	Magnetic Measurements, PTB Braunschweig, Bundesallee 100, D-38116 Braunschweig, Germany
Lüdtke-Buzug, K.	Institute of Medical Engineering, University of Lübeck, Ratzeburger Allee 160, D-23538 Lübeck, Germany
Luerkens, P.	Philips Research Laboratories Aachen, Weißhausstraße 2, D-52066 Aachen, Germany
Ludwig, F.	Institut für Elektrische Messtechnik und Grundlagen der Elektrotechnik, TU Braunschweig Hans-Sommer-Str. 66 Braunschweig, D-38106 Braunschweig, Germany
Lyer, S.	Section for Experimental Oncology and Nanomedicine (Else Kröner-Fresenius-Foundation-Professorship) at the ENT-Department of the University Erlangen-Nürnberg, Waldstr. 1, D-91054 Erlangen, Germany
Magnani, M.	Department of Biomolecular Sciences, University of Urbino, Via Saffi 2, Urbino, 61029, Italy
Markov, D.	Philips Research Europe, High Tech Campus 34, Eindhoven, 5656 AE, The Netherlands
Minard, K.R.	Biological Monitoring & Modeling, Pacific Northwest National Labs, 902 Battelle Blvd, P.O. Box 999; MSIN P7-58 Richland, WA 99352, USA
Müller, R.	Department of Bio NanoPhotonics, Institute of Photonic Technologies, Albert-Einstein-Straße 9, Jena, D-07745, Germany
Neumann, K.	Department of Otorhinolaryngology, Head and Neck Surgery, Martin Luther University, Halle-Wittenberg, D-06907 Halle, Germany
Odenbach, S.	Institute of Fluid Mechanics, Technische Universität Dresden, D-01062, Dresden, Germany
Otto, J.	Department for Surgery, Medical Faculty RWTH Aachen University, D-52074 Aachen, Germany
Port, M.	Guerbet Research BP 57400, 95943 Roissy CDG, France
Post, H.	Bruker BioSpin MRI GmbH, Rudolf-Plank-Str. 23, D-76275 Ettlingen, Germany
Rahmer, J.	Philips Technologie GmbH, Forschungs-laboratorien, Röntgenstraße 24-26, D-22315 Hamburg, Germany
Ramaker, K.	Division of Mucosal Immunology, Research Center Borstel, D-23845 Borstel, Germany
Rauwerdink, A.M.	Thayer School of Engineering, Dartmouth College, 8000 Cummings Hall. Hanover, NH 03755, USA
Raynal, I.	Guerbet Research BP 57400, 95943 Roissy CDG, France
Raynoud, J.S.	Guerbet Research BP 57400, 95943 Roissy CDG, France
Richter, H.	Physikalisch-Technische Bundesanstalt, Abbestrasse 2-12, D-10587 Berlin, Germany
Robert, P.	Guerbet Research BP 57400, 95943 Roissy CDG, France
Robic, C.	Guerbet Research BP 57400, 95943 Roissy CDG, France
Röckendorf, N.	Division of Mucosal Immunology, Research Center Borstel, D-23845 Borstel, Germany

Roepke, E.	Department of Otorhinolaryngology, Head and Neck Surgery, Martin Luther University, Halle-Wittenberg, D-06907 Halle, Germany
Ross, G.	Magnet-Physik Dr. Steingroever GmbH, Emil-Hoffmann-Str. 3, D-50996 Köln, Germany
Rousseaux, O.	Guerbet Research BP 57400, 95943 Roissy CDG, France
Rückert, M.A.	University of Applied Sciences Wuerzburg-Schweinfurt, Ignaz-Schön-Straße 11, D-97421 Schweinfurt, Germany
Ruhland, B.	Department of Obstetrics and Gynecology, University Clinic of Schleswig-Holstein, University of Lübeck, Ratzeburger Allee 160, D-23538 Lübeck, Germany
Sattel, T.F.	Institute of Medical Engineering, University of Lübeck, Ratzeburger Allee 160, D-23538 Lübeck, Germany
Schilling, M.	Institut für Elektrische Messtechnik und Grundlagen der Elektrotechnik, TU Braunschweig Hans-Sommer-Str. 66 Braunschweig, D-38106 Braunschweig, Germany
Schmale, I.	Philips Research Europe, Sector Medical Imaging Systems, Röntgenstr. 24-26, D-22335 Hamburg, Germany
Schmitz-Rode, T.	Applied Medical Engineering, Medical Faculty, Helmholtz-Institute, RWTH Aachen University, D-52074 Aachen, Germany
Schoen, I.	Department of Otorhinolaryngology, Head and Neck Surgery, Martin Luther University, Halle-Wittenberg, D-06907 Halle, Germany
Schütz, G.	Bayer Schering Pharma AG, Cardiovascular Imaging & Contrast Media Research Muellerstrasse 178, D-13353 Berlin, Germany
Sfara, C.	Department of Biomolecular Sciences, University of Urbino, Via Saffi 2, Urbino, 61029, Italy
Slabu, I.	Applied Medical Engineering, Medical Faculty, Helmholtz-Institute, RWTH Aachen University, D-52074 Aachen, Germany
Sobik, M.	MIRA Institute for Biomedical Technology and Technical Medicine, Low Temperature Div., University of Twente, P.O. Box 217, 7500 AE Enschede, The Netherlands
Steinhoff, U.	Physikalisch-Technische Bundesanstalt, Berlin, Abbestrasse 2-12, D-10587 Berlin, Germany
Ten Haken, B.	MIRA Institute for Biomedical Technology and Technical Medicine, Low Temperature Div., University of Twente, P.O. Box 217, 7500 AE Enschede, The Netherlands
Tietze, R.	Section for Experimental Oncology and Nanomedicine (Else Kröner-Fresenius-Foundation-Professorship) at the ENT-Department of the University Erlangen-Nürnberg, Waldstr. 1, D-91054 Erlangen, Germany
Trahms, L.	Physikalisch-Technische Bundesanstalt, Berlin, Abbestrasse 2-12, D-10587 Berlin, Germany
Sobik, M.	MIRA Institute for Biomedical Technology and Technical Medicine, Low Temperature Div., University of Twente, P.O. Box 217, 7500 AE Enschede, The Netherlands

Velders, A.H. MESA Institute for Nanotechnology, Supramolecular Chemistry and Technology, University of Twente, P.O. Box 217, 7500 AE Enschede, The Netherlands

Vogt, F.M. Clinic for Radiology and Nuclearmedicine, University Hospital Schleswig Holstein, Ratzeburger Allee 160, Lübeck, Schleswig-Holstein, D-23538 Lübeck, Germany

Walczak, P. Departments of Radiology, Biomedical Engineering, and Chemical & Biomolecular Engineering; Cellular Imaging Section, Institute for Cell Engineering, Johns Hopkins University School of Medicine, Baltimore, MD, USA

Wawrzik, T. Institut für Elektrische Messtechnik und Grundlagen der Elektrotechnik, TU Braunschweig Hans-Sommer-Str. 66 Braunschweig, D-38106 Braunschweig, Germany

Weaver, J.B. Department of Radiology, Dartmouth Medical School, Dartmouth-Hitchcock Medical Center, Lebanon, New Hampshire 03756, USA

Weizenecker, J. Department of Electrical Engineering, University of Applied Science, Moltkestraße 30, D-76133 Karlsruhe. Germany

Wiekhorst, F. Physikalisch-Technische Bundesanstalt, Berlin, Abbestrasse 2-12, D-10587 Berlin, Germany

Woywode, O. Philips Healthcare, GTC Development, Philips Medical Systems DMC GmbH, Röntgenstraße 24-26, D-22315 Hamburg, Germany

Wu, Y. Department of Physics, Case Western Reserve University, 10900 Euclid Avenue, Cleveland, OH, 44106, USA

Yao, Z. Department of Physics, Case Western Reserve University, 10900 Euclid Avenue, Cleveland, OH, 44106, USA

Zeisberger, M. Department of Spectroscopy and Imaging, Institute of Photonic Technologies, Albert-Einstein-Straße 9, Jena, D-07745, Germany